Praise for Kausler's first two editions

"Represents a Herculean effort to educate patients. It is an ambitious work that collates years of collected medical and psychiatric data into a dictionary format. The book defines and discusses several hundred symptoms, organs and problems encountered by our aging population as well as those confronting persons involved in their care. It is an educational and informational resource, easy to read, practical and useful."—*Chicago Medicine*

"[This book] is a valuable resource for both lay persons and practitioners who wish to acquire nontechnical expertise in aging. . . . [It] is comprehensive and clearly presented, strikes a nice balance between an emphasis on basic and applied issues, and is appropriately grounded in theory and research on the biological and psychosocial aspects of late adulthood. . . . It should be quite useful for some time to come."—*Contemporary Gerontology*

"Intended for general readers, this volume clearly explains various aspects of aging in nontechnical language. Topical coverage is very broad, and the selection of subjects appears to reflect both currently popular areas and the authors' own interests. . . . Recommended for general readers, undergraduates, and practitioners looking for basic information."—*Choice*

The
Essential
Guide
to Aging in the
Twenty-First Century

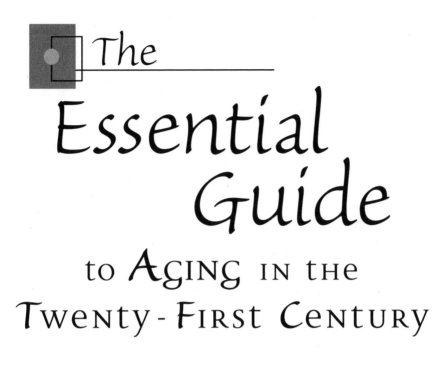

The
Essential
Guide
to Aging in the Twenty-First Century

Mind, Body, and Behavior

Donald H. Kausler

Barry C. Kausler

Jill A. Krupsaw

University of Missouri Press   Columbia and London

Library of Congress Cataloging-in-Publication Data
Kausler, Donald H.
  Aging in the twenty-first century : an everyday guide to health, mind, and
behavior / Donald H. Kausler, Barry C. Kausler, Jill A. Krupsaw. — 3rd ed.
    p. cm.
  Summary: "This third edition of The Graying of America has been retitled,
revised, and expanded. In concise, nontechnical language, it offers mid-
dle-aged and senior readers useful information on the effects of aging on
health, the mind, and behavior"—Provided by publisher.
  Includes bibliographical references and index.
  ISBN 978-0-8262-1707-3 (alk. paper)
  1. Older people—United States—Encyclopedias. 2. Aging—United
States—Encyclopedias. 3. Old age—United States—Encyclopedias. 4.
Gerontology—United States—Encyclopedias. I. Kausler, Barry C., 1961–
II. Krupsaw, Jill A. III. Kausler, Donald H. Graying of America. IV. Title.
  HQ1064.U5K30 2007
  305.2603—dc22

                                                    2007004142

∞™ This paper meets the requirements of the
American National Standard for Permanence of Paper
for Printed Library Materials, Z39.48, 1984.

Designer and Typesetter: *foleydesign*
Printer and Binder: Thomson-Shore, Inc.
Typeface: ITC New Baskerville

contents

Preface / vii

Introduction / xi

Alphabetical Entries / 1

Index of Entries and Cross-References / 483

Index of Entries by Broad Topics / 507

preface

The third edition of *The Graying of America*, renamed *Aging in the Twenty-First Century*, joins the second edition in providing important new information about human aging and its effects on physical health, mental health, cognitive or mental functioning, and behavior. As was true for the first and second editions, our intent in the third edition is to convey that information to the general public. Consequently, the third edition again offers an easily read guide to the many topics that interest and concern older people and those who love them and may need to care for them.

The five years since the second edition have been especially productive ones in terms of the amount of new research that adds greatly to our understanding of human aging. The third edition contains 588 entries, in contrast to the 476 entries of the second edition. Of the entries in the third edition, 172 are new, in contrast to the 152 in the second edition. The remaining entries include 150 that were in the second edition, but have been revised and extended by adding important new information. The remaining 266 entries in the third edition are carried over from the second edition with relatively minor changes in their content. An additional 64 entries from the second edition were eliminated in the present edition.

The present new entries range from Activity Diversity (Cognitive Benefits) to Women's Health Initiative. Some older adults diversify their activities by adding to traditional physical and mental activities such actions as doing volunteer work and gardening. They have been shown to perform better on cognitive tasks than other older adults with little diversification. The Women's Health Initiative is a major fifteen-year study employing thousands of postmenopausal women. It has yielded important new information about several diseases, such as breast cancer and osteoporosis.

Research on the senses has moved in several new and exciting directions that should help seniors adjust better to problems they may encounter in their everyday lives. Older husbands with impaired hearing should realize that their affliction is adversely affecting their wives as much as it is affecting them. Their impairment hinders their communication with their wives—and effective communication is very important for women (*see*

Untreated Hearing Impairment [Effects on Spouses]). The husbands should give serious consideration to the use of hearing aids. In terms of visual research, visual impairment is likely to contribute to poor sleep for elders. Sunlight is important for maintaining the normal functioning of sleep-awake centers in the brain. Perhaps it would help elders sleep better if they increased the time they spent outdoors in the daylight.

Recent research should help seniors who are concerned about their memory proficiency better perform daily tasks requiring memory. Researchers discovered that memory functions best for seniors in the morning (*see* Time of Day and Memory Performance). If you are a senior and you need to give a talk, perhaps at your senior center, try to schedule it in the morning when your memory works best. More evidence has appeared in the past five years to reveal that memory functions better than many elders believe it does. One of the problems that does hinder memory functioning for many elders is the negative view they have about their own memory. Elders with this negative view perform more poorly on memory tasks than elders who do not have that view (*see* Negative Stereotype and Memory). Elders who have this negative stereotyped view of aging and are concerned about their memory should consider receiving counseling to rid themselves of that view, rather than undergo memory training.

There are many new entries dealing with health issues. Included are a number on frailty and disability. Frailty seems to be a greater health problem in late adulthood than is obesity (*see* Frailty [Incidence and Causes]). There are also a number of new entries on nursing homes. Especially important is one that provides information on what to look for if you need to find a quality nursing home for a loved one (*see* Searching for a Quality Nursing Home).

Taste is an example of an old entry that has received a major revision. "Everything tastes the same" is a familiar refrain for many seniors. The age-related decline in smell has been widely accepted as the cause for the "tastelessness" of many seniors. However, recent evidence indicates that taste itself is not completely blameless. Elders have been found to have difficulty in discriminating among increasing concentrations of salt. For example, it takes more than doubling the concentration of salt for many elders to detect an increase in saltiness. This suggests why many elders increase the amount of salt in their food in order to detect the presence of salt. Doing so places them in danger of health problems created by consuming too much salt (*see* Salt Intake).

Senior Centers is a second example of an old entry that received a major revision. Included is information noting a decline in attendance at centers in recent years. Also included are the results of a study identifying the probable reasons for the decline and giving recommendations for steps that may be taken to reverse the decline.

Other examples of old entries that received important new information are Aspirin, Cardiovascular Diseases, Claudication (leg cramps), Divorce, Dizziness, Medical Records, and Smoking. The new information about claudication is included in the new entry Peripheral Arterial Disease and Claudication. Information about heart-valve dysfunction and brain aneurysms has been added to the entry Cardiovascular Diseases, and information about digital medical records to the entry Medical Records.

INtRODUCtION

I n 1870 the first census of people in the United States who were 65
years of age or older was conducted. It was estimated that about 1.2
million people (3 percent of the total population of 40 million) were
"old." The years since 1870 have seen a remarkable phenomenon—the
graying of America. The years between 1960 and 1980 were especially dramatic ones in their contribution to the graying phenomenon. From 1960
to 1980 the total population of the United States increased about 19 percent, but the population of people age 65 and older increased by about 35
percent. In 1980 there were about 25 million people age 65 and older. The
phenomenon has not diminished since 1980. In 2000 it was estimated that
there were 35 million Americans who were 65 and older (about 13 percent
of the total population). By the year 2030 it is estimated that the number
of people age 65 and older will be about 65 million (about 20 percent of
the total population).

The graying of America has brought with it an ever increasing need to
understand what happens as we age. Organisms do age, and the human organism is no exception. Aging actually begins at birth and continues throughout life. Aging is as inevitable as death and taxes. What makes human aging
unique is that we alone are aware of our own aging and have the ability to
understand what occurs with aging and therefore anticipate its consequences.

Our understanding of aging is augmented by research on aging. The past
30 years have been especially productive ones for research on the biology,
psychology, and sociology of aging. This research has provided an enhanced
understanding of how aging, both normal and abnormal, affects our health,
our mental abilities, our personalities, and our social behaviors. The outcome has been to replace many myths about aging with knowledge derived
from research.

Our objective in the third edition, as it was in earlier editions of this book,
is to convey this information about aging to the general public in language
that is nontechnical. We hope it helps seniors better understand their own
aging and will help younger adults better understand what is happening to
their parents and other relatives as they grow older—and what is in store
for themselves in the future. This edition differs from the earlier editions

by having many new entries and many expanded old entries that report the major developments in aging research during the past five or six years.

The format of this edition is the same as that of the earlier editions. The many entries are arranged in alphabetical order. Also comparable with the earlier editions is the inclusion of two indexes. The first lists the main topics as well as subtopics with many cross-references. The second index identifies broad areas of research, such as memory, with specific entries relevant to that area listed under it (for example, Time of Day and Memory Performance). This organization is to facilitate the finding of information for readers interested in a particular area of aging research.

A cautionary note must be sounded. Aging research is usually characterized by the reporting of averages for different age groups, with an indication of the variability around those averages. In some cases, research reveals that, on average, elderly adults perform at a level below that of younger adults. For example, this may be true for some components and functions of memory. However, it is important to realize that many elderly adults perform at a level that exceeds that of many younger adults, even though the *average* performance for elderly adults may be below that for younger adults.

The information reported in our entries is derived from numerous sources. Much of the information about adult age differences in mental functioning, personality, and social behavior was taken from research reports in major psychological and sociological journals dealing with human aging. They include the *Gerontologist, Journals of Gerontology: Psychological Sciences and Social Sciences, Psychology and Aging, Developmental Review, Human Development, Educational Gerontology, Experimental Aging Research,* and the *International Journal on Aging and Human Development.* Additional information about aging, health, and disease came from such mainstream medical journals as the *New England Journal of Medicine* and journals specializing in geriatric medicine, such as the *Journal of the American Geriatric Society* and the *Journals of Gerontology: Biological and Medical Sciences.* Among the other important sources of information were two AARP publications, *AARP the Magazine* and *AARP Bulletin,* newspaper columns by Dr. Paul Donohue, recent textbooks on human aging, and more advanced technical books. Both the journals and the books are likely to be found in either a university library or a medical school library, and they should be available to you for further reading on the various topics covered in this book. A partial listing of the books is given below.

Textbooks

Cavanaugh, J. C., and F. B. Fields. *Adult Development and Aging.* 5th ed. Belmont, Calif.: Thomson Wadsworth, 2006.

Einstein, G. O., and M. A. McDaniel. *Memory Fitness: A Guide for Successful Aging.* New Haven, Conn.: Yale University Press, 2004.

Erber, J. T. *Aging and Older Adulthood.* Belmont, Calif.: Thomson Wadsworth, 2005.

Park, D., and N. Schwarz, eds. *Cognitive Aging: A Primer.* Philadelphia: Psychology Press, 2000.

Advanced Technical Books

Birren, J. E., and K. W. Schaie, eds. *Handbook of the Psychology of Aging.* 6th ed. San Diego: Elsevier Academic Press, 2005.

Craik, F. I. M., and T. A. Salthouse, eds. *The Handbook of Aging and Cognition.* 2nd ed. Mahwah, N.J.: Erlbaum Associates, 2000.

Kausler, D. H. *Learning and Memory in Normal Aging.* San Diego: Academic Press, 1994.

Maddox, G. L., et al., eds. *The Encyclopedia of Aging.* 2nd ed. New York: Springer, 1996.

Rowe, J. W., and R. L. Kahn. *Successful Aging.* New York: Pantheon Books, 1998.

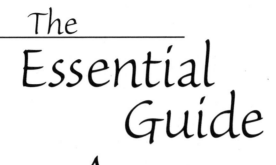

The
Essential
Guide
to Aging in the Twenty-First Century

A

AARP

The American Association of Retired Persons (as of January 1, 2000, its official name became AARP) was founded in 1958 by Dr. Ethel Andrus, a retired California educator. It was originally known as the National Retired Teachers Association. Its membership grew dramatically over the years, now exceeding thirty million people age fifty and older. It is the largest organization in the United States devoted to the needs of older people (its motto is "To serve, not to be served"), and it has become what many believe to be this country's most powerful congressional lobby. Its lobbying efforts have been especially effective for issues involving Social Security. AARP is active in many other areas of concern in gerontology (for example, helping older automobile drivers learn how to compensate for some of their declining abilities; see the Index of Entries and Cross-References for other examples).

In addition, AARP publishes a bimonthly magazine, *AARP the Magazine*, that has one of the largest circulations in the United States. Part of AARP is the Andrus Foundation, which is a major source of funding gerontological research, especially research directed at discovering ways of improving the welfare of older people. The address of both AARP headquarters and the Andrus Foundation is 601 E Street Northwest, Washington, DC 20049. AARP's Web site for information about a number of its programs is http://www.aarp.org.

Abilities (Physical and Mental) and Activity

Running, jumping, throwing a baseball: these are all physical abilities nearly all of us possess—but in levels of skill that vary from low to very high. Few people are truly competitive in a marathon race, and few of us could even complete one. Virtually none of us could challenge Carl Lewis in jumping or Nolan Ryan in the speed of throwing a baseball. These are all examples of physical abilities. Individual differences clearly exist at all age levels. The average levels of such physical abilities do change with normal aging. In general, they tend to decline, but the extent of the decline depends on many other factors besides aging itself. Certainly, health and regular exercise are critical factors. There is considerable evidence to indicate that physical abilities remain at a much higher level for those elderly adults who are in good health, are physically active, and who have been longtime regular exercisers (*see* Exercise [Relationship to Physical/Mental Performances]). Although it is highly unlikely that an elderly adult will win the Boston Marathon, it is true that many elderly adults do complete a marathon race. Muscle strength in elderly people can be increased, especially by following a training program that requires the appropriate exercise.

A number of physical abilities are specific to those individuals who acquired them through learning and practice early in life. Typing and playing the piano are examples. There is also evidence revealing that such skills are retained at a relatively constant level well into late adulthood, provided good health is retained and the skills have been practiced regularly and intensively over the years. This is the case for professional typists (*see* Expertise) and for professional pianists (*see* Motor Skill Learning).

Most of us also possess a number of mental abilities, such as reasoning ability, spatial ability, and verbal ability. There are large individual differences in the amount of ability at all age levels. Average levels of most mental abilities change with normal aging. Some decline modestly with aging, whereas others remain relatively constant, and still others may even increase by late adulthood.

Among those abilities that decline are components of what psychologists call fluid intelligence (*see* Intelligence). Spatial ability is an example. However, we know that elderly adults who had a high level of spatial ability as young adults continue to have a high level as elderly adults, relative to other elderly adults and even to most young adults (*see* Spatial Ability). Reading ability is another example of an ability that shows modest declines with normal aging. Elderly adults do read, on average, more slowly than younger adults, and they also demonstrate less comprehension of what they read, but only when the material contains complex phrasing (*see* Reading and Reading Skills). We also know that some of the declines in late adulthood can be reversed by appropriate interventions, such as training and practice (*see* Memory Training; Plasticity Theory; Transfer of Learning/Training). Whether "mental exercise" of various kinds (for example, playing chess, bridge, or other challenging mental games) aids in retaining mental skills is still an unresolved issue (but they surely can't harm you mentally; *see* Activity [Mental] and Mental Performance). Also largely unresolved is the role that might be played by lifelong physical exercise in maintaining these abilities at the levels achieved earlier in adulthood (*see* Exercise [Relationship to Physical/Mental Performances]).

Those abilities that remain relatively constant, and often increase in amounts, are components of what is called crystallized intelligence (*see* Intelligence). An example is wisdom, an ability that clearly increases from early to late adulthood (*see* Wisdom). Other examples are verbal ability and general knowledge. On average, elderly people score higher than younger adults on vocabulary tests and tests of general knowledge about the world (*see* Intelligence; Verbal Ability; Wechsler Intelligence Tests).

Abnormal Aging

People who age abnormally function at levels well below those of people who age normally. Abnormal aging is used in reference either to major problems in adjustment, as found in psychosis (*see* Psychosis) and clinical depression (*see* Depression [Incidence, Symptoms, Causes]) or to major problems in mental functioning to the point of dementia (*see* Alzheimer's Disease; Multi-Infarct Dementia; Senile Dementia). Dementia is character-ized primarily by memory problems that exceed greatly those found in normal aging (*see* Age-Associated Memory Impairment), problems in ori-entation to time and place, and attentional problems.

Accidents (at Home)

The incidence of accidents at home is the greatest for children and elderly adults. Not only is the rate of home accidents (falls, burns, accidental poison-ing, and so on) greater for people age sixty-five and older than for younger adults, but the incidence of disability and death resulting from such acci-dents is also increased. The high incidence in late adulthood undoubtedly is the consequence of decreased visual ability, decreased mobility, and decreased balance, relative to earlier adulthood.

Accidents (at Work)

Older workers have a lower frequency of minor accidents and temporary injuries on the job than do younger workers. A large 1981 study of work-ers' compensation records reported that the highest injury rate was for workers age twenty to twenty-four years and that the lowest rate was for workers age sixty-five and older. At the same time, time off from work as a result of these injuries is greater for older than for younger workers. Injuries resulting in death or disability are more frequent for younger workers. A major factor in the age difference in injury rates is job experi-ence. A large proportion of job injuries occur during a worker's first year, regardless of the worker's age. In addition, less qualified people tend to be removed from jobs before they reach an advanced age. Thus, most older workers are those who benefit from experience and those who have demon-strated their competence on the job.

Accidents (Automobile)

In recent years the number of automobile drivers who are sixty-five and older has been steadily increasing. Also steadily increasing has been the average number of miles driven annually by people in this age range. Unfortunately, elderly drivers also have more accidents per mile driven and more fatalities per mile driven than any other age group except the youngest drivers.

The number of fatal crashes for drivers age seventy and older was nearly five thousand in 1997, and the number of fatal crashes has increased by more than 40 percent since 1987. Drivers age sixty-five and older are more than one and a half times as likely to die from accidents as drivers between the ages of fifty-five and sixty-four from comparable injuries. Drivers seventy-five and older are more than two and a half times as likely to die from accidents as drivers between the ages of fifty-five and sixty-four from comparable injuries. Elderly drivers also have the highest fatality rate for pedestrians involved in automobile accidents—about one-fourth of pedestrian fatalities involve elderly adults.

Elderly drivers also experience more traffic violations per mile driven than any other age group. Older adults are less likely to be involved in accidents involving excessive speed, reckless driving, or intoxication than are younger drivers. Accidents involving older drivers are more likely to be caused by failure to see traffic signs, failure to yield the right-of-way, making unsafe turns, stopping unnecessarily (causing rear-end collisions), and improper highway entrance and exit. Interestingly, the incidence of accidents involving pilots of private planes who are in their sixties and seventies is less than the incidence of such accidents for younger pilots.

Driving an automobile is primarily a visual task. It is estimated that more than 90 percent of the information a driver must analyze is visual in nature. Aging is accompanied by declining proficiency in many components of vision (*see* Vision; Visual Disorders). Some of these declines are undoubtedly related to the greater accident-proneness experienced by elderly drivers, relative to younger drivers. Researchers at the University of Alabama at Birmingham recently provided convincing evidence that a primary factor in the high accident rate of elderly drivers is the shrinkage that occurs with aging in the *useful field of vision*. The useful field of vision is the extent of the visual periphery needed to perform the visual task at hand. Objects in the periphery must be detected by a driver in order for the driver to shift attention and focus on them. The researchers found that those elderly drivers with an especially large amount of shrinkage of the useful field of vision accounted for 95 percent of the intersection accidents surveyed in their study. Another visual function that is especially important in driving is the estimation of the velocity of an automobile being observed. Elderly adults are more likely to underestimate that velocity than are younger adults. Such underestimation is surely another major contributor to the high rate of accidents for elderly adults, especially accidents involving intersection crossings and merging a car into a line of traffic. Unfortunately, tests of the useful field of vision and vehicular velocity are not included in the visual tests administered to elderly drivers when they renew their driver's licenses. Another visual problem likely to cause a problem for elderly drivers is the greater time needed, relative to younger drivers, for refocusing from near to far objects and vice versa. The greater time needed to shift from focusing on the instrument panel to cars in front of the driver or to signs on the road may mean that the older driver will miss seeing important information.

An especially serious problem for elderly adults is driving when they have a cataract. The researchers at the University of Alabama at Birmingham found that elderly drivers with cataracts, relative to those without cataracts, were two and a half times more likely to have a history of fault crash involvement in the previous five years.

Difficulty with attention is another problem confronting many elderly drivers, one that may also be an important contributor to their high accident rate. Elderly adults, in general, have difficulty ignoring irrelevant sources of information while they are trying to attend to sources of relevant information (*see* Selective Attention). Drivers need to focus their attention on the flow of traffic (the relevant source of information) and tune out attention to the radio or words from a passenger (or, alas, a cell phone) (irrelevant sources of information). Failure to be selective in attention could lead to an accident, such as rear-ending the car in front of the elderly driver.

Visual and attentional impairments are not the only contributors to the driving accidents experienced by elderly drivers. Reaction time is slower for elderly adults than it is for younger adults (*see* Reaction Time). When events in a driver's pathway call for rapid braking of the car, it is likely that an elderly driver will respond more slowly than a younger driver, thus increasing the risk of an accident. Mental processes are also involved in the effective driving of an automobile. At times, decisions must be made as to when it is safe to pass another vehicle, the appropriate speed for given driving conditions, and so on.

Memory is not spared as a component of safe driving. Remembering that a specific road sign indicates an upcoming curve surely signals a reduction in speed. Similarly, one needs to remember especially dangerous intersections and approach them cautiously. Even mildly mentally impaired elderly adults are clearly at a greater risk than normally aging elderly drivers, given their poorer orientation and memory functioning. Yet some of these individuals are still driving automobiles. A study in New Jersey indicted that one-fourth of the outpatients in a dementia diagnostic clinic were still driving. Of these drivers, more than 75 percent had a history during the past year of "abnormal" driving habits, as indicated by such incidents as getting lost, having accidents, or receiving traffic tickets. Similarly, Canadian researchers discovered that patients in an outpatient clinic who met the criteria for dementia had about two and a half times as many crashes as age-matched normal adults. Especially a problem is the slowing down of processing or analyzing information that occurs in late adulthood (*see* Slowing-Down Principle). Elderly drivers may not analyze information fast enough to keep up with other cars nearby or with signs warning about a hazard ahead of the driver. Fortunately, Dr. Karlene Ball of the University of Alabama at Birmingham has developed computerized driving scenes that train older drivers to process information at a faster rate. She has found that not only do older drivers improve their speed on this task, but they also transfer it to driving in the real world.

Researchers at Washington University in St. Louis have devised a two-minute test to identify mentally impaired elderly adults who are likely to be accident prone. The test requires the taker to identify ten traffic signs. In an early use of the test 74 percent of the drivers with mild or moderate dementia were correctly identified by their performance on the test.

There are other physical conditions that seem to place elderly drivers at a greater risk than younger drivers either in terms of accidents per se or in terms of injuries from automobile accidents. For example, researchers at Yale University found that elderly drivers who walked little and had foot abnormalities had worse driving experiences than other elderly drivers who walked regularly and had no foot abnormalities.

Researchers in Florida reported that elderly women are twice as likely as elderly men to stop driving voluntarily. In a large sample of community-dwelling, ambulatory people age seventy and older, about 17 percent had voluntarily stopped driving. More than 30 percent of the people who were no longer driving cited health concerns as the reason for not driving. Researchers at Yale University found that diminished physical activity and reduced income were also factors contributing to the cessation of driving for a sample of elderly adults in New Haven, Connecticut.

A very sensitive, frequently debated issue is whether drivers should receive more thorough testing for license renewal when they reach a designated age. Should these drivers be required to demonstrate their competence for operating an automobile by means of tests other than a routine vision test? Such testing has been proposed by various states from time to time, most recently in California. Sensitivity enters the picture by the charge that selective testing is a form of age discrimination and the practice of ageism. Of course, this issue could be resolved by requiring people of *all* ages to undergo vigorous testing whenever they renew their licenses.

In 1991 there were seven states (California, Connecticut, Delaware, Nevada, New Jersey, Oregon, and Pennsylvania) that required physicians to report patients with apparent serious driving impairments. There were eight other states that authorized, but did not require, physicians to make these reports. Researchers in Massachusetts have demonstrated that reliable ratings of elderly drivers by competent observers can be made when they are required to drive in traffic. These ratings were found to correlate fairly substantially with scores on a mental test—the less the mental competence and alertness of the elderly driver, the poorer the driving ability as measured by performance on the test drive.

Older adults who are concerned about their declining skills should consider taking a course offered by AARP (*see* Drivers [Improving Their Skills]). Drivers who complete the course are eligible for an insurance discount in many states. *See also* Handedness.

Action Memory

"Did I turn out the lights in my car when I left it in the parking lot?" "Did I turn off the stove before leaving the kitchen?" "Was it last week Tuesday or Wednesday that I mowed the lawn?" In each of these questions, the person is testing his or her memory for actions or activities personally performed during daily living. It is not unusual to discover that our memory of our own performances is often impaired. That is, we sometimes have trouble remembering what actions we did perform or remembering when those actions were performed. The remarkable thing, however, is that we do have rather good memory of our own actions, even though we are unlikely to have the intent to remember them. We don't ordinarily say repeatedly to ourselves, "I locked the door" while making a deliberate attempt to commit that action to memory. That is, our memory for actions performed is usually incidental rather than intentional.

Of interest in gerontology is the extent to which action memory diminishes in proficiency from early to late adulthood. Elderly adults report most frequently that they have trouble remembering whether they turned off the stove or left the door unlocked. How accurate are their self-reports? Researchers have brought action memory into the laboratory by having participants of different ages perform a series of simple actions, such as clapping their hands and placing a cup on a saucer. After the series is completed, memory is then tested by either trying to recall the actions or by trying to recognize those that had just been performed from a list of actions. Several interesting findings have emerged from studies using this procedure. Participants who know their memory will be tested after the series has been completed score no higher on a recall test or a recognition test than do participants who are unaware of the subsequent memory test. That is, incidental memory is as proficient as intentional memory, just as it is for actions performed in the everyday world. This is true regardless of the participants' age. Both elderly and young participants have virtually perfect recognition memory scores. They have no difficulty recognizing which actions had been performed and which actions in the list had not been performed.

However, there is an age difference in the number of actions recalled, a difference attributable largely to adults who are age seventy and older. They recall, on average, only about 60 percent of the actions performed, whereas both young adults and adults in their sixties recall about 75 percent of the actions. Interestingly, elderly adults tend to recall more actions they regard as being less difficult to perform than actions regarded as being more difficult to perform. The opposite is true for younger adults. There is little difference for either young adult or elderly participants between the recall of unfamiliar actions (for example, placing a straw in your ear) and familiar actions (such as placing a straw in a glass).

The age difference in recall of actions may partially be the result of the greater difficulty experienced by elderly adults than by younger adults in retrieving information that has been stored in memory. It is also likely that actions are encoded (that is, converted into a memory trace) more thoroughly by younger than by older adults. Sufficient information about actions is probably encoded by elderly adults to permit eventual recognition of what they had been doing, but it may not be enough to permit recall of a number of those actions.

Are there interventions that improve the recall of one's own actions? To date, this is largely an unexplored topic. No one has determined, for example, whether elderly adults who have been regular, long-term exercisers have better action memories than elderly adults who have lived less physically active lives (see Exercise [Relationship to Physical/Mental Performances).

However, researchers at the University of Missouri at Columbia have discovered what may be an effective mnemonic for somewhat improving recall of actions (perhaps as much as 20 percent) regardless of age. Young adult and elderly participants were required to recall after every few actions those that had just been performed. That is, short-term recall was required for each action in the series. Short-term recall was especially beneficial to later long-term recall if there was a brief retention interval during which the participants performed some interfering activity, such as counting backward from a designated number. Short-term recall of actions seems to be beneficial to later long-term recall only if it is both somewhat effortful (as it is after an interval filled with an interfering activity) and successful.

Older adults who wish to improve recall of their own actions in the everyday world should try this short-term retrieval procedure. For example, if three successive actions are turning off the lights in the dining room, letting out the dog, and shutting off the garden hose, try recalling these last three actions performed after you have turned off the garden hose. It should help you to recall later when you have entered the bedroom that the lights are off in the dining room, that the dog is still outside, and that the hose is off.

Of further interest is the age difference in temporal memory for actions performed in the laboratory (*see* Temporal Memory). Here the demand is on remembering *when* an action is performed and not on remembering what action was performed. Age differences for temporal memory are tested by having participants perform a series of actions; they then reconstruct the temporal order in which they were performed. In several studies, substantial age differences, favoring young adults, have been found in the proficiency of making these time-oriented judgments. Temporal memory, whether for actions performed in the laboratory or for words viewed sequentially in a list, appears to be a highly age-sensitive form of memory.

Activities of Daily Living

It is estimated that more than 80 percent of the behavior of older people occurs in the home. Moreover, about one-third of each day is spent on behaviors termed the *activities of daily living* (activities for maintaining normal home living). A survey of healthy elderly people living independently in the community revealed that, on average, they spend daily 53 minutes on personal and health care activities, 77 minutes on eating, 68 minutes on housework and home maintenance, 69 minutes on cooking, and 22 minutes on shopping.

These averages are somewhat different for impaired older people (that is, those receiving in-home services). For example, they were found to average 71 minutes daily in personal and health care activities and only 38 minutes on housework and home maintenance. For what may be considered optional activities, the unimpaired and impaired elderly people were found to be fairly equivalent in the average daily time spent reading (59 and 52 minutes, respectively) and watching television (205 and 210 minutes, respectively). However, a major difference was found in the average time spent resting and relaxing (128 minutes for the unimpaired and 200 minutes for the impaired).

Of further interest is the difficulty experienced by elderly people in performing the activities of daily living. A national survey indicated that the percentage of elderly people who expressed difficulty in performing an activity varied greatly with the nature of the activity. For example, less than 2 percent expressed difficulty in eating and less than 5 percent in using the toilet. By contrast, nearly 10 percent expressed difficulty in bathing and nearly 20 percent in walking. However, for all of these activities the percentage of elderly people who actually receive help to perform them was quite small (for instance, 6 percent for bathing).

Activities may be classified in several different ways. One way is to distinguish among *obligatory activities, committed activities,* and *discretionary activities.* Obligatory activities are those required for survival (eating and personal care), committed activities are those required for household management (home repair and housework), and discretionary activities are those engaged in during free time (sports and hobbies). Elderly adults tend to spend more time on obligatory activities and passive discretionary activities than on committed activities, with the least time spent on active discretionary activities (such as sports).

A distinction is also made between simple *physical activities of daily living* (for example, bathing) and more complex *instrumental activities of daily living* (housework, shopping, or visiting places outside of walking distance). Interestingly, researchers at the University of Alabama at Birmingham found that proficiency on both forms of activities is associated positively and highly with mental ability as measured by the Mini-Mental State Exam (*see* Mini-Mental State Exam). In addition, researchers at Johns Hopkins University School of Medicine discovered that performance by elderly adults on laboratory tests of both physical and instrumental activities of daily living correlated highly with performance on similar activities at home.

There is also evidence indicating that perception of one's own ability to perform instrumental activities of daily living (such perception is a form of what is called self-efficacy; *see* Self-Efficacy) is positively associated with one's belief about his or her ability to perform these activities (such as arranging transportation and taking precautions for personal safety). That is, the greater the self-efficacy of an older person, the greater the confidence that person has in his or her functioning. Perhaps improving elderly people's self-efficacy could lead to their improved functioning in regard to instrumental activities. Attentional flexibility as measured by the Trail Making Test (*see* Trail Making Test) has been found to be positively related to the proficiency of performing complex instrumental activities of daily living.

Researchers at the University of Chicago reported that people who are age seventy-five and older and who have visual impairments are nearly one and a half times more likely to have difficulty in performing the activities of daily living than are people of the same age who do not have such impairments. They also reported the absence of a relationship between hearing impairment and performance of daily activities for people in the same age range.

Elderly women with upper body disability have been found to have more difficulty in performing physical daily activities than elderly men with a similar disability. This is probably because dressing oneself usually requires more dexterity for women than for men. On the other hand, the reverse is true for lower body disability (that is, elderly men have more difficulty than elderly women). This sex difference may be related to the greater willingness of women than of men to seek assistance in performing activities requiring lower body strength.

Difficulty in performing such activities as light housekeeping and shopping have been found to increase with the severity of lower back pain in women. Estimates of the number of older people who suffer from lower back pain vary greatly, ranging from 24 percent in women and 18 percent in men age sixty-five and older (in a survey of rural Iowans) to 68 percent in a survey of older women with fractures (*see* Back Pain).

Limitations in performing the physical activities of daily living produced by diseases are greatest for elderly people with cardiovascular disease or arthritis. At risk of losing some ability to perform both physical and instrumental activities of daily living are elderly adults who have been hospitalized for an acute medical illness and have had problems in their mobility while in the hospital. They are likely to benefit from intensive rehabilitative therapy during both their hospital stay and later at home in order to regain normal functioning.

Mild and moderately mentally impaired elderly adults experience moderately greater difficulty in performing both forms of daily activities than mentally unimpaired elderly adults. Researchers in Boston found that nursing home residents given weight-training exercises (resistance training of major muscles related to functioning and mobility) for ten months showed significantly less decline in activities of daily living such as dressing, personal hygiene, and eating compared to participants in a control group.

Activity Diversity (Cognitive Benefits)

Activities are not restricted to mental and physical exercises. In fact, many older adults engage in such diverse activities as volunteering at a hospital, gardening, pumping gasoline into their automobile, and so on as well as playing bridge and engaging in physical exercise. Australian researchers followed a group of older adults (average age of seventy-seven years at the start of their study) for six years. The participants were interviewed at regular intervals to determine how frequently they engaged in twenty-four diverse activities. They were tested both at the start of the study and at the end of the study on a variety of cognitive tasks (for example, recall of objects in a picture and speed of processing information). Those who participated more frequently at the start of the study scored higher on the cognitive tasks than those who participated less frequently. In addition, after six years the more frequent participants experienced a significantly smaller decline in their cognitive performances than did the less frequent participants.

Activity (Mental) and Mental Performance

"Use it or lose it" is a statement often heard in reference to aging and the mind. The implication is that elderly people need frequent "exercise" of their minds or risk significant decline in their mental functioning. Do elderly adults who regularly engage in challenging mental activities, such as playing bridge, playing chess, and solving crossword puzzles, perform better on memory tasks and intelligence tests than elderly adults who are less mentally active in their everyday lives?

Research providing support for the positive effects of challenging mental activities on mental performance has focused largely on leisure or recreational activities. A logical analysis suggests that frequent reading of newspaper editorials is more stimulating than frequent reading of newspaper comic strips. Similarly, playing chess is more stimulating than playing canasta, and watching the Discovery Channel is more stimulating than watching reruns of old sitcoms. Using this view of stimulation, Canadian researchers found that older men who reported frequent participation in stimulating and challenging mental activities scored higher on an intelligence test than did older men who participated in less stimulating mental activities.

Similarly, in a study involving thousands of participants in the Chicago area (age sixty-five and older), those who engaged in frequent intense mental or cognitive activities in their daily lives, such as reading a book and visiting a museum, performed at a higher level on a memory task than those who engaged in frequent, less intense mental activity, such as watching television and listening to a radio. Participation in intense daily activities was found to be associated with more education, higher income, and male sex. In addition. researchers in California found that long-term skilled elderly bridge players score higher on memory tasks than do nonplaying elderly people (*see also* Work).

Researchers at the Rush-Presbyterian–St. Luke's Medical Center studied more than eight hundred Roman Catholic nuns, priests, and brothers to determine how participation in such common activities as reading newspapers, doing crossword puzzles, and going to museums relates to developing Alzheimer's disease. They found that the participants with the highest frequency of activity had a 47 percent reduction in the risk for the disease compared to those with the lowest frequency of activity.

The one exception to this positive evidence comes from several studies reporting that older adults who are currently college students perform no better on laboratory memory tasks than older people who have been away from an academic setting for many years. Taking college courses should surely qualify as a source of vigorous regular mental activity.

One could argue that those elderly people who engage in demanding mental activities were brighter throughout their lives than other older people. Current mental activity could contribute little to the better mental functioning exhibited by those who engage in it. However, especially impressive evidence for the potentially positive effects of a high level of mental activity late in life comes from a study conducted at Harvard University. Physicians older than age sixty-five who were still working as physicians scored, on average, much higher on a variety of mental tests than physicians of the same age who were retired. Similarly, in another study, professors who were in their sixties performed as well as professors in their thirties on tests that required comprehending and remembering textual material. Surely, professors "exercise" their minds regularly.

More research is needed to determine exactly the effects of mental activity during late adulthood on reducing, or even eliminating, mental decline with normal aging. In the meantime, why be half safe? Keep exercising your mind!

Activity (Physical)

In 1985 a number of men ranging in age from sixty-five to eighty-four were measured on time spent on physical activity and were measured again ten years later. The average time spent on physical activity daily decreased by 33 percent (twenty-eight minutes) during the ten years of aging. However, walking was largely unaffected by aging. That is, other physical activities were the ones showing the decline.

In another study nearly one-third of men and one-half of women were found to engage in no physical activity by age seventy-five. All elderly adults could improve the quality of their lives and prolong their lives by simply performing such physical activities as mowing the lawn, washing the car, and walking to the store. In a study in Wales two thousand middle-aged men were followed from 1979 to 1997. The amount and type of physical activity in an average week were determined. It was found that men who burned as little as fifty-four calories a day on such activities as landscaping had about the same life-saving health benefits as did men who burned many more calories a day. Of course, a structured physical exercise program may be even more beneficial (see Exercise [Relationship to Physical/Mental Performances]). In a study of thousands of nurses aged forty-six to seventy-one, it was found that even a modest loss of weight (as little as five pounds) leads to better physical functioning on such tasks as walking up stairs.

In addition, a Japanese researcher discovered that positive social influences from family members, friends, and health experts are related positively to the amount of physical activity for elderly adults, while negative social influences are related negatively to the amount of physical activity. The potential bad effects of diminished physical activity in late adulthood on physical health and physical functioning have been well established in a study conducted by researchers in Finland.

Activity (Productive)

Activity is considered to be productive when it produces goods or services, regardless of whether pay is received for it. Productive activities include housework, child care, volunteer work, and help provided for family members and friends, as well as work on salaried occupations. A common belief is that men and women become increasingly similar to one another in the kinds of productive activities they perform as they grow older. This does not seem to be true, however. Older men tend to do more paid work outside the home and more household maintenance work than do older women.

Interestingly, researchers at the University of Vermont found that paid work had no effect on the emotional experiences of either older men or older women. Older women tend to do more housework, more child care in the home, more caregiving outside the home, and more volunteer work than do older men. Married and unmarried older men and women appear to be similar in paid work outside the home. In general, older people who are in good health engage in more productive activity than do those older people who are less healthy. This is true for men and women, whether white or African American.

There are, however, some racial differences in productive activity for older people. African Americans are less likely to retire early from paid work than are whites. In terms of work around the house, older African American women and men tend to engage in equal amounts, in contrast to the pattern found for older white women and men (*see also* Participation in Voluntary Organizations and Volunteer Work).

Another kind of productive work is that conducted by residents of nursing homes. It has long been known that activities of various kinds are beneficial to the welfare of the residents. In fact, in 1987 Congress passed a bill that mandated nursing homes to provide activities for their residents if they were to receive federal funds. The problem, however, is to get the residents involved in activities. Residents do differ greatly in the time they spend in activities.

Researchers in Michigan observed residents in a number of nursing homes. They discovered that women tend to spend more time in activities than do men. They also discovered that nondepressed residents tend to spend more time in activities than do depressed residents and that the time spent on activities decreases as the degree of mental impairment increases. Not surprisingly, they also discovered that the least time was spent by those residents who needed the greatest assistance in performing the activities of daily living (*see* Activities of Daily Living).

Activity Theory

Activity theory is concerned with the conditions that promote a high level of satisfaction with life in late adulthood. It began in a rough form at the University of Chicago during the 1960s in opposition to the then popular disengagement theory, which stressed that withdrawal from social activity is the best condition for successful aging (*see* Disengagement Theory). Activity theory initially stated that optimal satisfaction occurs when elderly people continue as much as possible the activities of middle age and find substitutes for those activities that are prohibited by any declining abilities.

A more systematic theory was proposed in the 1970s by gerontologists at the University of Southern California. Their theory specified three forms of activity and ordered them in terms of the magnitudes of the effects each should have on life satisfaction. The first form is *informal activity,* such as activities with friends, relatives, and neighbors. The second is *formal activity,* such as participation in voluntary organizations. The third is *solitary activity,* such as leisure pursuits and maintenance of a household. Each form was expected to increase life satisfaction as the amount of that activity increased. However, the beneficial effects of informal activity were expected to be greater than the effects of formal activity which, in turn, were expected to be greater than the effects of solitary activity.

In a test of their own theory, the gerontologists at the University of Southern California found only partial support for the theory. Only informal activity was found to be positively related to the degree of life satisfaction, and then only moderately so. A more thorough test of the theory was conducted in the 1980s by researchers at the University of Miami. They too found informal activity to be moderately and positively related to the degree of life satisfaction. Informal activity has also been found to be positively related to longevity for people aged sixty-five and older.

The researchers at the University of Miami also found formal activity to be negatively related to life satisfaction—that is, the greater the amount of formal activity, in general, the less the degree of life satisfaction. Other research on life satisfaction in late adulthood has revealed that life satisfaction is affected by many conditions in addition to activity (*see* Life Satisfaction).

Acupuncture

Acupuncture is an ancient Chinese way of treating a disease or a painful condition by inserting needles into various parts of the body. There is some evidence to support the therapeutic value of acupuncture for elderly adults, at least for some health problems. For example, for patients with a particular foot problem, researchers in Sweden contrasted those patients receiving acupuncture with those receiving physiotherapy and occupational therapy over a ten-week period. Patients receiving acupuncture recovered faster and to a greater degree than patients receiving the more traditional therapy.

More convincing evidence for the therapeutic value of acupuncture comes from a study in Taiwan in which people age sixty and older who reported having sleep problems received acupuncture at several places on the body for five days a week over a three-week period. Compared to participants in a placebo control group, the participants receiving acupuncture reported a significant reduction in the frequency of awakenings and in night wakeful time (*see also* Sleep Therapy).

Convincing evidence was also obtained by German researchers who found that patients receiving twelve weeks of acupuncture therapy experienced an average of a 50 percent reduction in the frequency of migraine headaches. Seniors suffering from pain caused by osteoarthritis may receive relief from it by acupuncture. Researchers compared participants receiving twelve acupuncture treatments for their knees with participants receiving twelve fake treatments. After eight weeks knee pain and stiffness decreased by half its original level for 52 percent of the acupuncture participants and only 28 percent for participants receiving the fake treatment.

Adapting a Home for Elderly Residents

Elderly people often have reasons for wanting to make their homes more adaptable to their changing motor skills and sensory abilities. Changing the home to reduce the risk of falls is discussed in the entry on falls (*see* Falls). Manufacturers now have available special home items to make home living safer and more pleasant for elderly residents. They include doors on bathtubs to eliminate the difficulty of stepping in or out of the tub and adjustable-height kitchen sinks for use by spouses and visitors of different heights.

Adapting to Fading Eyesight

Many older adults have a life greatly altered by diminished reading ability brought about by visual impairment. These older adults need to find ways of adapting to fading eyesight so that they can maintain a reasonable degree of independence.

Researchers at McMaster University in Hamilton, Canada, identified three types of barriers confronting visually impaired men and women aged sixty-five to ninety-three. For each they asked the participants in their study how they adapted to the barrier. The first barrier was meal preparation. Adaptation consisted of using old recipes that they memorized, or they rehearsed new recipes until they were stored in memory. Some also used large-print measuring cups or cups with tactile markers. The second barrier was using the telephone. Here they memorized important numbers. Some also used larger-size keypads and a magnifier to read unfamiliar numbers in a directory. The third barrier was in conducting their financial affairs. Here they memorized buttons and instructions of bank machines and withdrew only small amounts of cash at a time. *See also* Visual Disorders (Coping with Macular Degeneration).

Adult Day-Care Centers

Adult day-care centers began to appear in the United States during the late 1960s, and they have increased greatly in numbers over the years. In 1974 there were only eighteen centers. By 1995 there were more than three thousand.

Adult day-care centers were patterned after those of Great Britain, where they have long been a part of geriatric health services. The centers in the United States provide a community care program for the frail elderly. Participants in a center's program are in residence during the day and return to their homes in the evening. The objectives of the program are to enhance the health and social functioning of the participants and to reduce the burden and stress on home caregivers by making time available for activities other than caregiving. Clients of adult day-care centers are less likely to be severely mentally impaired than are residents in a nursing home or recipients of respite care (*see* Respite Care). However, the results of a recent survey indicated that about 25 percent of the clients in adult day-care centers do have severe disturbances. It appears that day-care programs are steadily increasing the numbers of severely demented individuals they serve.

Researchers at the University of Michigan sampled the clientele and services of a number of centers. They discovered that there are two distinct types of centers (excluding specialized centers, such as those for people who are blind). The first type is affiliated with a nursing home or rehabilitation hospital. This type of center usually serves a clientele composed of physically dependent older people, most of whom do not have a mental disorder. The services provided may include nursing, therapy, diet regulation, and other health and social services. Financial support usually comes from sources other than the government (for example, client payment). The second type is affiliated with a hospital (but unlikely to be located in the hospital) or a social service agency. The clientele is likely to have a large representation from minority populations with minimal physical disability, but frequently with some degree of mental disability. Services usually include counseling, nutrition education, and transportation to and from the center. Funding is likely to be derived from governmental services, especially Medicaid.

Results from the Michigan study also revealed that both caregivers and clients are generally pleased with the services received at such centers. In addition, the cost of day care is usually much less than either full-time care in a nursing home or respite care outside a nursing home. It is not surprising that the number of centers has been increasing rapidly during the past decade.

Advance Directives

An advance directive enables elderly people to maintain control over their health care if they become physically or mentally incapable of choosing medical treatment options. The two most common forms of advance directives are living wills, which state in advance one's preference regarding life-sustaining treatment, and durable powers of attorney for health care, which authorize another person to make medical decisions when a patient is unable to do so. These two directives may also be combined. The Patient Self-Determination Act of 1990 requires that patients in institutions such as hospitals, nursing homes, and hospices be informed about advance directives and their right to accept or refuse treatment.

A recent study revealed that 90 percent of the patients surveyed supported the concept of an advance directive, but only 15 percent had actually arranged to have one. Researchers at the University of Minnesota have developed an intervention for use with elderly people that seems to work in terms of increasing the number who record an advance directive. The intervention involves interactions with a social worker who provides information and counseling about the merits of an advance directive.

What factors determine decisions about the use of life-sustaining treatment or its cessation? Researchers at the University of Southern California gave people ranging in age from twenty-four to ninety-three hypothetical situations involving potential life-sustaining treatment. The factors rated most important in determining the nonapplication of the treatment were the mental capacity of the patient and the pain suffered by the patient. The factors rated least important in determining nonapplication were the burden of care on family members, financial strain for the family, and the age of the patient. However, the oldest participants in the study rated these last three factors as being somewhat more important than did the younger participants.

Aftereffects (Visual)

An aftereffect is a sensory experience that persists after the originating physical source of that experience has ceased. A familiar aftereffect occurs when you stare for a minute or so at a piece of brightly colored paper and then turn your gaze to a piece of white paper. You will "see" on the white paper a patch of color that is the complementary color of the one patch at which you had been staring. Thus, if the paper was blue, you will "see" yellow (the complementary color of blue) as the aftereffect (or negative afterimage, as it is often called).

Of interest is the evidence indicating that the color aftereffect persists several seconds longer for elderly people than for younger people. Longer persistence in late adulthood is also found for other aftereffects. For example, if you stare at a rapidly rotating spiral figure for some seconds you will "see" the spiral continue to rotate for several seconds even though the physical rotation has terminated. In such instances, the aftereffect persists longer for elderly people than for younger people. The reason for the age difference in the persistence of aftereffects is unknown. However, a popular hypothesis is that more time is required for stimulation "to clear the nervous system" in late adulthood than in earlier adulthood (*see* Stimulus Persistence).

Age-Associated Memory Impairment

Diagnosis of a disorder of any kind is the all-important first step before an appropriate treatment can be applied to the disorder. The outcome of diagnosis is the classification of the client's or the patient's disorder. The currently popular classification for those normally aging individuals who have moderate memory problems, but the extent of the problem is not great enough to be considered abnormal or pathological, is age-associated memory impairment (AAMI). Everyday examples of moderate memory problems include forgetting where you placed your keys and whether you locked the door when you left your home.

This classification has largely replaced the earlier one of benign senescent forgetfulness. The diagnosis of AAMI is made on the basis of the client's performance on memory tests that have had wide clinical application. One such test is the Wechsler Memory Scale (*see* Wechsler Memory Scale). A client who scores well below the average typically earned by normally aging individuals (but still well above the scores earned by individuals with a pathological memory impairment) is diagnosed as having AAMI.

The diagnosis is usually made by a neuropsychologist. Neuropsychology is the branch of psychology that deals with the relationship among the brain, mental functions, and behavior. One of a neuropsychologist's specialties is the interpretation of psychological and psychiatric tests and the information provided in interviews of a client and family.

Diagnosis does not end with the classification of a client as having AAMI. Further information about the client is needed to determine the reason for the memory problem. Conceivably, the problem is a temporary one caused by a change in the client's physical or mental health. For example, a physical health problem may have required treatment with a medication that has moderate mental confusion as a side effect, with memory dysfunction (that is, memory working at a level below what it should be) as the primary symptom. In this case, a different medicine may be substituted for the original one, or the client may be assured that the memory problem is likely to be eliminated when the physical problem is eliminated and the medication is no longer needed.

Alternatively, the client may be in a state of depression as a result of some recent traumatic experience. In some cases, depression may adversely affect memory functioning. Once the depression is significantly reduced by therapy or by the passage of time, the chances are good that the memory problem will also be eliminated. If these extraneous health problems are ruled out, then it may be decided that the client has a memory problem that may benefit from participation in a memory training program. Older adults who are concerned about their memory, and possible ways of improving it, may want to purchase the book *The Memory Manual: 10 Simple Things You Can Do to Improve Your Memory after Age 50* by Betty Fielding (Word Dancer Press).

There is the possibility that for some seniors with AAMI, their mild forgetfulness is a predictor of later Alzheimer's disease. Researchers at Rush University Medical Center in Chicago discovered that autopsies of these individuals revealed that they already had some of the pathological brain changes associated with Alzheimer's disease.

AAMI is not to be confused with another classification commonly called mild cognitive dementia (MCD). Here the everyday memory problems are more serious. They may include failure to keep an important appointment and failure to remember having already asked a question of someone. The probability is high that someone with MCD will eventually develop Alzheimer's disease (*see* Senile Dementia).

Age Change versus Age Difference

"I'm not as fast as I used to be." If said by elderly people, this statement is probably correct. When elderly people have measurements of their reaction time, their average speed of responding is indeed slower than that of younger adults. To measure reaction time, participants listen for or watch for a cue of some kind (for example, a tone is sounded or a light goes on) and then perform a response, such as pushing a button, as rapidly as they can. Reaction time is the time elapsed between the onset of the cue and the execution of the requested response (*see* Reaction Time).

Our point is that the statement made by elderly people is true. They have had an age change in their speed of reacting. They were faster when they were younger, and there has been a progressive slowing of their reaction time as aging progressed. There also is an age difference in the speed of responding. A group of young adults averages faster responses than a group of elderly adults when individuals in both groups are given a reaction-time task to perform (a cross-sectional study; *see* Cross-Sectional Method). The *age difference* in this case results because of an age *change*. An age change means that individuals are changing over the course of their adult life span, such that their performance on whatever task is being measured (speed of responding in the example given) also changes. However, it is important to realize that not all age differences are the result of an age change.

A simple example should clarify the distinction between an age difference and an age change. Suppose we were to measure the height of every man between the ages of twenty and twenty-nine and also the height of every man between the ages of seventy and seventy-nine. Not surprisingly, we would discover that men in their twenties average several inches taller than men in their seventies. Thus, there is a rather large *age difference* in height. However, very little of this age difference is the result of an *age change.* The height of elderly men is about the same as it was when they were young men. It is true that a modest age change probably did occur. Some shrinking occurs with aging, a shrinking produced largely through the thinning of the cartilage between the bones of the vertebral column. However, the amount of shrinking is not nearly pronounced enough to account for the age difference of several inches in height.

Most likely, it is the difference in generations (defined by birth year) between currently young and elderly adults. Members of a later generation (such as people currently in their twenties) encountered, during their childhoods, health care and diet conditions that were more favorable to physical growth than members of an earlier generation (such as people currently in their seventies). In fact, the generational difference is part of a trend toward increasing height of young men over the centuries. Consider, for example, the average height of young men who lived during the Middle Ages. People are usually shocked when they visit a museum and see for the first time a suit of armor worn by a knight of that period. Most of today's fifth-graders would find the suit to be a tight fit!

The distinction between an age difference and a true age change is an important one in understanding the effects of aging on behavior. Not all age differences in behavior are the result of people changing with age. As an example, consider the age difference in the personality trait of introversion (being shy and not very outgoing). Some years ago elderly people were found to have test scores for the trait of introversion that were much higher than those of young adults. Does this mean that the elderly people were then much more introverted than they were when they themselves were young adults—and that they became more and more introverted as they grew older? The evidence from more recent aging research indicates that this is not the case (*see* Personality Traits). Introversion, like most other personality traits, tends to be stable from early to late adulthood.

Today's elderly adults were probably no less introverted when they were young adults than they are today. As with the height example, the critical factor responsible for the age difference in introversion found in early studies was a difference among generations in some environmental condition (social or physical or both) present during preadulthood, not aging itself. An age difference produced by some condition other than aging may very well not be present in the future, especially if that condition stabilizes for future generations. In fact, current cross-sectional studies show little difference between younger and older adults in their average test scores on a test of introversion. By contrast, if aging is the critical factor, then an age difference in behavior may well persist for future generations, unless something has been discovered that greatly reduces or even eliminates the aging process. This is surely the fate of speed of responding. As noted above, the age difference is the result of a true age change.

Age Discrimination at Work

A number of companies and industries attempt to eliminate workers who are over the age of sixty. Their objectives are to save on salary, medical coverage, and retirement benefits. However, since the late 1960s there has been the Age Discrimination in Employment Act (*see also* Work). Fortunately, the courts have been sympathetic toward older workers. Although the number of lawsuits filed with the Equal Opportunity Commission decreased by 20 percent between 1993 and 1997, those who sued for age discrimination were awarded an average of 90 percent more than those who sued on the basis of race, sex, or disability. In the years 1988–1995 the average award for age discrimination was $219,000 compared to $107,000 for sex discrimination.

Ageism

The term *ageism* was introduced in 1968 by Dr. Robert N. Butler, a prominent geriatric physician and the first director of the National Institute on Aging. Ageism refers to the then widely held (and still not completely eliminated) negative attitude toward elderly individuals. In effect, ageism means a negative stereotype is applied toward the entire population of elderly adults, a stereotype in which they are viewed as being senile, rigid in their thinking, grumpy, and having other undesirable traits and behaviors.

Of course, ageism is not the only negative stereotype that has characterized large segments of our population. Others include racism and sexism. The stereotypical perception of elderly adults, like other such stereotypes, is, of course, false. For example, senility is rare in our elderly population, there is no firm evidence to indicate that rigidity (that is, inflexibility) in thinking is more prevalent among elderly people than it is among younger people (*see* Rigidity), and most elderly people are pleasant rather than grumpy.

The existence of ageism has been frequently demonstrated in psychological studies. For example, when college students are asked to rate a "typical" twenty-five-year-old and a "typical" seventy-year-old on a number of personality characteristics, they apply more negative characteristics to the seventy-year-old individual than to the twenty-five-year-old individual and more positive characteristics to the twenty-five-year-old than to the seventy-year-old. Most depressing is the evidence that elderly adults are nearly as likely as young adults to apply the negative stereotype in evaluating their peers.

Similarly, when young adults are given a description of a fictitious person who is having a memory problem (such as forgetting a telephone number while dialing it), they are more likely to believe that the problem is a serious one and a sign of mental difficulty if the person is described as being elderly rather than young. People of all ages often have difficulty remembering all of the digits of a telephone number encountered for the first time. The good news is that elderly adults performing the same task are less likely than young adults to view minor memory problems as a sign of senility (*see also* Work).

A negative evaluation is also more likely to be given when participants of different ages listen to a fictitious audio interview for a supervisor's job in which the interviewee is identified as being old. Younger adults with less than a high school education are especially likely to believe that nearly all older people tend to be senile, lack sexual behavior, live in poverty, and feel miserable about their lives.

However, there is some evidence to suggest that the negative stereotype is assigned more often to the "old" old (people in their eighties and beyond) than to the "young" old (especially people in their sixties). Surely forgotten by those holding this pessimistic view of the "old" old are the many great recitals by Pablo Casals, Arthur Rubenstein, Vladimir Horowitz, and others at very advanced ages.

Why does ageism exist in our society? Part of the reason is the lack of valid information that many people have about aging's effects on human behavior (*see* Facts of Aging Quiz). The lack of information is then replaced by myths about aging, myths perpetuated by the steady diet of unflattering descriptions and portrayals of elderly people often found in folklore, literature, movies, television shows, and even the daily comics (*see also* Myths about Aging). Consider the contributions of folklore through such adages as "You can't teach an old dog new tricks" and "There's no fool like an old fool." Many jokes about elderly people emphasize mental and physical deficits. Elderly people have not fared much better in literature. Witness, for example, Shakespeare's famous description of old age in *As You Like It* as being "sans teeth, sans eyes, sans taste, sans everything." With regard to television, familiar figures are those like the much maligned grandfather on *The Simpsons* and Raymond's grumpy old father in *Everybody Loves Raymond*. For those watching television reruns, there's the elderly woman on *Golden Girls* who is often depicted as being foolish, tactless, and irresponsible.

There is another possible reason for ageism's presence in our society, one convincingly advanced by Dr. Butler. He argued that ageism gives many younger individuals a reason for avoiding elderly people. Since elderly people differ from themselves, there is an excuse for having little to do with them. By avoiding elderly people as much as possible, younger people are able to reduce their fears regarding their own aging.

Unfortunately, many younger people do shy away as much as possible from interacting with elderly people. Medical students have been known to express a negative attitude toward their future treatment of elderly patients, so much that very few express an interest in geriatric medicine. Even members of the clergy are not completely free of what has been called the YAVIS syndrome (the preference for *young*, *attractive*, *verbal*, *intelligent*, and *successful*—therefore affluent—clients).

Fortunately, there is evidence to indicate that the negative view of elderly people, at least the one held by many medical students, may be overcome by appropriate training. A number of medical schools now offer courses that deal with aging and with ways of improving communication with elderly people. Students who are trained in this way show a more positive attitude toward elderly people and a greater willingness to work with elderly people as patients. *See also* Ageism Exists in Some Words.

Ageism Exists in Some Words

The word *old* implies being debilitated and infirm—concepts that do not apply to many "older" people. The word *elderly* implies frailty and possibly disability. Dr. Erdman Palmore, a prominent gerontologist, suggests replacing these potentially offensive words with more positive or neutral terms, such as *senior* and *elder.*

How do older people themselves feel about such terms as *old* and *elderly*? Researchers at the University of Texas Southwestern Medical Center at Dallas discovered that the most-liked nouns are *senior citizen* and *retiree* (liked by 75 percent and 70 percent, respectively, of the older participants in their study). The most-liked adjectives are *retired* (73 percent), *senior* (71 percent), and *mature* (68 percent). The most-disliked adjectives are *old* (67 percent), *aged* (62 percent), and *geriatric* (59 percent).

Age Simulation

An age change in some ability or characteristic results in a different performance level for elderly adults, on average, than for younger adults on tasks that involve that ability or characteristic. It is often debatable, however, whether the observed age difference in performance actually results from a change with aging. This is especially true when the study reporting the age difference used the cross-sectional method (*see* Age Change versus Age Difference).

An alternative is to use the longitudinal method in which the same individuals perform both when they are younger and when they are older. However, the longitudinal method is usually impractical and has its own limitations (*see* Longitudinal Method).

An ideal way to determine whether aging causes an observed age difference in performance on a particular task would be to test young adults on the task and then "age" them in such a manner that the ability or characteristic required for performance on the task is believed to be much like that of an average elderly adult. This procedure is called age simulation.

Unfortunately, there are few abilities or characteristics that can be artificially and temporarily "aged." One that is, however, is the characteristic believed to be responsible for the greater illusory Müller-Lyer effect experienced by elderly adults than by young adults (*see* Illusions). The yellowing of the lens with aging permits less light to reach the eyes' retinas. This light reduction presumably plays a major role in determining the greater illusory effect for elderly people. The age change in the amount of light reaching the retina can be simulated by having young adults perform the illusory task while wearing goggles that diminish the amount of light reaching the retina. When this is done, the illusory experience of young participants approximates that of elderly participants (performing, of course, without the goggles). This correspondence strengthens the belief that the reduction in light illumination is one of the age changes responsible for the age difference observed in certain illusory tasks.

Agitative Behaviors by Nursing Home Residents

There are four types of agitative behaviors exhibited by many nursing home residents (and by nonresidents who reside at home): physically aggressive behavior, physically nonaggressive behavior, verbally aggressive behavior, and verbally nonaggressive behavior. The type of behavior exhibited is more likely related to the cognitive or mental health status of a resident than to his or her physical health status. Residents with depressive symptoms are likely to make constant verbally nonaggressive requests for help and complain frequently, whereas those with psychotic symptoms are likely to show physically and verbally aggressive behaviors.

Of interest to the possible treatment of agitation in nursing home residents is a discovery by Dr. Louis Burgio of the University of Alabama at Birmingham. He observed that disruptive residents never exhibited vocal agitation while sitting under a hair dryer. He subsequently tested the use of white noise (the sound of a bubbling brook) and found that agitated residents became less agitated when white noise was applied.

Providing stimulation in one form or another does seem essential in order to reduce agitation in nursing home residents. Three types of stimulation were each found to be effective in a recent study. The first consisted of exposure to the kind of music that relatives of a resident had identified as being liked by that resident. The second consisted of exposure to family-generated videotapes with content selected by family members. The third consisted of one-on-one social interactions with a trained research assistant (for example, reading, playing games, or engaging in conversation). Each intervention lasted for thirty minutes over two consecutive weeks. Verbally aggressive behaviors decreased by 31 percent with music, 46 percent with videotapes, and 56 percent with social interaction (there was only a 16 percent reduction in a no-intervention control condition). *See also* Alzheimer's Disease.

AIDS (Acquired Immunodeficiency Syndrome)

Although AIDS is usually considered to be a disease of young people, older adults have not been spared the disease. Approximately 10 percent of all cases in the United States are for adults age fifty and older. Since the early 1990s the number of cases of AIDS for people age fifty and older has increased twice as fast as it has for younger adults. Conceivably, some older adults erroneously think they are not at risk in unsafe sexual activity. Of course, AIDS that is transmitted by blood transfusion knows no age barriers.

Alcoholism (Incidence and Causes)

Self-reports indicate that elderly people consume fewer alcoholic beverages than do younger people and that members of the present generation of elderly people drink less now than they did when they were younger. In fact, a fairly large proportion of elderly people report that they abstain completely from drinking alcoholic beverages. However, the reliability of these reports may be questioned. Nevertheless, the results of a three-year study of people age sixty-five and older showed a decline in alcohol consumption over the period. About a third of the men and half of the women in the study abstained from drinking in at least one of the three years. Those who did not abstain from drinking usually had experienced a serious negative life event, such as the death of a close friend.

Many elderly people may underestimate their use of alcohol to avoid criticism. The incidence of alcoholism among elderly people is largely unknown. Estimates of the percentage of elderly people with alcohol-related problems range from 1 percent to 25 percent. In a recent national survey it was reported that 10 percent of people age sixty-five and older have at least five drinks at a time at least once a month, and 5 percent have that many each time they have alcoholic drinks.

It is believed that at least two-thirds of older alcoholics were problem drinkers when they were younger. Unfortunately, some elderly alcoholics may find it easy to hide their addiction. With no job to attend, they may sleep off a hangover, and they may not have a spouse or significant other who is aware of their problem. In addition, some elderly adults believe they will be sent to a nursing home if they admit to their addiction. Physicians may also think it is too late to do anything about an older adult's drinking problem, or they may dislike challenging an elderly patient who vehemently denies having a drinking problem.

Of further interest are the probable reasons that older people cite as causes for a serious drinking problem. Such problems are seemingly related to negative events in their recent lives or to the presence of long-standing (chronic) sources of stress or both. In a California survey, comparisons were made between problem drinkers and non–problem drinkers in the same age range (between the ages of fifty-five and sixty-five). Important sex differences were found. Male problem drinkers were more likely than female problem drinkers to report long-term financial problems and problems with friends.

By contrast, female problem drinkers reported fewer financial sources of stress but more family-related sources of stress, including with their spouses, than did male problem drinkers. In addition, female problem drinkers reported receiving less support from their spouses or significant others than male problem drinkers did from their spouses or significant others. The investigators noted that women may be more likely than men to perceive nurturing someone with a drinking problem to be part of their role within a family.

There were other important findings from the California survey. Sources of stress (that is, stressors) were found to be no more severe for older problem drinkers than for older non–problem drinkers. Thus, problem drinkers in general did not have more difficult stressors with which to cope, or manage, than non–problem drinkers. Nevertheless, problem drinkers displayed, on average, a different form of coping behavior than did non–problem drinkers. The problem drinkers tended to use avoidance forms of coping with stressors in which they either avoided thoughts about a problem or resigned themselves to the belief that nothing could be done about a problem. Excessive drinking is presumably part of their failure to acknowledge and overcome their problems. By contrast, non–problem drinkers tended to use approach-coping behaviors in which they dealt directly with an issue and tried either to resolve it or to restructure it to make it less stressful.

Researchers at the University of Southern California further found that caregivers of spouses or significant others with Alzheimer's disease who detached themselves from the situation and experienced a larger burden were more likely to become heavy drinkers than caregivers who directly confronted the problems encountered in caregiving.

AARP has available a booklet about alcohol use by older adults. To order a free copy, write to AARP, 601 E Street Northwest, Washington, DC 20049.

Alcoholism (Treatment)

Centers for the treatment specifically of elderly alcoholics are rare, but there are some Alcoholics Anonymous (AA) groups for older people. AA meetings are open to people of all ages, but older adults usually prefer meeting with people their own age. In general, alcoholics over age sixty-five respond better to treatment than do younger alcoholics.

Alcohol (Physical and Mental Effects)

Alcohol has different effects on older people than on younger people. The intake of the same amount of alcohol raises blood alcohol levels higher in older people than in younger people. Elderly people also metabolize and excrete alcohol more slowly than do younger adults. These effects mean that alcohol abuse may produce more serious physical problems for elderly abusers than for younger abusers. The physical consequences for elderly people are complicated further by the likelihood of their having a disease being greater than it is for younger people, and the adverse effects of alcohol abuse may be intensified by the presence of disease.

Researchers at Harvard University Medical School examined all causes of death for more than twenty thousand male doctors during a period of eleven years. They discovered that the risk of death was 63 percent higher for those doctors who had two or more drinks a day than for those who did not drink at all. The greater risk for the heavy drinkers was linked to the greater incidence of cancer, especially throat, gastric, urinary tract, and brain cancer. However, in a study of Japanese American men in Hawaii, it was found that moderate drinkers (fifteen to thirty-nine milliliters of alcohol daily) had a slight decline in mortality rate. In addition, evidence has been increasing to show that the hops in beer serve as a deterrent for tumor growth. Drinking a moderate amount of beer rich in hops, such as stout and ale, may have health benefits for seniors.

The evidence regarding the effects of alcohol on the mental functioning of elderly adults is conflicting. There is some evidence indicating that memory proficiency is affected adversely more for elderly adults than for young adults. However, elderly adults in France were studied over a four-year period, and those who drank red wine moderately had fewer mental problems than those who abstained. In addition, researchers in New Mexico found that older moderate drinkers scored significantly higher than abstainers on seven mental tests in a battery of nine such tests,

Long-term alcoholics with a history of twenty to thirty years of excessive drinking run the risk of suffering from Korsakoff's disease. The primary symptom of the disease is amnesia, especially anterograde amnesia (difficulty in acquiring new information and storing it). Other components of intelligence may be unaffected. Personality, however, is likely to be affected, as the sufferers of the disease tend to become apathetic and excessively passive in their behaviors.

Not all of the effects of alcohol use are negative. Alcohol tends to raise HDL cholesterol (the good cholesterol; *see* Cholesterol; Nutrition and Diet) levels, and moderate amounts may therefore reduce the risk of blood clots and heart attacks. People over age sixty-five who drink light to moderate amounts (no more than two drinks a day for men and one drink a day for women) seem to have a lower risk of heart disease, especially nonfatal heart attacks. The researchers at Harvard discovered that the doctors who had two to four drinks a week had a lower risk (22 percent) of death than those doctors who did not drink at all. There is even evidence indicating that a substance in red wines may help to prevent Alzheimer's disease.

Residents of nursing homes may benefit both psychologically and socially from the moderate use of alcoholic beverages, especially when the beverages are consumed in a group setting that relaxes the tensions of feeling institutionalized. For normally aging people, the use of alcohol may help to reduce the stress brought about by relatively minor negative events. However, alcohol use is likely to increase the effects of stress brought about by more important life events.

Allergies

The ability to control allergies decreases in late adulthood because elderly adults have a less efficient immune system than younger adults. Older adults with allergies need to keep their home air-conditioning functioning, and they should change filters often. This is true for automobile air-conditioners as well. They should also enclose their mattress in plastic and keep their pillows washed and covered. They should use polyester pillows rather than feather pillows. They should not have a carpet in their bedrooms because it may contain mites. If they have a dog or cat, they should vacuum thoroughly all carpets in their home at least once a week to remove hair. In the summer they should avoid plant pollens by spending most of their time in areas where the pollen count is low.

Alternative Medical Treatments

The use of alternatives to traditional medical practice (for example, acupuncture and herbal medicines) is increasing for elderly adults. Nevertheless, the use of alternative treatments is less likely than by younger adults. One reason for less use by elderly adults is the fact that Medicare does not cover most alternative treatments. In a survey of more than seven hundred Californians on Medicare, 24 percent reported use of herbal medicines, 20 percent had had chiropractic treatments, 15 percent used massage therapy, and 14 percent underwent acupuncture. Such treatments can have health benefits, but they can also cause harm. For adverse effects of herbal medicines and their safe use, contact the American Botanical Council at http://www.herbal.org. *See also* Acupuncture.

Altruism (Adult Age Differences)

Altruism refers to helping others, either in the form of a donation or an intervention to aid someone in trouble. In gerontology, elderly people have commonly been viewed as the needy recipients of altruistic acts and not as the givers of these acts. Elderly people have traditionally been regarded as being less altruistic than younger people. Several possible reasons have been given for the presumed decline in altruism in late adulthood. One is that elderly people conserve their limited resources to improve their own lives. Another is that many elderly people are, in effect, repaying society for its lack of concern with their own problems.

However, there is evidence to indicate that altruism may actually increase from middle age through late adulthood. Part of that evidence comes from interviews with elderly people that revealed that most elderly people do have a strong interest and orientation toward altruism, as is apparent from their frequent contributions as volunteers for nonprofit organizations (*see* Participation in Voluntary Organizations and Volunteer Work).

More impressive evidence comes from a clever study conducted by researchers at the University of Detroit. They set up a donation booth with a canister for monetary deposits in various shopping centers and malls. Large posters in the booth indicated that the donations were for infants born with birth defects. The percentage of donors was greatest in the age range of sixty-five to seventy-four, with the next greatest percentage being for people seventy-five and older. The percentage of donors for younger adults (twenty-five to thirty-four years old) was much smaller. However, the amount of the average donation, as might be expected, was less for the oldest donors than for younger donors (the largest average amounts were for people in the age range of forty-five to sixty-four). The diminished economic resources of people in the postretirement years certainly accounts for their limited monetary donations.

The researchers conducted a second study in which economic status would not be a determiner in either the willingness to be a donor or the amount actually donated. The situation was much like that of the first study except that now donors were asked to pull a lever in the booth, with a poster noting that local merchants would donate five cents to the charitable fund for each pull. In terms of the percentage of donors, the outcome was the same as that of the first experiment: the percentage was highest for the oldest people. In terms of the amount of donation (now expressed in number of pulls of the lever), the outcome was quite different from that of the first experiment—the average amount was greatest for the oldest donors. There were no economic constraints placed on the oldest donors. There is good reason to believe that altruism actually *increases* rather than declines in late adulthood. *See also* Altruism (Health Benefits for Seniors).

Altruism (Health Benefits for Seniors)

Older adults are more altruistic than younger adults both in terms of giving to charities and in terms of giving social support to family members and friends. Researchers at Rutgers University discovered that the altruistic behavior of many seniors has positive effects on their physical health. The participants in their study were more than one thousand community-dwelling seniors (average age of seventy-four) who were diverse both racially and socioeconomically.

The researchers measured the extent to which the participants both gave social support to family members and friends and received social support from family members and friends. They found that the participants who gave greater social support, both materialistic and emotional, had less health problems (such as blood pressure or sleep problems) than participants who gave less social support. The positive health effect for giving support was independent of race and socioeconomic status. By contrast, the amount of social support received had no effect on health problems. *See also* Altruism (Adult Age Differences).

Alzheimer's Association

The Alzheimer's Association was founded in 1980, with headquarters in Chicago. Until 1989 it was known as the Alzheimer's Disease and Related Disorders Association. It is a privately funded, voluntary organization with hundreds of support groups and chapters for people coping with sufferers of Alzheimer's disease. The association's goals include the following: supporting research into the causes, treatment, and prevention of Alzheimer's disease; providing assistance to families with a relative who has Alzheimer's disease; making the general public better educated and informed about Alzheimer's disease; and promoting legislation at the local, state, and federal levels that responds to the needs of patients with Alzheimer's disease and their caregivers.

The national office offers grants for funding new investigations into the causes, treatment, and prevention of Alzheimer's disease, and it publishes a quarterly newsletter. The association is responsible for the now national observance of November as Alzheimer's Disease Month. There is a nationwide twenty-four-hour telephone hotline for providing information about Alzheimer's disease (1-800-272-3900) and for helping families find a support group and other forms of assistance. The address of the association is 919 North Michigan Avenue, Suite 1000, Chicago, IL 60611.

Alzheimer's Disease

The existence of both presenile dementia (in people in their forties or fifties) and senile dementia (usually among people in their seventies or older) has been known for centuries. However, it was not until 1907 that the first neurological diagnosis of dementia as a brain disorder was made. Dr. Alois Alzheimer, a German neurologist, had a patient with presenile dementia who died at age fifty-one. Postmortem analysis revealed massive atrophy of her brain, in particular the presence of numerous small bodies of protein (called senile plaques; *see* Brain and Aging) composed of bits of dying or dead neurons and neurofibrillary tangles (filaments that are wrapped around one another) within the bodies and axons of neurons scattered throughout the brain.

At the time it was believed that presenile dementia differed from senile dementia in terms of the brain changes responsible for each. Senile dementia was considered to be the result of "hardening of the arteries" or stroke, and presenile dementia was attributed to unknown causes. Only presenile dementia was given the name Alzheimer's disease. In the late 1960s it was discovered that the brain changes present in many cases of senile dementia are very similar to those present in presenile dementia. Consequently, senile dementia in which known causative factors (for example, a stroke) could be ruled out and for which postmortem examination revealed massive senile plaques and neurofibrillary tangles also became known as Alzheimer's disease.

It is estimated that more than 10 percent of the population of American adults age sixty-five or older has Alzheimer's disease. The percentage increases after age sixty-five, with nearly 50 percent of the population age eighty-five and older having the disease. About 40 percent of new entries to nursing homes are clients with Alzheimer's disease, and at least 80 percent of all nursing home residents are believed to have the disease. However, about 70 percent of patients with Alzheimer's disease live at home. The Alzheimer's Association estimates that there are one hundred thousand or more deaths annually from Alzheimer's disease. The duration of the disease after diagnosis ranges from eight to twenty years. The presenile form of the disease (affecting people in their forties and fifties) is much rarer. In general, patients with early Alzheimer's disease live for a number of years after the onset of the disease, whereas older victims are likely to live only a few years after its onset.

Diagnosis of Alzheimer's disease presently can be made with certainty only after death when analysis of the brain confirms massive atrophy of the brain and large amounts of senile plaques and neurofibrillary tangles, especially in the cerebral cortex and hippocampus (*see* Brain and Aging). Consequently, individuals strongly suspected of having Alzheimer's disease are likely to be diagnosed as having senile dementia of the Alzheimer's type (SDAT), with the realization that the true disease may eventually be discovered after postmortem analysis to be something other than Alzheimer's disease.

A diagnosis of SDAT is based on results of both neurological tests and mental tests (for example, the Blessed Mental Status Test and the Mental Status Questionnaire; *see* Blessed Mental Status Test; Mental Status Questionnaire). There is always the danger of misdiagnosis with mental tests in that the mental problems present in the early stages of Alzheimer's disease are somewhat similar to those found with severe depression.

Recent advancements in examining the living brain, such as computed axial tomography (CAT) scans, positron-emission tomography (PET) scans, and magnetic resonance imaging (MRI) have thus far not been very effective in enhancing the early diagnosis of SDAT, although such tests do reveal the progressive atrophy of the brain and its functioning as the disease progresses in severity. Researchers at the University of California at Los Angeles recently reported that PET scans may be especially valuable in detecting early brain degeneration in individuals possessing a gene related to Alzheimer's disease. Diagnosis is complicated further by the fact that a fairly large percentage of individuals with Alzheimer's disease (perhaps as large as 20 percent) have dementias that are increased further by multi-infarct dementia (stroke-induced dementia; *see* Multi-Infarct Dementia).

An important area of research is the search for diagnostic tests that will identify Alzheimer's disease early, that is, before actual symptoms of the disease appear. The hope is that by the time a reliable test has been found, researchers will have discovered means of intervening with the progression of the disease. The result could be many cases in which the disease's occurrence has been prevented.

Several tests or procedures have shown some promise of serving eventually as an early diagnostic test. One is the use of a smell identification test. Incorrect responses on the test seem to predict the risk of later Alzheimer's disease for patients with mild mental impairment. There is even the possibility of a behavioral predictor of later Alzheimer's disease. For example, a study of nuns by researchers at the University of Kentucky (*see* Nun Study) revealed that those with poorer language skills early in adulthood were more likely to show later Alzheimer's disease than nuns with superior language skills in early adulthood.

Atrophy of the brain is especially pronounced in the cerebral cortex, the hippocampus, and other brain areas associated with memory functioning and other mental operations in Alzheimer's sufferers. A major problem is the severe decline in the amount of acetylcholine, a neurotransmitter chemical linked to memory functioning, present in the brain (*see* Brain and Aging). This decline appears to be caused by massive destruction of neurons in a structure called the nucleus basalis of Meynert located at the base of the brain, neurons that seem to be critical in the production of acetylcholine.

The most prominent mental symptom of Alzheimer's disease is the progressive and severe decline in memory functioning. The severity of the decline is especially pronounced for the various forms of episodic memory (*see* Episodic Memory). Both short-term and long-term memories decline greatly in proficiency, and the decline may be seen in memory for noncontent attributes of episodic events (for instance, their frequency of occurrence and their spatial locations, as well as the content of those events).

Semantic memory is also affected, but to a lesser extent than episodic memory (*see* Lexicon; Semantic Memory). Individuals with Alzheimer's disease have difficulty naming pictures and objects, and their word associations differ greatly from those of normally aging people (*see* Word Associations), although it is uncertain whether it is the actual knowledge of words that is lost with the disease or difficulty in gaining access to words that is affected by the disease. There is some evidence to indicate that the rate of progressive decline in mental functions over time is greater for those with an earlier onset of the disease than for those with a later onset.

Individuals with Alzheimer's disease are also characterized by disorientation in terms of time and place, and various personality disorders are likely to be present, especially depression and inappropriate social behavior. Approximately 30 percent of patients with Alzheimer's disease are believed to have severe depression in addition to their mental impairment. An even larger percentage have some form of depressive symptoms. Researchers at the University of Washington discovered that 70 percent of their sample of more than five hundred community-dwelling Alzheimer's disease patients had symptoms of anxiety, and more than 50 percent had symptoms of both anxiety and depression.

As the disease progresses, individuals with the disease become increasingly incapable of performing the activities of daily living (for example, feeding themselves and personal hygiene), thus requiring considerable caregiving either at home or in a nursing home. The researchers in Washington found that the presence of anxiety correlated significantly not only with impairment in the activities of daily living but also with other behavioral problems such as wandering and verbal abuse.

Some patients also have paranoia, that is, pronounced delusions or false beliefs about events in their world. Especially likely are delusions of persecution in which the patients believe they are being robbed or are being spied on. Such delusions add to the concerns and problems of the patient's caregivers. Patients with delusions tend to be older and female and have a later onset of the disease than patients without delusions. They also tend to have more severe cognitive impairment. In some cases the delusions may diminish with repeated reminders by caregivers that there is no factual basis for these beliefs.

One of the most prominent physical symptoms for severely impaired individuals is agitation (*see* Agitative Behaviors by Nursing Home Residents). Agitation consists of inappropriate verbal, vocal, or motor behavior that may be abusive toward others, such as cursing or hitting caregivers. Studies have indicated that more than half of nursing home residents scream at least once a day. The frequency of screaming has been found to be related to such factors as the degree of the ability to perform the activities of daily living and the degree of mental impairment.

Another prominent physical symptom is wandering behavior (*see* Wandering). Wandering does seem to have a positive effect for some patients with Alzheimer's disease. Some evidence indicates that wandering may reduce negative aggressive behaviors when individuals are permitted to wander freely in a protected environment. The problem with wandering is that individuals may escape the so-called protected environment and enter areas that may be dangerous to their well-being. Exits from protected areas may occur at any time during the day or night, but they are most likely to occur within a few hours after eating a meal. Researchers in Ohio discovered that nursing home residents with Alzheimer's disease may best be discouraged from leaving a secured area by concealing the exit door behind a cloth panel.

Problems in performing complex motor tasks are present, even for patients with mild Alzheimer's disease. Thus, motor impairment is part of the overall functional decline with the disease. Not surprisingly, patients who continue to drive have an increased risk of automobile accidents (*see* Accidents [Automobile]).

Another potential physical risk with Alzheimer's disease is the occurrence of increased illnesses that require hospitalization. Past evidence regarding the incidence of hospitalization has been conflicting. However, a major study by researchers at Columbia University yielded convincing evidence for an increased risk of hospitalization, especially from infections, that is associated with the disease. Their evidence indicates further that the greater risk of medical problems requiring hospitalization is not related to the mental state of Alzheimer's disease patients, nor is it related to lack of physical care.

The cause(s) of Alzheimer's disease remains largely unknown. There is the possibility of a genetic defect on a particular chromosome that encodes information about a specific brain protein. When incorrectly encoded, the result is the production of a protein fragment called beta-amyloid that may be responsible for the massive degeneration of the brain found in Alzheimer's disease by clumping together to form plaques that interfere with neuron functioning.

It appears that early Alzheimer's disease may be inheritable, although why the onset of the disease is delayed until middle age is unknown. Inheritance may also be involved in later onset of the disease. Researchers at Duke University Medical Center identified a gene, called APDE-4, that appears to play a role in causing the disease. They found that the more copies of this gene possessed by an individual, the greater the risk of having the disease—and the earlier the onset of the disease. The discovery of this genetic factor holds great promise for an eventual cure for the disease.

Also suspected of being a causative factor is a viral infection that has yet to be determined. At one time a popular theory was that aluminum toxicity was important in causing Alzheimer's disease. However, there is no evidence indicating a relationship between the extent of use of aluminum in daily life (for example, cookware) and the occurrence of the disease.

Another possibility is that the disease is caused by an inadequate diet. The disease is much less prevalent in China and perhaps other Eastern countries as well than in the United States. The diet in these countries differs greatly from that of most Americans. Especially believed by some experts to be a critical part of the diet for enabling many people in these countries to avoid Alzheimer's disease is bean sprouts (that is, soybean sprouts). There is also speculation that the disease is related to the decline in insulin consumption that increases as the disease progresses, and that the disease may actually be a form of diabetes.

The most prominent current theory is that chunks of a protein called beta-amyloid are cut from plaques in the brain by the enzyme gamma secretase. These chunks then interfere with neural functioning. The search is on for a substance that will prevent this from happening.

A cure for the disease has yet to be found. At one time it was believed that injections of acetylcholine or its artificial equivalent would greatly reduce the memory problems of victims of the disease by replenishing the diminished supply of this critical neurotransmitter. The results of clinical trials with drugs such as lecithin, which aid in the synthesis of acetylcholine, proved disappointing. Tacrine is another drug that has been used as treatment for the mental difficulties encountered by patients with the disease. The results of clinical trials with the drug yielded conflicting results. Exelon is a drug that may aid in slowing down the progression of symptoms of dementia, but whatever effectiveness it has may be limited to the dementia that occurs for some patients with advanced Parkinson's disease (*see* Parkinson's Disease).

Alternatives to tacrine for improving cognitive functioning in patients with Alzheimer's disease include an extract from the leaves of the ginkgo tree (*see* Ginkgo). In a double-blind study (that is, neither the patient nor the researcher knew if the patient received ginkgo or a placebo), a slight benefit was found for performance on mental tests, but mainly for patients with the least impairment. Other herbal treatments have also been proposed. For example, one is the use of the moss extract huperzine A. However, there is little evidence to support its effectiveness in slowing down the progression of Alzheimer's disease.

There has been hope for the use of estrogen (hormone) replacement therapy as a treatment for Alzheimer's disease. It is well known that more women than men suffer from the disease, and the treatment given to women could serve to reduce the disparity. However, there is no evidence to indicate that the therapy slows down the progression of the disease's symptoms. In addition, other evidence has indicated that the hormone treatment may actually increase the risk of dementia by increasing the risk of a stroke that leads to dementia.

What may turn out to be the most important new treatment is a vaccine discovered in research with mice. Researchers found that mice given the vaccine showed a significant reduction in the levels of beta-amyloid plaques. The hope is that the vaccine will do the same for the human brain (that is, prevent plaques in people with a high risk of Alzheimer's disease and destroy plaques in people who have the disease). However, there are problems confronting its future use. First, it is unknown if the vaccine will work with human beings the way it does with mice. Second, the role played by plaques in causing Alzheimer's disease remains unknown (destroying plaques may not eliminate the disease). Finally, potential negative side effects of the vaccine remain unknown. Clinical trials with the vaccine have yet to be conducted, and they are at least six years in the future.

Although the mental symptoms of Alzheimer's disease are presently immune to treatment, some of the behavioral dysfunctions (for example, personal care and eating) may be at least partially improved by the effective use of behavioral modification procedures (*see* Psychotherapy). In some cases, depression may be treated by the drugs used to treat depression in normally aging adults, and some of the personality symptoms may be treated by other drugs.

For more information about Alzheimer's disease, contact the Alzheimer's Disease Education and Referral Center. The address is ADEAR, P.O. Box 8250, Silver Springs, MD 20907. The telephone number is (301) 587-4352. *See also* Sleep Disorders.

Anagram Solving

Jumble is a daily feature in many newspapers in the United States. Players of the game have to unscramble several strings of letters to turn them into words. Strings of letters that translate to words are called anagrams. Are elderly adults likely to be good at playing *Jumble*? The answer is yes and no. Researchers at the University of Arkansas found that elderly adults who solve crossword puzzles regularly do not differ from young adults in their proficiency of solving anagrams. However, elderly adults who infrequently solve crossword puzzles are, in general, less proficient anagram solvers than young adults.

Analgesics

See Pain Medications (Analgesics).

Androgyny

Psychological androgyny refers to both feminine and masculine characteristics integrated in the same individual. An androgenous person is one who has avoided being bound by rigid gender roles often associated with his or her sex. Of interest is the possibility of changes in androgyny during various periods of adulthood. A popular theory of androgyny stresses that men and women retain their traditional male and female roles, respectively, through the parenting years and then become more like each other in late adulthood. That is, elderly men and women become more like one another in terms of a blend of masculine and feminine characteristics.

However, there is evidence from two studies, one conducted in the 1970s and one in the 1980s, that the trend toward androgyny is more characteristic of elderly men than it is of elderly women. The percentage of androgynous men in the samples studied was found to increase from 20 percent to 30 percent in the forty-one-to-sixty-year age range and from 30 percent to 40 percent in the sixty-one-and-older age range. By contrast, the percentage of androgynous women in the sixty-one-and-older age range was only 10 percent to 30 percent. The percentage of men classified as being predominantly masculine in their characteristics decreased from 40 percent to 50 percent in the forty-one-to-sixty-year age range to 20 percent to 30 percent in the sixty-one-and-older age range. The percentage of women classified as being predominantly feminine in their characteristics increased from about 40 percent in the forty-one-to-sixty-year age range to about 70 percent in the sixty-one-and-older age range.

The two studies were conducted nearly ten years apart; thus, the older individuals surveyed were from different generations or cohorts. The fact that the outcomes were very similar for these widely separated cohorts suggests that the change toward increasing femininity for both older men and older women may represent a true age change and is not an effect attributable to cohort or generational differences (*see* Age Change versus Age Difference; Time-Lag Comparison)

Anemia

Anemia is a condition in which there is a reduction of the number of red blood corpuscles or of the total amount of hemoglobin or both. The result is insufficient oxygen being delivered to body tissues. *Anemia* is a generic term that includes a number of specific types of anemia. Two of the most common types are iron deficiency anemia and vitamin B12 deficiency anemia.

Iron deficiency anemia is the most common type of anemia. About 20 percent of women and 3 percent of men are iron deficient. Iron is an important component of hemoglobin, the component essential for red cells to carry oxygen. Oxygen is necessary for the normal functioning of every cell in your body. Iron is usually obtained from certain foods that we eat and from recycling old red blood cells. Iron deficiency usually results from too little iron in our diet or from poor absorption of iron by our body. Symptoms of iron deficiency anemia include a pale skin color, fatigue, irritability, shortness of breath, and brittle nails. Treatment consists of taking oral iron supplements, especially on an empty stomach. Milk and antacids may block the absorption of iron.

Vitamin B12 deficiency anemia is caused by a deficiency of vitamin B12.

The main sources of this vitamin are meat, eggs, and dairy products. There are several types of vitamin B12 deficiency anemia. The most common type is pernicious anemia. Causes of the disease include a diet low in vitamin D (for instance, a strict vegetarian diet), chronic alcoholism, and the lack of intrinsic factor (a protein secreted by cells in the stomach that vitamin B12 must bind to in order to be absorbed by your body). The disease may be detected by the presence of various neurological tests. The disease may also cause loss of appetite, diarrhea, and difficulty walking. Treatment consists of B12 injections and a balanced diet. *See also* Angiodysplasia.

Angiodysplasia

Angiodysplasia is a condition occurring most often in adults in their sixties and seventies. Webs of fragile blood vessels form on the lining of the digestive tract, usually the colon. They bleed easily, and may lead to anemia. An application of heat to the vessels may serve to seal them.

Antiaging Products—Do They Really Work?

Efforts to combat aging and the diseases associated with aging did not end with Ponce de León's futile search in the 1500s for a magical fountain of youth. Antiaging substances have existed for centuries. Until recently, however, antiaging substances were herbs and other natural matter rather than products derived from scientific research. These new products have created a multibillion-dollar industry.

The new products usually claim that they make it possible to slow down aging, or, in some cases, even reverse aging. Analyses of these products by distinguished groups of gerobiologists clearly refute these claims. There seems to be little scientific evidence to support the antiaging claims of these products.

On the other hand, animal research has indicated that greatly restricting the amount of calories consumed daily may extend longevity. However, as noted by the gerobiologists, there is no evidence to indicate that severe caloric reduction would have the same effect on human beings. To be effective, the restriction would have to be at a level most people would find intolerable. Most people seem to prefer quality of life over quantity of life.

But the search for a fountain of youth goes on nevertheless. For example, researchers at Washington University in St. Louis are exploring testosterone (male sex hormone) therapy as a way of rejuvenating older men.

Antioxidants

The cells of our bodies require oxygen to generate the energy our bodies need. During this process, toxic substances known as free radicals are produced. According to a long-standing biological theory of aging (*see* Why Aging? [Biological Theories of Aging]), free radicals are believed to cause many of the illnesses and biological declines that occur in late adulthood. That is, free radicals travel through the body and produce damage to vital cell structures.

Although the evidence to support the free-radical theory of biological aging is not strong, there has been considerable interest recently in substances called antioxidants that defend the body against oxygen's presumably harmful effects by reducing the amount of free radicals. Among these substances are beta-carotene and vitamins C, E, and K. Beta-carotene is found in deeply colored orange and green fruits and vegetables, such as carrots, sweet potatoes, broccoli, spinach, oranges, apricots, and cantaloupe. Vitamin C is found in citrus fruits, strawberries, peppers, broccoli, and cauliflower. The best sources of vitamin E are fatty foods, such as vegetable oils, nuts, and seeds. However, a normal diet would not include the large amounts of these foods necessary to produce sufficient vitamin E to serve as an antioxidant. Consequently, it is not unusual for physicians to recommend that elderly patients supplement their diets with vitamin E capsules. Nevertheless, it is antioxidants in such foods as blueberries that seem to help to reduce the risk of cancer and perhaps Alzheimer's disease.

In support of the health benefits gained from daily supplements of vitamin E, British researchers found that they lowered the risk of heart attacks by more than 70 percent for people with bad hearts. Similarly, Finnish researchers found that vitamin E supplements are associated with a moderate decrease of heart pain. Of further interest is the so-called French paradox. The paradox is that French people have a low rate of heart disease despite eating a high fat diet. The low rate may result from the antioxidants found in the red wine they drink often (*see also* Portion Size and Heart Health). There is also evidence indicating that vitamins C and E reduce the risk of prostate tumors. *See also* Grape Juice; Why Aging? (Biological Theories of Aging).

Anxiety

Are you about to take the test to renew your driver's license? Are you feeling uneasy, nervous, and tense and dreading the future event—in other words, experiencing anxiety? Psychologists distinguish among three forms of anxiety: trait anxiety, state anxiety, and clinical anxiety (that is, an anxiety disorder or neurosis).

Both trait anxiety and state anxiety are general characteristics of normal individuals (in other words, they are not clinically abnormal). They both may affect behavior in many kinds of situations. Individuals high in trait anxiety are likely to be anxious throughout their lives in many kinds of situations, even those that are only mildly threatening to individuals with lower trait anxiety. State anxiety is more transitory and depends on situations that are threatening to one's self-esteem. When faced with an examination, some people become much more anxious than others; they have a high degree of state anxiety. They are likely to feel very nervous and agitated and to have various physical signs of their anxiety, such as heavy perspiration and irregular breathing. There is considerable evidence to indicate that there are no adult age differences in either trait anxiety or state anxiety, at least as anxiety is measured by psychological tests. That is, the scores of older adults on these tests differ very little from the scores of younger adults. The absence of any pronounced increase in anxiety, in general, during late adulthood is demonstrated further by the fact that the incidence of an anxiety disorder (a clinically significant form of neurotic anxiety that is especially debilitating to the affected individual) is quite low for elderly people.

A high level of either state or trait anxiety is likely to hinder performance on the task being performed while the anxiety is present. By contrast, a moderate amount of anxiety could improve performance by forcing increased concentration on the task at hand. The age differences that do exist in anxiety are seemingly too insignificant to affect age differences in performance on either laboratory or everyday tasks. However, elderly people who believe they are being handicapped by excessive anxiety are as likely to benefit from training in relaxation as are younger people.

Aphasia

Aphasia is a disorder involving either the expression of speech (expressive aphasia) or the comprehension of speech (receptive aphasia). The disorder is caused by a lesion in the brain usually resulting from a stroke or head injury. The lesion for expressive aphasia is usually in a segment of the left frontal lobe known as Broca's area. The lesion for receptive aphasia is usually in a segment of the left temporal lobe known as Wernicke's area.

Aphasias in elderly people are more likely to be receptive than expressive. Language impairment in aphasia can often be treated effectively by speech therapy. At one time it was believed that elderly people were far less likely to benefit from speech therapy than younger people. However, recent studies have challenged this belief and have reported little relationship between age at the onset of an aphasia and the extent of recovery achieved by therapy.

Arithmetic Ability

Numerous studies have indicated that if there are age differences in the accuracy of simple arithmetic operations, such as addition and subtraction, they are slight. However, older adults are slower than younger adults in completing simple arithmetic problems. In terms of solving fairly simple word problems, there is also little effect of aging on accuracy, at least through the midseventies. Our reference is to solving simple problems in which all of the elements are physically present (for example, when participants are given 534 and 28 as addends and are asked to give the sum). Researchers at the University of Missouri at Columbia found further that elderly adults retrieve information about arithmetic from memory as efficiently as younger adults do (for example, answer "True or false—2 x 3 = 5"; the answer, of course, is "false"). Moreover, elderly adults tend to be superior to young adults in solving simple subtraction problems and in their knowledge about multiplication.

On the other hand, it is a different matter when one or both addends must be held mentally while mentally summing the two. Here there does seem to be a decided disadvantage for elderly adults. The size of the disadvantage is especially apparent when both addends must be "held in the head" while summing them. There are occasions when we may be tempted to use mental arithmetic. Consider shopping in the supermarket for two items, and you have only two dollars with you. One item costs ninety-eight cents and the other eighty-five cents. Do you have enough money with you to make both purchases? (Be sure to add the sales tax, if needed.) Why rely on your mental addition? People of all ages (but especially elderly people) should carry a pocket calculator to do arithmetic when shopping, or have a small notebook and a pen so that they can do their shopping arithmetic with physically present numbers.

Army Alpha and Army Beta Intelligence Tests

The Army Alpha test was the first widely used group verbal (reading ability needed to take the test) intelligence test. Among the abilities it tested were analogies, numerical ability, and reasoning. The test was developed during World War I as a selection device for finding army officer candidates among enlisted men and for assigning soldiers to services they were deemed intellectually fit to perform. The test was administered to nearly two million men during the war. The results from this testing provided the first clear indication of adult age differences in scores on an intelligence test. A progressive age-related decline in scores was found from officers in their twenties to officers in their fifties. Later use of the test with civilians demonstrated further age-related declines beyond the fifties. Age-related declines were also found to vary greatly among the various subtests of the Army Alpha, suggesting that the mental abilities measured by these subtests vary greatly in the extent to which they are affected by normal aging.

The Army Alpha test requires reading ability in English. During World War I military personnel were aware that many recruits would be either illiterate or foreign born and unable to read English. Consequently, a nonverbal (no reading ability required to take the test) group intelligence test, the Army Beta, was developed with the Army Alpha. The Army Beta test included subtests such as mazes, digit symbol substitution, and number checking.

Arousal

When frightened, angry, or otherwise highly emotionally excited, a number of physiological changes occur in our bodies as the adrenalin (also known as epinephrine) begins to flow. Stimulation from the brain during times of excitement activates the secretion of adrenalin from the adrenal glands, which are located on top of each kidney. The physiological changes produced by the adrenalin include an increase in heart rate, an increase in breathing rate, and other changes that collectively result in a state known as physiological arousal.

Psychologists have long known that the intensity of arousal produced by a stressful or demanding situation affects one's performance in that situation. As the intensity of arousal increases, performance on a task at hand is likely to increase in proficiency. However, this is true only until some optimal level of intensity is reached. Beyond that optimal level, performance on the same task is likely to decrease in proficiency. For levels of arousal below the optimal level, people are said to be underaroused, and for levels above the optimal level, they are said to be overaroused. In either case, performance on the task confronting them is likely to be less than optimal.

The peak time for optimal arousal for older adults occurs in the morning, and for younger adults it is in the evening. In agreement with this age difference in peak times, performance scores on such tasks as word span are greater for older participants when tested in the morning than when tested in the evening. The reverse is true for younger participants (*see* Time of Day and Memory Performance).

For more than forty years gerontological psychologists have debated whether elderly adults are characterized by underarousal or overarousal when they are asked to perform demanding and difficult tasks. Much of the difficulty in resolving the issue of underarousal or overarousal arises from the fact that there is no single measure of arousal that adequately serves to evaluate its intensity. There are a number of separate measures that have yielded different outcomes when applied in aging research.

One of these measures is the amount of free fatty acids in the blood. Use of this measure has indicated that elderly people, in general, become overaroused when performing a demanding task. The evidence comes from studies in which elderly participants receive either a drug known to reduce the level of free fatty acids in the blood (and therefore a decreased arousal level) or a placebo (that is, a neutral substance) in advance of practicing a difficult learning task. Participants receiving the drug perform at a much higher level than participants receiving the placebo, presumably because the debilitating effects on performance of overarousal present for the placebo participants are removed for the drug participants.

Another measure of physiological arousal is that of the skin's electrical conductance level. Research with this measure has suggested that elderly people tend to be underaroused when confronted by a demanding task (for instance, a difficult learning task).

Arousal is also used in reference to the brain's activity level, particularly activity of the cortex. Cortical activity is indicated in terms of the brain's electrical output, and it is measured by means of electroencephalography. There is clear evidence of cortical underarousal on the part of elderly people in general. Most important, there is also evidence to indicate the importance of integrating cortical arousal with physiological arousal to achieve effective performances on demanding tasks. Such integration seemingly occurs to a lesser degree for elderly people than for younger people.

The diminished integration of the two forms of arousal probably presents a greater problem to elderly adults than does the actual level of either physiological or cortical arousal. However, there is little evidence to support this position, evidence that is badly needed if this speculation is to be accepted as valid. Of course, the absence of an acceptable means of measuring adult age differences in physiological arousal continues to be a problem.

Arthritis

The most prevalent chronic disease in late adulthood is arthritis, affecting nearly 50 percent of people age sixty-five or older (and about 25 percent of people in the forty-five-to-sixty-four-year age range). Overall, it is estimated that nearly forty-three million people in the United States have some form of arthritis; there are more than one hundred kinds. Each form of arthritis involves joints, but other parts of the body may be affected as well. The Centers for Disease Control and Prevention predict that by the year 2020 there will be sixty million people in the United States with some form of arthritis.

Arthritis is a chronic disease that for many affected people lasts the rest of their lives. More than three million Americans have severe limitations of their activities of daily living (dressing, bathing, and so on) caused by arthritis. Leisure activities are also likely to be limited. Elderly adults who do not replace leisure activities that can no longer be performed with other activities are the least likely to adjust to their condition and the most likely to have problems with their well-being.

The two most common forms of arthritis are rheumatoid arthritis and osteoarthritis. Rheumatoid arthritis affects more than two million people in the United States, with women more likely to have the disease than men. It involves inflammation of joints and their capsules and ligaments. The onset of the disease usually occurs between the ages of twenty and sixty; thus, many elderly people already have the disease before old age. However, onset of the disease may occur after age sixty. The incidence of late onset is about the same for men and women. Stiffness and pain are commonly found in the fingers, wrists, and ankles. Rheumatoid arthritis is a progressive disease in that the symptoms often increase in intensity with the duration of the disease. In some patients the symptoms show cycles of remission followed by recurrence. The reason for the disorder in the body's immunological system that causes the disease is not fully understood, and a cure has yet to be found. There are procedures for reducing the pain and increasing body movements, including drugs that control the immune system (for example, Enbrel) and exercise.

People with rheumatoid arthritis are prone to develop heart disease. Treatment with a newer class of drugs called TNF inhibitors appears to lower the risk of cardiovascular disorders.

Early diagnosis and treatment of the disease is important for affected persons to continue living a productive lifestyle. Early treatment can limit joint damage, resulting in less loss of movement and work time.

Osteoarthritis (or degenerative joint disease) is most often found in people older than age fifty, and it affects more than sixteen million Americans. It is characterized by the breakdown of joint tissue and the loss of the protective cartilage of joints, usually with little inflammation of the joints. It is commonly found in the hands, hips, spine, and knees. Pain occurs with movement of the affected joints, and it may also occur during rest as the pain progresses. Contributors to osteoarthritis are obesity, injury, and degeneration from wear and tear over time.

Pain and discomfort from osteoarthritis may be assessed by the Osteoarthritis Severity Scale Items. Those with the disease rate on a five-point scale the intensity of pain and stiffness occurring with rising, standing, and walking. There is no known cure for osteoarthritis. Treatment of symptoms include exercise, physical therapy, moist heat, and drugs—for instance, medications containing acetaminophen, such as Tylenol Extra Strength (but *see* Pain Medications [Analgesics]), or nonsteroid anti-inflammatory drugs (NSAIDs), such as aspirin. Such treatment often allows victims of the disease to live relatively pain-free and active lives.

Fibromyalgia is a disease often confused with osteoarthritis. It often affects people over age fifty, especially older women. Three to six million Americans have the disease. Its symptoms are chronic fatigue, stiffness, and constant pain in the muscles, the tendons connecting muscles to bones, and the ligaments connecting bone to bone. There is no known cure. Stretching, walking, and water exercises are recommended for reducing the pain. Applications of heat and cold, massages, whirlpool therapy, and ultrasound therapy may also help to reduce the pain. The medicine Mirapex may help some patients. For more information, contact the National Institutes of Health Web site at http://www.nih.gov.niams.healthinfo/ fibromyalgia.htm or write to the National Arthritis and Musculoskeletal and Skin Diseases

Clearinghouse, National Institutes of Health, 1 AMS Circle, Bethesda, MD 20892-3675.

Gout is a rarer, but fairly well-known, form of arthritis (it affects about one million Americans, mostly men). Gout is caused by uric-acid salt deposits in joints, especially those of the feet and hands; the big toe is the most frequent site. Joints affected by these deposits are painful, swollen, and tender. Gout usually appears between the ages of forty and fifty-five, and the intensity of the symptoms is likely to increase with increasing age. Certain drugs are used to reduce symptoms during acute stages of the disease. After the pain subsides there are medicines (for instance, indomethacin) that help to reduce uric-acid production. Dietary restrictions are very important in reducing the frequency and duration of acute symptoms. Foods to be avoided include liver, gravies, beans, peas, cauliflower, anchovies, sardines, and herring. Also to be avoided are alcoholic beverages.

Other diseases related to arthritis include polymyalgia rheumatica, mixed connective tissue disease (MCTD), and lupus. Polymyalgia rheumatica affects more than four hundred thousand Americans, usually older women. It causes muscle pain and neck, shoulder, and hip stiffness. MCTD and lupus are both autoimmune diseases. In autoimmune diseases the immune system produces antibodies that attack normal cells and tissues. MCTD occurs much more frequently in women than in men. It may resemble rheumatoid arthritis in producing joint pain. It may also cause difficulty in swallowing and, most seriously, pulmonary hypertension that could cause heart or lung failure. Lupus is a disease in which the body's immune system attacks healthy tissues rather than germs. The most common form is systemic lupus (or just lupus). It may attack many parts of the body, such as joints, kidneys, and lungs. Discoid lupus is less common. It attacks only the skin, causing raised red circles. It rarely becomes systemic lupus. For more information about lupus, contact the National Institutes of Arthritis and Musculoskeletal and Skin Diseases at http://www.nih.niams.gov or call 877-22-NIAMS.

There are arthritis centers located in medical schools and hospitals across the country. They have facilities for the diagnosis and treatment of arthritis and provide information about arthritis.

The natural medicines glucosamine chondroitin sulphate and MSM (methyl-sulfonyl-methane) have been widely publicized as ways of reducing damage to cartilage in those with osteoarthritis. There have been a few studies indicating modest improvements in diminishing pain and swelling caused by arthritis of the knee and hip for users of glucosamine chondrotin. However, other studies have failed to find improvements. Recent evidence indicates that when improvement has been found it is simply from a placebo effect, rather than from a beneficial effect caused by the substance itself.

Interestingly, there is limited evidence to indicate that writing about stressful experiences may improve symptoms of rheumatoid arthritis.

Researchers found that about half of the patients in their study who wrote for twenty minutes a day over three consecutive days had reduced pain that lasted for months. There is even evidence to indicate that wearing a gold ring helps to relieve the symptoms of arthritis. Patients with gold bands were found to have less arthritis in their ring finger and adjacent joints than in comparable joints in the other hand.

It is very important for people to take charge of their arthritis and seek prompt treatment if they have pain, swelling, or stiffness that persists for more than two weeks. They should join a support group, and they should set goals for lifestyle changes, especially beginning an exercise program recommended by an expert in arthritis. Information about advances in the understanding, diagnosis, and treatment of arthritis may be obtained from an arthritis center at a medical school or hospital or from the Arthritis Foundation. *See also* Activities of Daily Living; Disability (Adaptation); Leisure Activities.

Aspirin

A daily low-dose (baby) aspirin (eighty-three milligrams per tablet) may help to prevent a heart attack or stroke. However, recent evidence indicates that the benefit of a daily aspirin differs for older men and older women. For women, the aspirin seems to reduce the likelihood of a stroke but not the likelihood of a heart attack. For men, it reduces the likelihood of a heart attack but not the likelihood of a stroke. For older men, at least, taking an aspirin immediately when experiencing a heart attack may save their lives.

However, aspirin is not medicine's perfect panacea. Aspirin may cause gastric bleeding, and it may cause acid reflux. Acid reflux is a form of heart-burn in the esophagus that occurs frequently for some adults. Its long-term persistence could result in serious damage to the esophagus. There are medications to control its occurrences (consult your physician). If the med-ications are ineffective, there are certain activities that help to avoid acid-reflux occurrences. They include eating slowly, eating more frequent smaller meals, and avoiding laying down after eating a meal.

For more information about aspirin, you should read the article by Dr. Isadore Rosenfeld in the January 1, 2006, issue of *Parade* magazine. Most important, you should consult your physician before you start taking aspirin regularly.

Asset and Health Dynamics among the Oldest Old (AHEAD)

The AHEAD study began in 1993–1994 with interviews of more than seven thousand people who were representative of community-dwelling adults age seventy and older. The participants were followed for four years. By that time nearly two thousand had died. Among the information gained from the study were the difficulty participants had performing the normal activities of daily living (*see* Activities of Daily Living) and the presence of obesity, as defined by self-reports of height and weight (*see* Obesity [Effects on Longevity and Disability]).

Assisted Living Facilities

Twenty-five years ago the only options for elderly people living alone who were no longer physically functioning independently, but who were still cognitively unimpaired, were either to go to live with one of their adult children or to seek admission to a nursing home. Neither of these options was viewed favorably by most elderly people. Since then, several alternatives have emerged. One is what is called an assisted living facility (another is home care; *see* Home Care).

Assisted living (also called aging in place) consists of housing for frail elderly people that provides supportive services in a homelike environment. It stresses a consumer-focused model in which delivery of services is organized around the resident and not the facility. (Services made by choice of residents are available on a twenty-four-hour schedule.) It contrasts with a medically oriented model of care where residents are really patients cared for according to the facility schedule. Assisted living facilities vary in terms of type of residence (apartment or room), range of services (assistance to skilled nursing), level of privacy (shared room or private), and degree of independence (right to refuse services). The annual cost may be prohibitive for many seniors.

The Assisted Living Facilities Associations have identified the basic needs that facilities must have to ensure a high quality of life for residents. They include some form of independence, autonomy, privacy, and aging in place. Aging in place means providing health and personal care in the most homelike environment possible.

Gerontologists are concerned about other conditions that may affect residents' quality of life. They have found that an important condition is the presence of helpful and supportive staff members. Also needed are a positive social environment, active social participation, and stimulating involvement by family members and friends.

Researchers at the University of Maryland–Baltimore County surveyed 156 residents in thirteen different assisted living facilities to gain some idea of what factors determine the level of satisfaction residents have with their living conditions. They found that more satisfied residents tend to be happier individuals who are more functionally independent and have less education than other residents. Greater satisfaction was also found to be associated with several characteristics of the facilities, namely, smaller size, greater availability of personal space, and, interestingly, fewer sociorecreational activities.

Assistive Devices

Assistive devices are things that help people reduce the limitations they have when suffering from sensory or physical impairments or disabilities. Magnifying glasses, closed caption television, hearing aids, and walkers are familiar examples of assistive devices. They are especially important for older adults, given the fact that they are more likely to have limitations and impairments than are younger adults.

For seniors with visual impairment there are lighted magnifying glasses, books and popular magazines printed in larger letters, and playing cards larger than the usual size. Hearing aids are available in varying sizes and costs. Unfortunately, nearly two-thirds of the millions of Americans with hearing impairment do not use hearing aids.

A number of assistive devices improve the mobility of older adults with lower-limb impairments. One such device is a walker. Most walkers fall into three categories: walking frames (no wheels), two-wheeled walkers that do not roll too far away from the user, and four-wheeled walkers (however, the hand break is difficult to operate for seniors with arthritis in the hands).

Many seniors need to use a wheelchair. The X-braced folding wheelchair is especially popular with seniors because of its ease of storage and transportation. Seniors with little use of their arms and legs need to use a powered wheelchair.

Not to be overlooked are canes and crutches. These simple device have been effective for many years in reducing the number of hours of home care that physically impaired seniors require. *See also* Canes and Crutches; Walkers; Wheelchairs.

Asthma

Asthma is a breathing problem in which the breathing tubes are sensitive to smoke, pollen, dust, and other substances. When the tubes react, they become inflamed and narrower, thus making breathing more difficult. Although asthma is commonly associated with children, it does occur in older people as well. In fact, more than one million Americans age sixty-five or older have asthma. Their condition could be a recurrence of the disease they had as children, or it could be a first-time occurrence of the disease. The symptoms include a wheezing sound while breathing (sometimes only when the person has a cold), a cough that may last a week, shortness of breath, and tightness in the chest.

There are medications used to treat asthma effectively, as well as various devices to aid breathing during periods of attack. The standard medication for treating asthma has been steroids. However, they do have potentially serious side effects, such as heightened blood pressure and weight gain. A medication called rhuMAb-E25 received clinical trials in 1999. About one-fourth of the asthma patients tested were able to stop taking inhaled steroids, and about one-third of those taking oral steroids were able to stop taking them. If you believe you have asthma, consult your physician as soon as possible. For more information about asthma, call your local American Lung Association.

Attention and Stroke Recovery

Two-thirds of strokes occur in people over age sixty-five. The best-known symptom of a stroke is paralysis of one side of the body that limits motor or muscular functioning for that side of the body.

The ability to divide attention between two or more activities (*see* Divided Attention) has been identified as a critical cognitive ability relating to recovery from a stroke. The ability to divide attention is usually impaired after a stroke, and the extent of that impairment seems to be related to the extent of motor impairment after a stroke.

An effective intervention for improving the motor functioning of stroke victims may be to provide them with extensive training on divided-attention tasks. Such training has been found to improve attentional abilities and may lead to improved motor functioning for stroke victims.

Attention (Overview)

Open up a dictionary, and look up the word *attention*. You are likely to find a definition like "careful observation." This definition is too vague to be useful in understanding aging. Regardless of the definition, it is apparent that attention somehow plays an important role in our everyday lives. An indication of that importance comes from the many statements we hear or see that refer to attention in some way. "Probable cause of the accident—inattention of the driver in vehicle A." "Be on guard!" "Watch for any sign of movement by the enemy." "When is our next quiz? I was listening to that guy talking behind me, and I wasn't paying attention to the professor." "I heard this ad on my car radio while driving home today."

These statements are also an indication that there are different forms of attention. Watching for movement by the enemy is obviously different from listening to one individual while tuning out another. Moreover, both of these forms differ from listening to the radio while driving a car. "Watching for movement" is an example of *vigilance,* "tuning out the professor's voice" is an example of *selective attention,* and "listening to the ad while driving" is an example of *divided attention.*

Vigilance refers to monitoring a constant stream of like stimulation to detect a change in that stimulation. A military guard stationed near the enemy is on the alert to determine whether the steady silence of the night is interrupted by some unexpected noise. Similarly, a quality-control inspector on a production line watches for the rare occurrence of a defective product. Selective attention means directing attention to one source of stimulation in the immediate environment while ignoring other sources of stimulation. We are constantly bombarded by visual and auditory stimuli and often by stimuli from the other senses that are present in our environment. Our interest and objective at any given moment determine which of these stimuli are selected to receive attention and therefore enter our consciousness. Those that do receive attention are called relevant stimuli (for example, the guy's voice for the student); those occurring simultaneously are called irrelevant stimuli (the professor's voice for the student—but if the student's interest at the time had been different, the professor's voice would surely have been the relevant stimulus). Divided attention means literally what it says. We attempt to share our attention among several sources of simultaneously present stimulations. Thus, the driver listening to the car radio is sharing attention between two sources of stimuli, one visual, the other auditory. The visual stimuli from the road ahead are one source, and the ad on the radio is the auditory stimulus. As long as traffic is light, the driver will not find it difficult to divide attention between the two. However, with heavy traffic the driver may begin to ignore the radio (or, alternatively, tell a passenger to be quiet).

Psychologists believe that we possess some form of an attentional resource, one that has a limited capacity or capability for maintaining attention. That is, we can attend to only a limited amount of stimulation from our environment at any one time. Many researchers in the psychology of aging believe that this attentional capacity decreases somewhat with aging. Some forms of attention place little demand on this capacity (the attention needed to perform a simple vigilance task) and therefore are unaffected by normal aging. Other forms of attention, however, are very demanding and therefore more likely to be affected by aging (for example, dividing attention between two tasks, each of which is difficult to perform alone). Aging's effects on each of the three basic forms of attention are discussed in other entries. *See* Attention and Stroke Recovery; Divided Attention; Selective Attention; Vigilance.

Attitudes (Political and Social)

Attitudes express our feelings and behavioral tendencies for various groups of people, organizations, and social and political issues. They are usually measured by psychologists in terms of dimensions that are anchored by opposites, such as conservative at one end of the spectrum and liberal at the other end (with moderate in the middle). Some people fall at one extreme or the other, while others fall in the middle.

Gerontologists have most often studied age differences in attitudes toward social and political issues in which the opposites of conservative and liberal are truly applicable. These studies have typically indicated the presence of more conservative attitudes among older people than among younger people. For example, in one study, the participants, all faculty spouses at a university, were evaluated with respect to attitudes toward race, law enforcement, and patriotism. Overall, only 21 percent of the spouses in the fifty-and-older range were classified as being liberal on the basis of their attitude test scores, in contrast to 55 percent of the spouses in the twenty-to-twenty-nine-year range.

There is good reason to believe that such age differences are more the product of membership in different generations than the product of a true age change from liberalism to conservatism as one grows older. That is, members of earlier generations were more likely to have acquired conservative positions on many issues than were members of later generations. This may be seen, for example, in analyses of allegiance to political parties. Several years ago the proportion of elderly people who considered themselves Republicans was much greater than the proportion of young adults who considered themselves Republican. This does not necessarily mean that growing old converts Democrats into Republicans. The older Republicans were predominantly Republicans when they themselves were young adults. Other studies have revealed that age itself has little effect on attitudes toward economic and foreign policy issues.

As society and its standards change, the attitudes of many people are likely to change as well. A common belief is that elderly people are more rigid and less flexible in their ability to change their attitudes. However, this does not seem to be the case. As cultural changes occur over time, they are likely to influence older people to about the same extent as they influence younger people. This seems to be true, for example, for attitudes toward legalized abortion, businesses being open on Sundays, and so on. In fact, some evidence suggests that elderly adults may be more open to change than younger adults when presented with effective information that conflicts with their social or political attitudes. Some psychologists suspect that the declining cognitive abilities of some elderly adults may hinder their ability to resist arguments opposed to their existing attitudes.

Attribution

Attribution refers to the way you assign blame when something goes wrong in your life. To determine whether there are age differences in attribution, psychologists give participants statements such as "You give an important talk in front of a group, and the audience reacts negatively." The participants are asked to imagine that this experience happened to them, and then to rate on a scale from one to seven who is to blame for the experience they had. One end of the scale is defined as "totally due to others," the other end as "totally due to me."

They also rate themselves on two other seven-point scales. The first scale evaluates the stability of their attribution, and it is anchored on one end by "will never again be present" and the other by "will always be present." The other scale evaluates the global nature of their attribution (in other words, how general it is); it is anchored at one end by "influences just this particular situation" and at the other end by "influences all situations in my life."

Researchers have found that elderly adults are, on average, more likely than young adults to place responsibility for negative events on negative abilities that they possess. Elderly adults are, on average, also more likely than young adults to perceive the situation as being stable, that is, it will continue to be present in future encounters with the same situation. However, elderly adults have also been found to be less general than young adults in their attributions. As perceived by an elderly person, the responsibility for an audience's negative reaction to his or her talk probably rests with that person (for example, he or she had speech anxiety). Moreover, the negative audience reaction will probably occur whenever a talk is given by that person (that is, stability), but the person's anxiety would not affect other kinds of performances. By contrast, a young adult is likely to perceive his or her poor speech as being related to something like fatigue that is only temporary but would affect many other kinds of performances when it is present.

Autobiographical Memory

A familiar refrain of many elderly people is that they remember well events that happened to them years ago, but they have trouble remembering what happened recently. The memory of personally experienced events is known as autobiographical memory. Is it true that the remote memories of elderly people tend to remain remarkably preserved while their recent memories fade away quickly?

Memory research has indicated that this is not completely true. The standard method for testing autobiographical memory is to give participants a series of seemingly random words, with instructions to recall some personal memory in response to each word. The series may include such words as *book, sorry, fun,* and *surprised.* After all memory associations have been given, the participants are asked to date when each recalled event occurred. Surprisingly, the most frequently recalled memories to the words by elderly participants are recent ones, dating back to the past few years or only to the past few months. The next most frequently recalled memories are for events that occurred in early adulthood ("the reminiscence bump"). Midlife events are recalled much less frequently than either recent events or events from early adulthood. Events from early childhood are rarely recalled. The unavailability of memories from early childhood is also true for younger adults. The unavailability of very early memories is known as childhood amnesia.

The decline in memory from recent events to midlife events follows the course of normal forgetfulness. Recent events have yet to experience much interference from later events, the kind of interference that produces forgetting (*see* Forgetting). By contrast, midlife events have experienced considerable interference from years of intervening events. Why then the relatively high frequency of memories of events from early adulthood, events that surely have encountered more intervening events than those of midlife? One reason early events are recalled easily is that many of them are first-time events, a condition that makes them more readily retrievable. By contrast, midlife events are made less retrievable by being events that have happened frequently.

There is another reason as well. In a different procedure, elderly participants are asked simply to identify the events that were most important in their lives. The most frequently recalled important events are those of adolescence and early adulthood, with recent events having the next highest frequency. As with the individual word procedure, midlife events have the lowest frequency of occurrence. The events of adolescence and early adulthood appear to be especially significant ones in shaping the remainder of their lives. As such, they remain highly vivid and accessible to recall. Moreover, it is these events that are likely to be recalled and therefore strengthened further to resist forgetting when people reminisce about their earlier life (*see* Reminiscence).

Automatic Teller Machines (ATMs)

A survey of adults in Georgia reported that 86 percent of those between the ages of eighteen and thirty-five use ATMs, whereas only 33 percent of those between the ages of sixty-five and eighty do. The elderly adults who use ATMs are those who use technological equipment in general (such as VCRs or answering machines). The results of a study by researchers at the Georgia Institute of Technology indicated that more elderly adults would use ATMs if glare from the screen was reduced, if keys were aligned better with their functions, and if the written material was in larger print. These changes would undoubtedly not only increase the number of older users of ATMs but also reduce mistakes in their use by elderly people. *See also* Scams.

B

Baby Talk (Elderspeak)

Some young people feel that elderly people, both those living in the community and those living in nursing homes, are so incompetent that they have to talk baby talk (elderspeak) to them. That is, they speak loudly and in a high pitch, and they use words and expressions they would use with children. These changes in speech do not seem to aid comprehension by elderly listeners. However, sentences should be kept grammatically simple and devoid of subordinate clauses.

Back Pain

Millions of Americans suffer from back pain. Older adults are no exception. Usually, the pain is tolerable and goes away spontaneously. However, it often returns, and in some cases develops into chronic back pain. Common back pain is also called back strain or lumbago, and it may extend to the legs and buttocks.

Back pain usually occurs for no known reason. However, there are steps that may be taken to lower the risk of back pain. If you need to sit for a prolonged period, take a break and move around. Soft soles help, and women should not wear high heels. Sleep on a firm mattress. When seated, have your feet touch the floor, and have your knees slightly higher than your hips. Exercise that improves muscle tone in the lower back should help.

When suffering from back pain, bed rest does not help, but stretching exercises do help to relieve the pain. Ordinary pain medications such as Tylenol and Advil help to lower the pain. If pain is severe, you need to see a physician who will probably give you a prescription for an anti-inflammatory medication. Surgery is usually required only under certain conditions, such as a pinched nerve.

Balance Impairment and Cognitive Demands

Elderly adults, compared to younger adults, have a difficult time maintaining balance while performing simultaneously a cognitively demanding task (for example, reading a street sign on a dimly lit street corner). This is especially true of older adults who have been clinically found to be impaired in balance. Laboratory evidence in support of this adverse effect comes from studies in which balance is disturbed by the sudden movement of a platform while responding differently to two different tones. This is a contributing factor to the high risk of falls for older people with impaired balance (*see* Falls).

Barriers to Health in Older Men

Millions of older men will not eat vegetables, will not exercise, and will not participate in a senior health promotion program. Nor do older men visit a physician as often as older women do. When they do see a physician, they ask fewer questions and seek less information than older women do. Many older men see themselves as being self-reliant. Seeing a physician may be viewed as a sign of weakness. Health information just does not seem to apply to these men. They try to ignore a health problem they may be experiencing in the fear that addressing it will change their lifestyle. By ignoring it, it may go away. These men need effective role models and persuasive spouses and friends to remove these barriers to better health. *See also* Physicians (Communication with).

Bathing

Bathing for nonambulatory elderly adults presents a challenge. The easiest way for them to bathe is to use a roll-in shower stall. However, many of them enjoy a warm bath in a tub. There are a number of special bathtubs and devices for assistance while bathing in a tub. They include grab handles that clamp to the side of the tub and a bench that reaches from edge to edge. There are also power-lifting seats that raise and lower the body.

Bathing persons with Alzheimer's disease and other forms of dementia presents a problem to their caregivers. Demented people may dislike bathing because they view it as a form of assault. They are taken from their rooms, undressed, and scrubbed, perhaps without regard to their feelings. Disruptive behaviors are likely to be their only defense. Caregivers should decide first if a bath or shower is really necessary now. If it is, then they should structure the environment to make bathing a comfortable and pleasant experience. For example, they could play restful music in the background, minimize glare in the room, put scented oils in the water, and perhaps add bubble bath powder for some patients. In addition, they should approach the patient calmly and gently, and praise each form of cooperation (such as "You're doing great!").

Many elderly adults suffer from dry skin in the winter. There are ways to minimize this condition. Bathing once or twice a week is sufficient for most elderly adults in that they have reduced sweat glands. When they do bathe, it should be in tepid or warm water (hot water robs the skin of moisture). After bathing, they should then apply skin lotion containing lanolin.

Bed Rest

Many older adults take to their beds when they feel ill. What are the consequences of too much bed rest for community-dwelling older adults?

Researchers at Yale University followed a group of frail seniors and a group of nonfrail seniors (age seventy and older) for eighteen months. The amount of bed rest was measured monthly by a telephone interview in which participants were asked how many episodes of bed rest since the last interview (staying in bed for at least half a day due to illness, injury, or some other problem). The average amount of time spent in bed rest was 3.2 months for the frail participants and 2.4 months for the nonfrail participants.

For the nonfrail participants the number of months with bed rest was significantly associated with declines in performance of instrumental activities of daily living (for example, shopping and housework), physical activities (leisure activities), and social activities (such as visiting friends). For frail participants the amount of bed rest was significantly associated only with a decline in the performance of instrumental activities of daily living.

Unfortunately, many illnesses in late adulthood presently call for lengthy periods of bed rest in their treatment. Health professionals need to discover alternatives to bed rest in the treatment of many of these illnesses.

Bed Sores

Bed sores are ulcers in areas of the skin that are under pressure from lying in bed, sitting in a wheelchair, or wearing a cast for long periods of time. The pressure causes the blood supply to the affected area of skin to be cut off. When left unattended, the skin may break open and become infected. The sores occur most often on the buttocks or on the heels of the feet.

Elderly hospital patients and nursing home residents are especially susceptible to bed sores from lying in bed for long periods. They may occur after only a few hours of immobility. On the third day of hospitalization, more than 6 percent of patients age sixty-five or older have bed sores. To avoid the sores they should have their position in bed changed from their back to their right side then to their left side and than the back again. Their heads should not be elevated more than thirty degrees. It is important that they have good nutrition. Without it the skin becomes very thin and adds to the development of bed sores. The skin should be kept clean and dry.

Once bed sores occur, pressure should be removed from the affected area, and the wound should be covered with medicated gauze or other kind of dressing. Antibiotics may be needed. The specific treatment depends on the severity of the sores.

The occurrence of bed sores is significantly associated with increasing age, male sex, urinary and fecal incontinence, difficulty turning in bed, and poor nutritional status.

Beliefs about Aging Affect Physical Health

Many older adults share the negative beliefs with younger adults that aging is a time of physical impairment, memory problems, constant health problems, and so on. Do such negative beliefs affect the physical health of older adults who have them? Evidence gathered by researchers at the Yale University School of Medicine indicates that it does indeed.

More than six hundred people who were in their fifties or early sixties at the start of the study were followed for twenty-three years. Those with an early positive belief about their own aging lived on average seven and a half years longer than those with a less positive belief.

Older adults with a positive belief were also found to have better functional health (that is, mobility and the ability to perform successfully the normal activities of daily living). Functional health is a good indicator of an individual's overall physical health.

Seniors with a negative belief about their own aging appear to live a self-fulfilling prophecy of an expected negative outcome of their aging. This belief evokes behaviors that make the expected negative outcome more likely (for instance, little exercise and poor diet). By contrast, those with a positive belief appear to live a self-fulfilling prophecy of an expected positive outcome. As a result, they are likely to manifest behaviors that help them realize the positive outcome (such as regular exercising and proper diet).

Bifocals

Of the more than 160 million Americans who need glasses, 60 percent wear bifocals, trifocals, or progressives. Many of this percentage are elderly adults. More than half of people with bifocals have trouble adjusting to them. The adjustment problem is much less with progressives, the newest form of lenses that change gradually and invisibly from distance viewing at the top to reading at the bottom.

For elderly adults with bifocals there are ways to avoid feeling woozy while viewing near and far objects. For example, when reading a newspaper, fold it in half or in fourths, and keep your head and eyes still while moving the paper instead of your eyes. You should not look at your feet when you are walking. If your bifocals are new, wear them all day every day for the first week or so to get used to them.

Bingo

Bingo is a popular game for elderly adults, especially women. Some gerontologists believe that it is a waste of their time. However, Dr. Iseli Krauss of Clarion University has discovered that there are positive effects of playing bingo. Her research involved about two hundred people, half of whom were experienced bingo players, the other half inexperienced. She discovered that if elderly adults play bingo regularly, they maintain a high level of skill in the ability to divide attention (*see* Divided Attention) while searching for a number and a pattern of numbers simultaneously. Playing with only one to three cards probably does not do much for elderly adults, but playing with many cards provides mental stimulation. In addition, a researcher at Harvard University followed a group of people for thirteen years (they were sixty-five and older at the beginning of the study). After controlling for race, income, and health status, the researcher discovered that a social activity, such as bingo, lowered the risk of death just as much as exercise activity did.

Biological Age

A person's biological age may be expressed in two different ways. One is in terms of how that person's health status compares with the average health status at different age levels. If his or her health and biological functioning is comparable to the average seventy year old of the same sex, then that person's biological age would be seventy years. This would be the case whether the person's actual (chronological) age is sixty or eighty years. The second way is in terms of the number of years he or she is expected to live (*see* Life Expectancy) based on his or her health status. Thus, if a person's health status is comparable to the average seventy year old of the same sex, then his or her biological age is the number of remaining years the average seventy year old is expected to live.

Bladder Cancer

Bladder cancer occurs most often between the ages of fifty and seventy years. The incidence of bladder cancer is four times greater in men than in women. It is the fourth most frequently found cancer in men, and the ninth most frequent in women. A major risk factor is smoking, with the incidence of bladder cancer being five times higher in smokers than in nonsmokers. One way for elderly adults to lower their risk of bladder cancer is to make certain that they drink plenty of fluids daily.

Researchers at Harvard University provided evidence to show that drinking a lot of fluids (including water, juices, coffee, and even alcoholic beverages) reduces the risk of bladder cancer. Their study was conducted over ten years, and it involved forty-eight thousand men ranging in age from forty to seventy-five. Fluids are presumed to work because a high fluid concentration dilutes the concentration of cancer-causing substances in urine. In the same study it was found that eating broccoli and other cruciferous vegetables also reduced the risk of bladder cancer.

If the cancer is detected early, there is a good chance of successful treatment with minimal side effects. If the cancer has spread beyond the bladder, treatment is much more difficult.

Bladder (Overactive)

A bladder is considered to be overactive if a person is urinating at least eight times in twenty-four hours. Only about 20 percent of people with overactive bladder report it to their physicians. The number of elderly persons having overactive bladder is unknown, but they are more likely to have it than younger people. Elderly women are more likely to have it than elderly men. They could be helped by the medication Detrol, which has fewer side effects than many other medications.

Blessed Mental Status Test

The Blessed Mental Status Test is likely to be part of the battery of physical and psychological tests used in the diagnosis of senile dementia of the Alzheimer's type (that is, a diagnosis of suspected Alzheimer's disease). It has been widely used in clinical assessment since its introduction by Dr. G. Blessed and colleagues more than twenty years ago. The validity of the test's diagnostic accuracy has received strong support from the correlation found between scores on the test and the number of senile plaques found in the brain at autopsy (*see* Alzheimer's Disease).

The test consists of two parts. For the first part, a relative or close friend of a client is asked questions about the client's competence in dealing with practical tasks in the everyday world (in other words, his or her ability to perform common household chores). For the second part, the client is given a series of mental tasks that test his or her concentration, orientation, recent memory, and remote memory. For example, the client is asked when World War II occurred and to count backward from twenty.

Blood Pressure (High and Low)

Blood pressure is the force of blood pushing against arterial walls. When your blood pressure is measured, the top number is for systolic pressure, the bottom number for diastolic pressure. Optimal pressure is 120/80 (or less for each number), and prehypertension is between 120 and 130/ between 80 and 89.

High blood pressure, or *hypertension,* is considered to be over 140/90.

When so defined, about 54 percent of adults in the sixty-five-to-seventy-four age range have hypertension. It is estimated that 10 percent of Americans are taking medications to control high blood pressure (have your pressure checked and consult your physician about it). The medications include diuretics, ACE inhibitors, alpha blockers, alpha-beta blockers, vasodilators, and calcium channel blockers. Alpha blockers and vasodilators serve to relax muscles in blood vessels, allowing blood to flow more freely. Alpha-beta blockers do the same while also slowing the heartbeat.

Eating a lot of fresh fruits and vegetables may lower blood pressure, even with only slightly lower salt intake. French investigators demonstrated that a high fiber diet with six to eight daily servings of fruits and vegetables is especially conducive to lower blood pressure. Considerable evidence indicates that aerobic exercise lowers systolic blood pressure in older adults. However, its effectiveness in lowering diastolic pressure has not been firmly established.

Treatment of patients with diastolic heart failure includes reduction in sodium intake, cautious use of diuretics, and the correction of increased diastolic blood pressure.

For years physicians considered diastolic pressure (the lower of the two numbers) to be the one to be concerned about in terms of potential stroke or heart attack. However, recent evidence indicates that it is systolic pressure (the top number) that needs to be lowered to protect patients from a stroke or heart attack.

A lowering of systolic pressure (systolic hypotension) after eating a meal is a common condition for seniors. The incidence may be higher for older adults with Parkinson's disease or heart failure. It may result in dizziness, fainting, or even a stroke. The symptoms occur more often after breakfast and lunch than after dinner.

Treatment with medications is difficult. Nonpharmacological treatments are usually recommended. Included in some cases is lying down after a meal for an hour or two to prevent falling. Walking after a meal usually restores systolic blood pressure to what it was before its sudden lowering.

Low blood pressure, or *hypotension,* results from too little blood circulating to support normal blood pressure. Among the reasons for low blood pressure, also known as hypovolemia, are severe hemorrhaging caused by a wound and excessive urination. If hypovolemia is severe, an individual may experience shock, and death may occur unless a physician restores the volume of blood. *See also* Cardiovascular Diseases; Flaxseed: Hypertension and Mental Functioning.

Body Build and Body Characteristics

Height remains relatively stable until people reach their fifties. Between ages fifty-five and seventy-five, men tend to lose about half an inch to an inch in height, and women lose an inch to two inches. Several factors are responsible for the decrease in height. They include compression of the spine from loss of bone strength, the thinning of the cartilage found between the bones of the vertebral column, and, alas, the effects of bad posture over the years.

From early adulthood to middle age, most people gain weight (the familiar "middle-aged spread"). The main reason is that middle-aged people tend to eat as much (or more) as they did as young adults. At the same time, many become less active physically and therefore convert less food into energy. In addition, the rate at which people convert food into energy (basal metabolic rate) slows by about 3 percent every ten years. As a result, the caloric intake per day needed to maintain one's present rate decreases, on average, about 5 percent to 10 percent every ten years.

The fact that middle-aged people are unlikely to reduce their food intake means that they do not burn up enough food. Consequently, fat accumulates throughout their bodies, and, for many middle-aged people, their weight increases by 10 percent to 15 percent of what it was in their twenties. The weight gain may be especially in the stomach/abdominal area, resulting in the "middle-aged spread." An excessive amount of this gain (a measurement around the level of the navel of greater than forty inches for men and thirty-five inches for women) could be a warning sign of an impending heart attack and stroke. These individuals should be eating less and exercising more.

After middle age, the body's weight usually levels off and begins a slow progressive decrease as the body loses some bone, muscle, and fat. In late adulthood the ratio of lean body mass to fat declines, on average, resulting in a lower basal metabolic rate because the metabolic needs of fat tissue are less than those of lean tissue. As a result, fewer calories need to be consumed by older people even when they exercise regularly, and, of course, many of them do not.

The skin cells of older people live about half as long as the cells of thirty-year-old people (fifty days versus one hundred days), and they are replaced more slowly than are the cells of younger people. As the number of skin cells decreases, the skin becomes thinner and is more easily scratched or chapped. The skin also loses much of its elasticity as the substance elastin beneath the skin decreases. And it loses much of its firmness as the protein collagen decreases and loses much of its ability to hold moisture as the substance glycosaminoglycan decreases. The changes in the skin produced by aging are accelerated by tobacco smoke and pollution.

Light-skinned people often find their skin becoming even lighter as they age. This results from a decrease in the amount of pigment in the remaining cells. The skin of elderly people often contains "age spots" consisting of areas of dark pigmentation that resembles freckles. The number of moles in the skin is also likely to increase in late adulthood, and small red lines may appear in the skin as some blood vessels become dilated.

Varicose veins are not uncommon, and they do occur more often after age sixty-five than before that age. They appear as irregular swellings in veins, especially those in the legs, and wearing of special support hose may be required. They are often the result of years of many hours of regular standing, but they may also be caused by such conditions as heart disease, gout, and abdominal tumors. One way of treating varicose veins is through a procedure called sclerotherapy in which an injected material in the veins irritates their linings and fuses their inner surfaces. The disorder known as piles consists of varicose veins of the rectum. Spider veins are fairly common for women over the age of forty.

There is the tendency for older women to show sagging of the breasts. The sagging is caused by partial deterioration of the glandular tissues that produce firmness of the breasts and some stretching of the tissues connecting the breasts to their muscles. Measures may be taken earlier in life that may prevent, or at least reduce, sagging later in life. They include wearing supportive brassieres during pregnancy, breast feeding, and exercising. *See also* Strength and Stamina.

Body Mass Index

The body mass index (BMI) estimates the fat and muscle composition of a person's body. It is a better indicator of the person's physical condition than weight alone. The BMI is found by dividing your weight in kilograms by your height in meters squared. A BMI of 19–24.9 is considered excellent, 25–29.9 is overweight, and 30–39.9 is obese.

Body Odor

Older adults should be aware of the fact that unusual body odors may be a symptom of some disease. For example, an ammonia-like odor may result from a kidney disease, and an odor like polish remover from diabetes. Some medications may also cause an unusual body odor. This is the case, for example, for tamoxifen, a frequently used medication for breast cancer.

Boredom

Do you feel bored with your life and want to add some excitement to it? On the surface, you might expect to find that elderly people experience more boredom than do younger people, especially young adults. However, recent evidence suggests that this is not the case. Age differences in boredom were investigated by researchers at the National Institute on Aging with a large sample of individuals ranging in age over the adult life span. The participants responded to such statements as "I am seldom bored" and "I am always glad to find some excuse to take me away from work." Their responses indicated the extent to which each statement applied to them. Surprisingly, it was found that boredom tends to decrease with age, being greatest early in adulthood, after which it declines through middle age.

Most surprisingly, there was no tendency for boredom to increase after middle age. That is, boredom was no greater in late adulthood than in middle age—and for both middle-aged and older adults it was found to be well below the level experienced by young adults.

Closely associated with boredom is the need to find relief from it by seeking external or internal stimulation of some kind. The need for external stimulation was tested in the boredom study by having the participants respond to such statements as "At the amusement park I like to go on the most scary rides" and "I find sitting at home a nice way to pass the time."

The results were much like those found for boredom. The need for external stimulation was greatest for young adults and about the same for middle-aged and elderly adults. As the feeling of boredom decreases after young adulthood, the need for experiencing exciting events as an antidote for boredom decreases as well. The same outcome has been found by other researchers for the frequency of daydreaming, a form of internal stimulation used as an antidote for boredom. That is, elderly adults actually daydream less than young adults (*see* Daydreaming).

Bowels

Many people do not have a bowel movement every day. That is quite normal, as is having one every three days. This does not necessarily mean constipation. Constipation is defined by hard stools and straining to pass them.

However, chronic constipation is found in about 25 percent of people over age sixty-five. To avoid constipation elderly adults should eat at least 35 grams of fiber and drink eight 8-ounce glasses of water daily as well as walk for exercise. Researchers at the University of Pittsburgh found that elderly adults with chronic constipation show more signs of psychological distress than elderly adults without it.

Another bowel problem for many elderly people is irritable bowel syndrome (IBS). The symptoms are abdominal pain, bloating, and alternating diarrhea and constipation. It is estimated that half a million visits to physicians annually are for IBS and that more than three hundred thousand prescriptions are written annually for it. IBS is generally associated with overall poorer physical functioning and a lower quality of life. Tension may set off an attack of IBS. Certain exercises help to combat it, as do deep breathing techniques.

Perhaps the most serious problem is bowel incontinence or lack of bowel control. It is caused by malfunctioning of the sphincter muscle that surrounds the anus and controls bowel movements. In some cases, biofeedback (*see* Psychotherapy) may aid in restoring some of the sphincter's control. In other cases, surgery may be needed. *See also* Flaxseed; Physiological Functions.

Brain and Aging

Several years ago, a prominent gerontologist was asked at a meeting why age-related changes occur in mental functioning. He replied, "The brain rots." This is, of course, a gross exaggeration. At the same time, it cannot be denied that changes do take place in the brain with normal aging, and even greater changes take place with abnormal aging (for instance, in Alzheimer's disease). These changes are likely to affect mental functioning, but some forms of mental functioning are more affected than others.

Much of our knowledge of changes in the structure of the brain is derived from autopsies in which detailed studies are made of younger and older brains. These studies reveal that, on average, the brain decreases in weight by 5 percent to 10 percent from age twenty to age ninety, with the amount of decrease varying with the presence or absence of disease. Some areas of the brain show greater decreases in size than other areas. The volume of the brain also decreases by 15 percent to 20 percent. Researchers in Michigan found that shrinkage of the brain is greater for men than for women. As the brain shrinks, the amount of fluid between the brain and the skull increases. Between the ages of sixty-five and ninety-five, men average about a 30 percent increase in fluid, women only about 1 percent. The shrinkage is from loss of gray matter cells, and it occurs mostly in the frontal and temporal lobes. In general, brain mass decreases about two grams a year from age twenty-six to age eighty.

As you look down at the brain from an open skull, you see a number of swelling-like areas known as gyri and a number of "valleys" (fissures or sulci) between the gyri. The gyri tend to become smaller in the aging brain, and the sulci become wider.

It is estimated that the human brain contains ten to twenty billion neurons (nerve cells) at the point of its maximum growth. How many neurons die and are not replaced as aging occurs is highly speculative. Some estimates are that twenty thousand nerve cells are lost per day after age thirty; other estimates have the loss as one hundred thousand neurons per day after age thirty. Other neurons that do not die may, nevertheless, become less functional in late adulthood as the pigment lipofuscin accumulates in them and interferes with their functioning.

Changes in neurons with aging include the appearance of neurofibrillary tangles within the bodies and axons (that extension of a neuron along which neural messages are transmitted to make contact with the dendrites of other neurons) of some neurons and the presence of vacuoles (spaces) in the fluid surrounding the nucleus of some neurons. Senile plaques, consisting of hard clusters of dead or damaged neurons, are present in the aging brain; they too interfere with the normal functioning of the neurons near them. Recent evidence indicates that the protein nicastrin plays a critical role in forming these plaques. Other neurons may lose some of their dendrites (extensions that receive neural messages transmitted by axons from other neurons at points called synapses), thus diminishing the amount of neural information that may be received by those neurons.

An especially important change in the aging brain is the decrease in the amounts of neurotransmitters, both in the cerebral cortex (the gray matter you would see if you looked down on an opened skull) and in other areas. Neurotransmitters are chemicals that bridge the gap between the axon of one neuron and the dendrites of other neurons, making possible the transmission of neural information from neuron to neuron. These neurotransmitters include acetylcholine, norepinephrine, dopamine, serotonin, and gamma-aminobutyric acid.

Acetylcholine is of particular importance in maintaining normal memory functioning, as is norepinephrine. Dopamine is a primary neurotransmitter in those areas of the brain controlling motor or muscular movements. Extreme declines in its production lead to Parkinson's disease. Serotonin is found in those areas of the brain controlling arousal and sleep. Decline in its presence seemingly account for many of the sleep problems encountered by a number of elderly people. Gamma-aminobutyric acid is concentrated largely in the thalamus, a bundle of neurons beneath the cerebral cortex that is involved in sensory functioning. Its reduction seemingly accounts for some of the sensory problems in elderly adults that are not explained by declining functioning of sense organs themselves.

There is evidence indicating that a protein known as nerve growth factor (NGF) is important for the normal functioning of cholinergic neurons, that is, those neurons that use acetylcholine for transmission across synapses, and therefore for normal memory functioning. NGF is important in helping nerve cells to grow and divide. There seems to be a diminished supply of nerve growth factor in aging brains, a decrement that is especially pronounced for people with Alzheimer's disease. Scientists at the University of California at San Diego have discovered that transplanting NGF into the brains of aging monkeys restored seemingly inactive neurons to normal functioning. Eventually, this procedure may be applied to aging human brains to restore normal functioning.

Areas and structures of the brain are affected differentially by normal aging. One of the earliest structures adversely affected by aging is the *hippocampus,* a small bundle of neurons located beneath the cerebral cortex. It has long been known that the hippocampus plays a major role in transferring information from short-term storage to long-term storage. Lesions to the hippocampus often lead to major problems in registering new information in long-term memory. Neuronal loss and diminished amounts of acetylcholine in the hippocampus seemingly account for the difficulty of many elderly adults in registering new information in permanent memory.

Neuronal loss or dysfunctioning with normal aging seems to be less pronounced in the *prefrontal area of the cerebral cortex* (the front of the brain). However, other parts of the frontal lobes tend to age faster than do most other parts of the brain. This area of the brain is involved in the retention of very old memories and in many higher-level mental operations (such as reasoning). Pronounced neuronal dysfunctioning in this area may result in what is called *frontal lobe deficit,* characterized by difficulty in decision making, slowness of thought, and difficulty in controlling impulses.

At the back of the brain are the *cerebellum, medulla,* and *pons.* The cerebellum is involved in maintaining body equilibrium and in smoothly coordinating muscular movements. Neuronal loss appears to be fairly severe in this area, sufficient in some elderly adults to result in impaired body balance (thus increasing the risk of falls) and the loss of some muscle tone that, in turn, results in greater susceptibility to muscular fatigue. Neuronal dysfunctioning in this area may also result in the tremors found in some elderly people (for instance, the shaking apparent while they try to make a deliberate movement of the hand). Evidence is also accumulating to implicate loss of neurons in the cerebellum as a major factor in the difficulty older people have in a form of learning known as classical conditioning (*see* Classical Conditioning). By contrast, normal aging seems to result in little neuronal loss or dysfunctioning in that area of the brain that controls gross body movements (the *basal ganglia*). The medulla controls critical biological functions, such as breathing and heartbeat, and the pons is involved in sleep and waking.

The brain is separated into two large hemispheres, the *left and right cerebral hemispheres,* that have different, specialized functions. The left hemisphere controls movements for the right side of the body, and the right hemisphere for the left side. Similarly, the left hemisphere determines feelings of touch from the right side of the body, the right hemisphere for the left side. Moreover, for most people, verbal thought processes are controlled by the left hemisphere; spatial and imaginal thought processes are governed by the right hemisphere.

Of great interest in gerontology is the possibility that the right hemisphere ages at a faster rate than does the left hemisphere. We know that verbal ability remains well preserved in late adulthood (*see* Verbal Ability), while imaginal ability shows, on average, fairly substantial declines with normal aging (*see* Imagery). Biological evidence in support of differential rates of cerebral aging has been conflicting, and the issue of differential hemispheric aging remains unresolved. In fact, the most recent, and one of the best, studies by researchers at the University of Southern California found no support for differential rates of aging.

Most of our knowledge of aging's effects on the brain has come from postmortem examinations. In recent years three new devices have permitted examinations of the living brain. The first is called *computed axial tomography (CAT)* scanning. An X-ray source sends a narrow beam of X-rays through an individual's head to a detector on the other side of the head. The source and the detector are then rotated one degree for another beam to be projected through the head. This one-degree-at-a-time process continues through 180 one-degree rotations. The amount of X-ray absorbed at each point in the given slice of the brain being examined is transmitted to a computer that translates these amounts into a picture of the slice's neural structure. The individual can then be moved along the axis of rotation, and a "picture" of another slice is taken.

For normally aging elderly adults, these "pictures" reveal increases in the fluid-filled spaces of the brain. However, these "pictures" have not been very revealing in identifying specific areas of the brain where atrophy has occurred that may then be related to specific mental and behavioral declines. CAT scans have not been very helpful in the early diagnosis of Alzheimer's disease. However, as the disease progresses in severity, CAT scans do show an atrophied brain with enlarged cortical sulci and enlarged cerebral ventricles.

The second device is called *positron-emission tomography (PET)* scanning. The procedure requires the release or emission of positively charged particles (positrons) during an individual's neural activity. A radioactive isotope is injected, which interacts with activated neurons and causes the emission of two gamma-ray photons that travel in opposite directions. These photons are delivered to a computer that constructs a "picture" of the metabolism occurring in the area where there is ongoing neural activity. Thus, PET scans provide information about neural functioning rather than neural structures.

To date, PET scans have not provided any major new insights into the brain changes that occur with normal aging. Apparently, changes in brain glucose and oxygen metabolism are slight with normal aging. Moreover, measures of brain metabolism of elderly adults have not been found to correlate highly with scores on various mental tasks. However, PET scans do reveal pronounced reductions in the rates of glucose and oxygen metabolism in various regions of the brain for patients with severe impairments as a result of Alzheimer's disease. Research with CAT and PET scans is still in its infancy. There is great hope that future advancements in the technology of each scanning procedure will lead to major discoveries about the effects of both normal and abnormal aging on the brain.

Perhaps the most promising procedure for offering new insights into the effects of both normal and abnormal aging on the brain is offered by the third device, *magnetic resonance imaging (MRI)*. MRI is used on soft tissue, such as the brain and other organs. The procedure is based on the fact that soft tissues are rich in water. During scanning the person being scanned lies inside the cylindrical heart of a large circular magnet. The magnet generates a magnetic field that causes hydrogen atoms of water molecules to line up like little magnets. Generators emit radio waves that rattle the hydrogen atoms. When the waves stop, the atoms realign under the magnetic field, and they give off their radio signals. From these signals images of the tissues are constructed. The standard MRI is used on brain structures to show activation during different kinds of neural activity (for example, holding information in short-term memory).

Aging of the brain occurs at different rates for different individuals. Declines in the brain's functioning with normal aging are likely to occur faster and be greater for individuals with lengthy histories of bad health practices, such as smoking and excessive drinking of alcoholic beverages. Declines are also likely to occur more slowly and to be less extensive for those individuals who have been lifelong regular exercisers.

Our focus has been on the adverse effects of aging on the brain. However, positive changes may also take place in the brain during late adulthood. Transmission across synapses may be enhanced by the increased branching of dendrites found in many old brains. The brain does show considerable plasticity or resiliency in recovering from atrophied areas of the brain. Such plasticity may be related to various factors, such as good health practices and living a mentally active and stimulating life. Much remains to be discovered about how lifestyles affect the brain's structures and functions.

Neurogenesis is the creation of new brain cells. This can be accomplished by stem cells (primitive unspecialized cells) that morph into mature brain cells. This was demonstrated on the hippocampus by researchers at the Salk Institute in California. *See also* Nutrition and Diet; Plasticity Theory.

Breast Cancer

The American Cancer Society reports that more than two hundred thousand women are diagnosed with breast cancer annually, and more than forty thousand breast cancer patients will die. In general, the risk of breast cancer is higher for older women than for younger women (the incidence of breast cancer increases steadily after age fifty), for women who have never had children, for women who had menopause at either an early age or a late age, for women with a higher educational and socioeconomic level, and for women who have consumed excessive amounts of alcohol. Breast cancer also occurs more often in women who have a family history of the disease and in women who have already had the disease.

The first gene linked to breast cancer, BRCAT, was identified in 1994. It causes about half of familial breast cancers. When this gene is defective, the woman involved is susceptible to both breast and ovarian cancers.

It is estimated that the death rate from breast cancer for women age fifty and older could be reduced by at least 30 percent if all women, starting at age forty, received an annual film mammography (or digital mammography for women under age fifty) and clinical examination to determine whether lumps are present in the breast. Medicare will pay 80 percent of the approved amount for one mammogram every year for female Part B beneficiaries. There are encouraging signs, however. The percentage of women aged forty and older who had a mammogram in the previous two years increased from 29 percent in 1987 to 70 percent in 2000. In addition, all women should perform breast self-examinations each month to detect any suspicious lump.

Once breast cancer is diagnosed, several alternative treatments are available. They all involve surgery in some form, usually followed by either chemotherapy, radiation therapy, or medication (drug) therapy. Surgery may consist of a radical mastectomy in which the affected breast is removed along with all of the underarm lymph nodes and the chest muscles; a modified mastectomy in which the affected breast and lymph nodes are removed, but not the chest muscles; or a lumpectomy in which only the tumor is removed from the affected breast. At one time it was believed that a lumpectomy could result in more secondary cancers (that is, forms other than breast cancer) than a mastectomy. However, the greater risk may not be true, especially when a lumpectomy is combined with radiation therapy.

There have been several recent advances in radiation therapy. It is now possible to target beams that kill cancer tumors at the site of the tumor rather than the entire breast. This procedure reduces the treatment to five days instead of six weeks. Canadian researchers are developing a procedure for implanting radiation seeds inside the breast to kill stray cancer cells. In addition, in 2006 the Food and Drug Administration approved a new machine (Xoft Inc.'s Axxent Electronic Brachytherapy System) that delivers radiation through a miniature X-ray system.

The drug tamoxifen (trade name Nolvadex), an antiestrogen medication, has been found to be effective for many postsurgery women in avoiding recurrences of the cancer. There is unlikely to be a benefit from the drug beyond five years of use, and its continued use could lead to other forms of cancer. Moreover, researchers at Duke University Medical Center reported in 1999 that extended use of tamoxifen could lead to a reversal of its effect such that it may help the breast cancer to grow. Tamoxifen has also been found to reduce the incidence of breast cancer by 45 percent for women who are at risk of developing breast cancer.

It is recommended that a switch from tamoxifen to the drug arimidex be made after several years of tamoxifen. Arimidex may provide more cancer protection than staying with tamoxifen. Both tamoxifen and arimidex work by reducing a patient's level of estrogen. Estrogen, if left untreated, serves as a kind of fuel for breast cancer to grow. Tamoxifen works by blocking estrogen receptors in cells. Arimidex works by cutting down on the production of estrogen. Other estrogen-blocking drugs for the treatment of early-stage breast cancer are aromasin, femara, herceptin, and raloxifen (*see also* Osteoporosis), a drug likely to be approved by the FDA in 2006.

Herceptin has been found to be effective for preventing recurrences of the cancer for both early and late stages of breast cancer, especially for women who have the HER2 protein on the surface of their cancer cells (found in about one-fourth of breast cancers). Some experts believe it should be used in the early stages of all forms of breast cancer. However, other experts believe physicians should wait to prescribe it until additional evidence of its effectiveness is available. The drug was once believed to be a potential risk for heart damage. However, recent evidence has suggested that this may not be true.

In its advanced stages breast cancer often metastasizes to other organs of the body, resulting in probable death if not detected early enough for chemotherapy or radiation therapy. Researchers at Washington University in St. Louis have developed a clinical test for the early detection of metastatic involvement by the presence of mammaglobin, a protein secreted by breast tumor cells, in the blood serum of patients with the involvement.

A diet rich in protein from poultry and dairy foods (but not red meat) may reduce the risk of dying from breast cancer, according to the results of a study of 120,000 nurses. Cabbage, if eaten several times a week, has also been found to reduce the risk of breast cancer. Women who like their meat (hamburger, steak, bacon) cooked very well may be increasing their risk of breast cancer. In a study of nearly 1,000 women who ate all three meats cooked very well done it was found that their risk of breast cancer was more than four times that of women who ate the same meats cooked medium.

The importance of vitamin D in preventing breast cancer is apparent from evidence indicating that women who live in sunny areas and have a diet that includes foods and fluids containing vitamin D are less likely to develop breast cancer than women who live in less sunny northern areas and have a diet with less vitamin D content. Low levels of vitamin B12 also increase the risk of breast cancer for postmenstrual women. Exercise is an important means of reducing the risk of breast cancer. An hour or two a day of moderate to vigorous exercise may reduce the risk by 20 percent. Even exercise for two to four hours a week may reduce the risk by 10 percent.

There is an especially dangerous form of breast cancer called *inflammatory breast cancer*. There is no apparent tumor, just a rash and an altered appearance of the breast. It tends to come on suddenly and may not be detected by a mammogram. Chemotherapy is the usual treatment, followed by surgery if needed.

For more information about breast cancer, contact the National Institutes of Health, 9000 Rockville Pike, Bethesda, MD 20892, or call its toll free number, 800-4-CANCER.

Bruises

Elderly adults are especially susceptible to dark bruises. Aging skin thins, and blood vessels below the skin lose supporting tissue (*see* Body Build and Body Characteristics). As a result, even slight trauma may cause broken blood vessels. Elderly adults should avoid bumping their bodies as much as possible and avoid rubbing hard to dry after bathing. In addition, easy bruising could mean that an older adult's blood-clotting mechanism is not functioning as it should. A blood-clotting test by his or her physician would be in order. Many bruises appearing without a sign of injury could also indicate something is wrong with the body's blood-clotting system.

C

Cancer (General Information)

It is estimated that half of all cancers occur in people who are older than age sixty-five. Some kinds of cancer occur in both men and women; they include lung cancer, bladder cancer, colon cancer, stomach cancer, pancreatic cancer, skin cancer, and oral cancer. Breast cancer occurs primarily in women. The kinds of cancer that occur only in women are cervical cancer, ovarian cancer, and uterine cancer. Prostate cancer and testicular cancer, of course, occur only in men.

Gene profiling for breast cancer has served to identify which women with an early stage of the cancer may avoid unnecessary chemotherapy. A similar gene profiling is being developed to identify which patients with an early stage of lung cancer may also avoid unnecessary chemotherapy.

Being diagnosed as having cancer of any kind is undoubtedly a stressful event. Unknown, however, is the role, if any, that stress may have had in leading to cancer. Some studies have found that people with cancer report major stressful events in their lives before they were diagnosed as having cancer. However, other studies have found no relationship between prior stress and eventual cancer.

Of interest in gerontology is the possibility of age differences in making decisions about treatment once a diagnosis of cancer has been made. For example, are older people more or less likely than younger people to seek a second medical opinion about their diagnosis? Is there an age difference in the amount of information gathered about different treatments before a decision is made as to which treatment to have?

The results of a survey conducted by researchers at Pennsylvania State University suggest that there are indeed important age differences in the decision-making process. The participants were women ranging in age from eighteen to eighty-eight, each of whom had recent breast cancer. Younger women were more likely to seek a second medical opinion than were older women; the average age of the women who sought a second opinion was forty-eight, whereas the average age of the women who did not seek a second opinion was fifty-eight. Younger women were also found to take longer to decide on the treatment they wanted than were the older women: the average age of the women who took weeks before deciding was forty-six years, whereas the average age of the women who made their treatment decision within a day of the diagnosis was fifty-six years. On the other hand, age was found to be unrelated to the choice of treatment that was selected.

For more information about cancer, call the American Cancer Society at 800-ACS-2345 (the Web site is http://www.cancer.org). Also, you may write to Cancer Information Service (CIS), National Cancer Institute, Building 31, Room 10A16, Bethesda, MD 20892, or call 800-4-CANCER. *See also* Alcohol (Physical and Mental Effects); Why Aging? (Biological Theories of Aging).

Canes and Crutches

Osteoarthritis and other diseases (*see* Arthritis) may affect the legs of many seniors to the point that locomotion is very difficult. Problems with locomotion, in turn, may hamper the ability to perform many of the activities of daily living (*see* Activities of Daily Living). In some cases the use of a cane or crutches may provide sufficient help for locomotion to make performance of those activities possible. This could mean less reliance on formal or informal (family members) home care.

Carbon Monoxide Poisoning

Nearly five thousand people are treated annually in hospital emergency rooms for carbon monoxide poisoning. The fact that carbon monoxide is odorless makes it especially dangerous. The poisoning usually results from poorly or improperly vented organic fuel heaters. Homes should be equipped with carbon monoxide detectors that set off an alarm when the gas is present. The lower economic status of many elderly people makes them especially vulnerable to poorly functioning heaters and to the absence of detectors. For more information, write for a copy of *Carbon Monoxide—the Silent, Cold Weather Killer* from the American Industrial Hygiene Association, AIHA Publications, 2700 Prosperity Avenue, Suite 250, Fairfax, VA 22031 (enclose a self-addressed, stamped envelope), or visit its Web site at http://www.aiha.org.

Cardiovascular Disease and Mental Performance

The effects of aging itself on mental functioning and mental performances are complicated by the frequent presence of diseases in elderly people. Lowered mental functioning in many elderly people may be the consequence of disease rather than the product of normal aging. The clearest evidence of the negative effects of disease comes from studies of elderly people with cardiovascular diseases, particularly hypertension.

In the early 1970s a large group of people in the sixty-to-sixty-nine-year age range had thorough physical examinations. On the basis of these examinations, the individuals were classified into three groups: normotensive (normal blood pressure), mildly elevated (blood pressure slightly above the normal range), and hypertensive (blood pressure significantly above the normal range). These individuals were all administered the Wechsler Adult Intelligence Scale at the beginning of the study and again after ten years. There was no significant change in scores on those components of the test measuring crystallized intelligence (for instance, vocabulary and general information; see Intelligence; Wechsler Intelligence Tests) for any of the three groups. The normotensive group also showed no change in scores on the components of the test measuring fluid intelligence.

By contrast, the hypertensive group, on average, showed a significant decline in fluid intelligence test scores. Interestingly, the group with mildly elevated blood pressure showed significant improvement in fluid intelligence test scores, suggesting to some researchers that mild increases in blood pressure may enhance intellectual functioning. Why is there a decline in fluid intelligence with more severe elevations of blood pressure? Researchers have speculated that persistent high levels of blood pressure may add to the decline in functioning of some areas of the brain brought about by normal aging, especially the hippocampus (see Brain and Aging).

A more recent longitudinal study has followed groups of normotensive and hypertensive individuals who were in their forties when the study began. Neither crystallized nor fluid intelligence test scores showed a significant decline during a ten-year period for either group unless the hypertensive individuals had other medical complications (for example, myocardial infarction; see Cardiovascular Diseases).

The adverse effects of hypertension on intellectual functioning are seemingly not manifested until the affected individuals are in their sixties. In agreement with this conclusion, researchers at the National Institute on Aging found that older chronic (existing at least ten years) hypertensive men had subtle changes taking place in their cerebral glucose metabolism and even greater fluctuations in subcortical nuclei. These changes imply that cognitive declines are likely to be beginning.

Cardiovascular Diseases

About sixty-one million Americans have some form of heart or cardiovascular disease. Almost six million hospitalizations a year are due to heart or cardiovascular disease of some kind. Although heart and cardiovascular diseases are found in younger adults, they are more prevalent in elderly adults, and more frequently in elderly men than in elderly women. The most common heart disease in late adulthood results from the muscles of the heart receiving insufficient oxygen because of obstructions in the coronary arteries. It is called *ischemic heart disease* (the word *ischemic* means deprived of blood), or coronary heart disease, and is found in about 20 percent of men and about 12 percent of women age sixty-five or older. The disease can lead to a *myocardial infarction* (heart attack; an infarction is a blockage of a blood vessel, resulting in a loss of supply of blood to the part of the body served by that vessel). The symptoms of a heart attack are variable among elderly people. Chest pain is generally less common than when a heart attack occurs in younger people.

The American Heart Association reported that about 75 percent of deaths from sudden cardiac arrest occur at home. Someone else at home may have to apply emergency cardiac pulmonary resuscitation (CPR). The association's guidelines recommend that CPR consist of thirty chest compressions to two breath applications. Compression tends to increase blood flow within minutes after the heart stops functioning.

In very old people the infarction is likely to be a "silent" heart attack in the sense of the absence of pain and discomfort. Unfortunately, many people age sixty-five and older may not receive care (such as clot-dissolving drugs) as fast as do younger people after a heart attack. As a result, older people who have a heart attack are twice as likely to die after a year than the younger victims who did receive fast treatment. The usual drug for preventing clotting is Lovenox. It could, however, cause severe bleeding. A new drug that is presently being tested, Arixtra, seems to be as effective as Lovenox in preventing clotting, but it also has a much lower risk of causing severe bleeding.

There are important steps to take to reduce the risk of a heart attack. A study of middle-aged nurses revealed that those who exercised regularly, controlled their weight, and had only an occasional alcoholic drink reduced their chance of a heart attack by 82 percent. However, the difficulty of such self-control is apparent from the fact that only 1 percent of the nurses followed all of these rules. In addition, there is a new procedure with magnetic resonance imaging (*see* Brain and Aging) that may offer a means of detecting potential heart attacks. The procedure analyzes blood vessels supplying the heart to measure the thickness of clots in the arteries and to determine the nature of plaques in arteries.

Dysrhythmias or *fibrillation* (irregular heartbeats in which the heart's muscle contractions are random rather than rhythmic) are common in older people. Either the atrial or the ventricular chambers of the heart may be involved. The irregularities can be serious and may cause sudden death. There are medications that control fibrillations, provided they are detected and treated promptly. Atrial fibrillation may be corrected by surgical removal of a pulmonary vein, and venticular fibrillation by application of machines called defibrillators (*see* Defibrillators).

If the reduction of blood flow to the heart and the amount of oxygen reaching the heart are great enough, chest pains known as *angina* may occur. The pain of angina has been described by some sufferers as a burn-ing sensation and by others as a pressure or tightness that may spread from behind the breastbone to the back and arms. Angina most often occurs after physical exertion or after an intense emotional experience, and it is usually relieved within ten minutes. Patients with angina, regardless of age, are commonly treated by such medicines as nitroglycerin and beta-blockers (drugs that counter the effects of adrenaline [epinephrine] on the heart).

Congestive heart failure occurs when the heart is unable to sustain the needs of organs and muscles. A failing heart keeps working, but it does it less effectively. Consequently, blood backs up in the veins and lungs. The result could be the accumulation of fluids in the legs, abdomen, and lungs that can be life-threatening. Congestive heart failure is present in more than three million people, and it contributes to about three hundred thou-sand deaths per year, largely of elderly people. It is the most common cause of hospitalization for people over age sixty-five. Symptoms include swelling of the feet, ankles, and legs; weight gain; persistent coughing; fatigue; breathlessness; and difficulty in breathing while asleep.

Unfortunately, some elderly people believe that these symptoms are sim-ply part of growing old and are not an indication of a serious health prob-lem. Medications may control these symptoms once they are diagnosed and prolong the lives of individuals with congestive heart failure. Diuretics that draw excess fluid from the body may be used to reduce tissue swelling, and digoxin (a form of digitalis) may be used to strengthen the heartbeat in people with moderate to severe heart failure. A new pacemaker device called a venticular resynchronizer synchronizes the right and left ventricles of the heart so that they pump at the same time, making pumping more forceful. Other forms of treatment include rest, a proper diet, and drugs such as ACE and beta-blockers.

The heart's difficulty in providing the blood supply needed by organs and muscles may be caused by one or more of the heart's four heart valves being diseased. *Heart-valve disease* means that a valve is not functioning properly. There may be difficulty in opening a valve (or valves) all the way (a condition called stenosis) or in closing a valve all the way. Consequently, blood does not move through the heart chambers as well as it should be moving.

During open heart surgery, one or more valves may be repaired or replaced. Repair consists of sewing a ring around the valve to tighten it. If the damage to a valve is too great for repairing it, replacement of the valve is required. One kind of valve is a mechanical one. If this kind of valve is used, the patient will need lifelong therapy with an anticoagulant (blood thinner) to prevent blood clots around the valve. An alternative is a biological valve taken from a pig, cow, or human donor. This type of valve needs replacement more often than a mechanical valve. The heart receiv-ing surgery must not beat during the surgery. A heart-lung machine is used to keep the patient's blood flowing. Drugs such as Aprotinin are needed to reduce bleeding during the surgery.

When the heart is extensively diseased, a heart transplant may be needed. The patient's heart is removed and replaced by a healthy heart that is attached to the blood vessels serving the heart.

Disorders of the circulatory system beyond the heart include *atherosclerosis* and *hypertension*. Atherosclerosis is one form of a general class of cardiovascular disorders known as *arteriosclerosis* (the hardening of the arteries or their loss of elasticity) that is more common in late adulthood than in early adulthood. Atherosclerosis is characterized by the presence of pronounced fat deposits along the inner wall of arteries and the thickening of the inner walls and the resulting interference that occurs in the flow of blood through the arteries. The walls may eventually bulge (an *aneurysm*) and rupture. The risk of blood clots is increased for women who are on estrogen replacement therapy.

Many older people have abdominal aortic aneurysms (an estimated 1.5 million older Americans). Unfortunately, only about 200,000 of them are aware of their presence. If the aneurysm is smaller than four to five centimeters, surgery is usually not performed. An ultrasonography test is made every six months to determine if the aneurysm's size requires repair.

An aneurysm large enough to risk bursting (larger than five centimeters) usually requires repairing the artery before it does burst, which probably results in death. Surgery is the traditional procedure. A large incision is made in the chest or abdomen, and blood flow is temporarily directed around the aneurysm. The aneurysm is surgically removed and replaced by a graft. An alternative procedure, endovascular aortic repair, may be used instead, especially for older and sicker people. A stent graft is directed by a catheter inserted in an artery to the inside of the aneurysm where it patches the damaged part of the aorta. Some people have experienced problems with this procedure, and not all aneurysms can be repaired by it.

Another potentially life-threatening aneurysm is a brain (or cerebral) aneurysm. It is an abnormal bulging of an artery in the brain. It may occur in people of all ages, but it occurs most often in people ages thirty to sixty. About one in fifteen people in the United States is likely to have a brain aneurysm.

People with an unruptured brain aneurysm often experience no symptoms. If they do, they may include, among others, peripheral-vision deficits, decreased concentration, and loss of balance and coordination. People with a ruptured aneurysm may experience, among others, a terrible headache, neck pain, and blurred or double vision. Diagnosis of a ruptured aneurysm is usually made by computed axial tomography (CAT scan). The traditional treatment of a ruptured aneurysm involves surgically removing a segment of the skull to reach the aneurysm and then placing a tiny clip on the aneurysm to stop the blood flow. To prevent rupturing, an alternative treatment called endovascular therapy may be employed. The aneurysm is reached by a catheter that travels to the brain after being inserted in a femoral artery. Tiny platinum cells reach the aneurysm to prevent rupturing.

Atherosclerosis of the coronary arteries, that is, the arteries that nourish the heart muscle itself, may be so severe that a coronary bypass is needed in which an artery from another part of the body (usually the leg) is transplanted to replace the affected (clogged) coronary artery. Daily higher doses of vitamin E after bypass surgery may result in less narrowing of the heart arteries and a lower risk of heart disease. Alternatively, a procedure known as *angioplasty* may be performed. It involves the inflation of a small balloon inserted in the affected artery to open it and increase blood flow through it. In some cases, application of a Rotor Rooter–like device may be required. In other cases, a stent (a small piece of metal) may be placed in the artery to support the inflation achieved by angioplasty.

Tests such as an electrocardiogram and stress test (running on a treadmill) yield too many false positives and false negatives to reliably detect blockage in the heart's arteries. Recent advances with computed axial tomography (*see* Brain and Aging) have made it much easier to identify the extent to which the arteries that nourish the heart are blocked and need very early treatment. Advances are also being made with magnetic resonance imaging (*see* Brain and Aging), with a nuclear stress test (which includes taking pictures of the heart's arteries by a radioactive tracer), and with a cardiac cath test (injecting a dye into the heart muscle).

A risk with angioplasty is the possibility of clotting within the first twenty-four hours after the procedure. To avoid such clotting the patient is usually given anticlotting drugs during the procedure. In a number of angioplasties the opened vessel closes again within six months, requiring another angioplasty. However, the chance of needing a second angioplasty is greatly reduced if the patient is treated with an appropriate drug.

The accumulation of some fat deposits in the arteries seems to be part of normal aging. The presence of excessive amounts may lead to atherosclerosis. A heart attack is linked to such factors as smoking and elevated serum cholesterol levels that could be controlled by appropriate health habits (for instance, not smoking, eating a modified diet, and getting regular exercise). The presence of excessive triglycerides in the blood is a risk factor for heart disease. Triglycerides are fat deposits that are found naturally in your body and in some foods. A level of 200 to 500 found in a test of your blood is considered high and a reason for concern. A high level may be the result of obesity, a sedentary lifestyle, inadequate diet, uncontrolled diabetes, a problem with your thyroid gland, excessive alcohol consumption, and some medications. If there is a problem, you need to consult with your physician for steps to be taken to lower the level (*see also* Peripheral Arterial Disease and Claudication).

Veins may also cause health problems, especially for older adults. Phlebitis is one of the most common problems. It consists of inflammation and a blood clot in a vein, usually one in a leg (but occasionally in an arm) that may cause considerable pain. If the inflammation is in a vein near the surface, the disorder is probably not serious, and should go away in a few weeks. However, a deep vein phlebitis may be serious. Parts of the clot in the vein may break off (called an embolus) and travel to the lungs where they may restrict blood flow to the lungs. If the clot is large enough, it may cause a pulmonary embolism and eventually death. Deep vein phlebitis is usually treated with blood-thinning medications.

Hypertension refers to excessive arterial blood pressure (systolic pressure more than 140 mm Hg or diastolic pressure more than 90 mm Hg; *see also* Blood Pressure [High and Low]). Hypertension, or high blood pressure, is life-threatening because it implies reduced blood flow to vital organs and increased risk of heart attack, stroke, or kidney failure. Medications such as diuretics are used to treat high blood pressure by ridding the body of excess fluid and sodium. Obesity, smoking, and excessive consumption of alcohol are all likely to increase the risk of hypertension in older people. There is some evidence indicating that certain pain medications (known as non-steroidal anti-inflammatory drugs, or NSAIDS) may increase blood pressure in elderly adults if they are taken at high dosages for long periods of time.

The warning signs of a heart attack include chest pain, usually in the center of the chest, perhaps with a squeezing sensation or a burning feeling (which could be mistaken for heartburn) that may radiate to the lower jaw, neck, and either the shoulder or arm. People, especially women, do not always have the typical signs. If someone suspects a heart attack, he or she should call emergency assistance immediately.

The death rate from a heart attack alone has decreased by more than 50 percent since the 1960s. Further progress, however, is hindered by the myth that after surviving a heart attack, the risk of another heart attack disappears. The risk of another attack does persist, as does the risk of heart failure given the weakened heart muscles from the attack. More women (about 20 percent) have a second heart attack than men (about 16 percent). Drugs that dissolve blood clots can reduce heart muscle damage if they are administered quickly after the onset of symptoms of a heart attack. Low doses of aspirin daily are commonly recommended by physicians for those who had a heart attack (at least for men; *see* Aspirin). Evidence is available to show that red grape juice and aspirin (at least for men) help to prevent heart attacks by slowing down blood clotting.

On the other hand, women who were on estrogen replacement therapy (hormone replacement therapy) that combines estrogen and progestin (*see* Estrogen Replacement Therapy [Hormone Replacement Therapy]) were found in the Women's Health Initiative Study (*see* Women's Health Initiative) to have 29 percent more heart attacks than women who were not on the therapy. In another study it was found that estrogen-only therapy had no effect on the likelihood of a heart attack.

Researchers at the University of Alabama at Birmingham Medical School found that one-third of four hundred thousand heart attack sufferers went to the hospital without chest pain. These painless patients were more than twice as likely to die as those with chest pain because physicians failed to make a fast diagnosis.

For more information about cardiovascular diseases, visit the American Heart Association's Web site, http://www.americanheart.org. *See also* Hypertension; Hypertension and Mental Functioning; Stroke.

Cardiovascular Diseases (Psychological Interventions)

Exhibiting frequent anger has been linked to heart disease. Research has revealed that group therapy for patients with heart attacks reduced by 44 percent second heart attacks over a four and a half year period compared to patients receiving only medical treatment. The therapy consisted of modifying Type A behaviors (*see* Retirement [Involuntary]) as well as counseling about risk factors for heart attacks.

Caregivers (Early Adulthood)

In some cases caregivers are under the age of twenty-one. They provide primary caregiving assistance (for example, bathing, dressing, feeding) for a parent or parents with problems ranging from dementia to drug abuse. In one study of early adult caregivers it was found that when interviewed between the ages of twenty-three and fifty-eight they reported more positive mental health signs than negative mental health signs, and they rarely showed evidence of depression.

Caregivers (Elderly Parents)

Elderly parents who function well themselves often serve as caregivers for adult children with disabilities of various kinds. Researchers at the University of Wisconsin at Madison surveyed several hundred mothers (average age sixty-five) of such adult children (average age thirty-three).

Elderly mothers of adult children with mental illness (such as schizophrenia) reported higher levels of frustration and lower levels of gratification from caregiving than did elderly mothers of mentally retarded adult children. More emotion-focused coping with stress strategy was used by mothers of adult children with mental illness than by mothers of adult children with mental retardation (*see* Stress and Coping with Stress). The use of a problem-focused coping strategy was found to yield a positive sense of well-being for mothers of adult children with mental retardation but not for mothers of adult children with mental illness.

There are several reasons for these differences. Social interactions are usually fewer and families are less cohesive when mental illness is the reason for caring for an adult child than when mental retardation is the reason. Leaving home during the day to work or to attend a day-care center is more likely for adults with retardation than for adults with mental illness.

Caregivers (Family and Friends)

According to a survey by the National Alliance for Caregiving, there are more than twenty-two million households in the United States that report caregiving, and there are about twenty-five million caregivers. Both functionally disabled and mentally impaired individuals are the recipients of caregiving. The average age of the recipients is seventy-seven years, and the average duration of caregiving is four and a half years. The help provided by caregivers enables their patients to remain noninstitutionalized.

In a national survey of caregivers, 75 percent were women, 65 percent provided services for one parent, 26 percent for two parents, and 9 percent for three parents (their own plus a partner's parent). The average age of the caregivers was fifty. Most important, 56 percent of the caregivers reported helping an elderly parent more than twelve hours a week by providing such services as cooking meals and regulating the administration of medicines.

Adult children serving as caregivers are usually the same sex as the disabled person. Because those needing care are more likely to be mothers than fathers, the number of daughters serving as caregivers greatly exceeds the number of sons. The estimate is that daughters make up nearly 40 percent of caregivers. The stress experienced by caregivers is less, in general, the closer they are in age to the affected individual. This accounts in part for the general success of friends as caregivers—they are closer in age to the recipient of care.

Researchers at the University of California at Berkeley found that the positive effects of outside employment for caregivers (for instance, a sense of achievement) outweighed the negative effects (such as increased fatigue). Although the recipients receive fewer hours of care, they also are likely to receive significantly more hours of help from other sources.

Caregiving understandably places a considerable burden on the caregiver. The consequences of this burden, and the discovery of ways to reduce the consequences, have been widely studied in recent years by gerontologists. The incidence of depression among caregivers is high (perhaps as high as 50 percent of the caregivers), although the extent of the depression has been found to be no greater for those caring for greatly impaired individuals than for those caring for less impaired individuals.

Researchers at Ohio State University found that caregivers of persons with Alzheimer's disease continue to show significant depression for at least two years after the death of the person receiving the caregiving. In general, female caregivers appear to be more depressed than male caregivers, and wives as caregivers appear to perceive themselves as being more burdened than do husbands as caregivers. Spouses serving as caregivers who score high on the trait of neuroticism (*see* Personality Traits) and low in mastery of situations (that is, low in internal locus of control; *see* Control over Life's Events) tend to experience more strain and depression than spouses scoring low in neuroticism and high in mastery.

Caregivers, in general, who score high on optimism rate themselves as feeling less stress and less depression than those with lower scores on optimism. Interestingly, training caregivers of patients with Alzheimer's disease to decrease the depressive symptoms of those patients (for example, by emphasizing pleasant events) has been found to reduce the depressive symptoms of the caregivers as well.

Spouses who are caregivers of patients with Alzheimer's disease have been found to have significantly worse mental health, but better physical health, than spouses of patients with Parkinson's disease. Closeness of a caregiver to a patient with either a functional disability or a cognitive impairment appears to be unrelated to depression experienced by the caregiver. Differences in depression between white and African American spouses as caregivers tend to be slight. Some studies have reported no difference, while others have reported less depression for African American caregivers.

When daughters serve as caregivers, the subjective burden tends to be less if there is a stronger attachment to their mothers. In general, daughters experience the fewest negative effects of caregiving for their mothers when the mothers live separately. For two-generation households (mother and caregiving daughter, no grandchildren), daughters provide more care and experience fewer negative emotional effects than in three-generation households (grandchildren present in the home).

Daughters who exhibit mastery of caregiving through the use of a problem-focused coping strategy exhibit less depression than daughters who use an emotion-focused coping strategy, which results in greater depression. Daughters whose husbands provide little support for the impaired parent generally experience more stress and poorer health and less satisfaction with their marriages than daughters whose husbands provide greater support.

On the other hand, sharing caregiving responsibility with a sibling results in less stress and less depression than going it alone. For daughters, the duration of caregiving usually has little effect on their satisfaction in caregiving unless there is an increase in the amount of care needed. Daughters who also have roles as mother, wife, and employee generally experience increased stress as a caregiver if stress increases for any one of their three roles. Many offices and services are open only in the daytime and only on weekdays, thus forcing caregivers to take time off from their jobs if they need to conduct business with these agencies.

Adult sons usually become caregivers for their mothers only if a sister is unavailable. When a sister is unavailable to serve as a caregiver, a son is likely to rely on his wife for major assistance, and he provides relatively little care himself. Researchers at the University of Michigan found no difference in care received by parents-in-law compared to parents when either daughters-in-law or sons-in-law served as caregivers.

The frustration experienced by caregivers by the disruption of their own life plans is apparently greatest at the onset of the symptoms of the person receiving the care, and often decreases over time as the caregivers develop routines for providing care, even though the need for care increases during that period. It is not unusual to discover that caregivers have emotional symptoms other than depression, such as anxiety, guilt, and psychosomatic disorders.

Support groups have become a major means of trying to reduce the stress experienced by caregivers and to help them to develop the skills needed to cope with their duties. A support group consists of several caregivers who are led in their meetings by either a professional gerontologist or by one of their peers. The group usually meets for six to eight weekly sessions, with each session lasting about two hours. The members of the group are usually trained to use one another as a support system or network. Members of the group are encouraged to share their feelings and caregiving experiences with other members of the group and to maintain contact with other group members after the meetings have been completed.

If the support group consists of caregivers for persons with Alzheimer's disease, then the group meetings are likely to provide information about the nature of the disease and its stages. The group members may also be trained to give their recipients exercises in memory and problem solving to help slow down the decline in their abilities as much as possible. However, after analyzing the results of many studies on interventions designed to reduce stress for caregivers, researchers at the University of Southern California concluded that group interventions are less effective than individual interventions in which a caregiver is given professional counseling and other forms of psychological assistance.

Because of the stress and distress often experienced by caregivers, they should explore the services and facilities available in their communities to help them with their caregiving responsibilities. Finding and joining a support group is one possibility. Both the caregiver and the person receiving the care are likely to benefit. An alternative is to seek individual counseling and training in problem solving. Another possibility is the use of respite care services available in their community (*see* Respite Care). Again, both the caregiver and the recipient are likely to benefit. Researchers at John Carroll University found that long-term male caregivers were much more likely to use respite care than short-term caregivers. Those who used respite care used the free time effectively for their own otherwise limited enjoyment (for example, golfing or walking). Engaging in social interactions for fun and recreation has also been found to reduce the burden of caregiving experienced by many family caregivers.

A promising way of coping with the anger that may often follow the frustration of caregiving has been introduced by Dr. Dolores Gallagher-Thompson and her associates at the Veterans Administration Medical Center in Palo Alto, California. They have developed an intervention program that teaches wives or daughters who are caregivers the skills needed to manage their frustrations without producing intense anger. The skills include learning to relax during periods of extreme stress and learning to be appropriately assertive with the recipients of their caregiving.

A promising psychoeducational intervention has been devised by researchers in Minnesota. The intervention consists of seven weekly two-hour sessions attended by primary caregivers and their families. The sessions stress education, family support, and skill training. Preliminary results have indicated that caregivers reduce their negative reactions to disruptive behaviors by the patient, and they perceive themselves as having less burden in their caregiving role.

Family members and friends of someone likely to need caregiving in the near future are likely to be concerned about their new role in life and how they should handle it. Help for them may be on the way. Several resources in Michigan have established a "caregiver college" that offers a program designed for family caregivers. Seven sessions are given in each term in which professionals cover such topics as safety, nutrition, incontinence, and caregiver stress. Similar programs are likely to spread to other states.

Unfortunately, many family caregivers ultimately have to decide that the caregiving recipient must be placed in a nursing home. In a major study, caregivers of elderly patients with dementia were followed for two years. No patient characteristic, severity of the dementia, or characteristic of the caregiver predicted time of placement in the nursing home. However, families scoring high on negative family feelings, high on emotional closeness, and low on family efficiency placed their patients in a nursing home significantly earlier than other families. Apparently, negative family feelings are only increased by caregiving, and emotional closeness may be viewed by the caregiver as being disrupted and eventually destroyed by caregiving. Families that are efficient and good planners experience less stress and therefore have a lower burden from caregiving.

There is a very helpful manual on caregiving that is edited by Dr. Chandra Mehrotra of the College of St. Scholastica in Duluth, Minnesota, and may be obtained by writing to him. The manual covers such topics as managing stress, communicating with the patient, and where to get help. *See also* Stress and Coping with Stress.

Caregivers (Hassles in Administering Medications)

Caregivers commonly have the responsibility of administering medications to those in their care. In so doing they frequently encounter hassles in trying to complete the chore. Interviews with twenty-three family caregivers of patients over age sixty-five who took medications daily and depended on their caregivers to manage their medication regimen discovered that hassles fall into three categories: scheduling problems (29.5 percent), administration problems (31.9 percent), and safety issues (38.6 percent). Scheduling problems included giving medications on time and keeping prescriptions filled.

Caregivers (How African American and White Caregivers Differ)

In general, African American caregivers of family members with Alzheimer's disease have been found to experience more benefits from their caregiving than do white caregivers. One of the reasons for the racial difference appears to be the greater religiosity of African American caregivers in general. Apparently, religious interventions to help caregivers may increase benefits received by many African American caregivers but are unlikely to affect many white caregivers. In addition, African American caregivers tend to be less upset by a patient's difficult behavior than are white caregivers.

Caregivers (Long-Distance)

It is estimated that more than 25 percent of caregivers give their care by long-distance (for example, by telephone). They make arrangements with a geriatric-care manager for home-care services delivered by a home-health-care worker. For those considering providing long-distance care they should contact the care recipient's home state agency on aging and inquire about reliable home-care services. If possible, they should meet the home-health-care worker before committing to his or her service.

Caregivers (Negative Reactions of Recipients of Care)

Individuals with physical impairments (for example, from a stroke or from an accident) often express negative reactions toward the caregiving they receive from a spouse or significant other. Researchers at Portland State University found that about two-thirds of recipients reported negative reactions related to too little care or poor quality care. More than half of them expressed the view that they were overly dependent on the caregiver, and more than 25 percent believed they could never return the favor. Negative reactions may lead to depression and a feeling of incompetence for the recipients.

However, the researchers also found that negative caregiving behaviors, such as resentfulness, discourteousness, and criticism, are fairly rare (about 10 percent of the caregivers in the study). The problem of negative reactions on the part of the recipients of care would seem to be in what may be their distorted perceptions of the care they are receiving. Caregivers should seek help from professional mental health experts in resolving this problem.

Caregivers (Paid Workers)

Adult children, especially daughters, have traditionally been the main source of caregivers for disabled elderly people. However, as the number of women entering the labor force has increased, the availability of daughters for caregiving has decreased. The demand for paid caregivers has consequently increased. The majority of paid caregivers have been middle-aged minority women without a high school education. As the educational level of future generations of these women increases, the number who accept low-paying jobs like caregiving will decrease. Caregiving in the home usually pays much less than nursing assistants in hospitals are paid, and the benefits are also much less for those working in homes.

There have been various attempts to fill the void in home-care workers. For example, attempts have been made to train welfare recipients as caregivers, but without much success. Men, in general, are not interested in caregiving, and young people are considered to be too immature to serve as caregivers. Given the likely future increase in the number of physically and mentally disabled older people and the emphasis on home care in preference to institutionalization, more innovative ways are needed to make home caregiving a more attractive occupation.

Some possibilities have been explored in demonstration projects sponsored by the Ford Foundation in several cities. Overall, these projects were successful in reducing the turnover among home caregivers and in increasing on-the-job longevity. Some components of the projects were relatively inexpensive. For example, in one of the cities, both experienced and novice employees received training in home-care skills, and they received several status symbols (for instance, identification badges like those of nursing assistants in hospitals) to boost their morale. However, other components, such as providing health insurance benefits for the participants, did require a much larger expenditure. In the long term, continuation of such projects would require subsidies by either private or governmental agencies. They may well be worth the cost.

Caregivers (Positive Effects of Caregiving)

Perhaps the most common experience of family members who serve as caregivers is stress. However, the fact that caregiving can, and often does, have positive emotional effects should not be ignored. A survey by researchers at the University of Southern California revealed that a third of the families involved in caregiving report more positive than negative changes in their lives during the course of caregiving. The positive changes included increased closeness among the family members (for example, among siblings). Some spouses of elderly people with Alzheimer's disease even reported an improvement in their marital relationship. *See also* Grandparents Raising Their Own Grandchildren.

Caregivers (Secondary)

The primary caregiver of someone with Alzheimer's disease is usually that person's spouse. The secondary caregiver is usually an adult child of the patient. The secondary caregiver helps the primary one in a number of ways (for instance, financial support and even direct physical care of the patient). Primary and secondary caregivers often differ in their perceptions of the primary caregiver's ability to deal with the patient's dementia and about the degree of the patient's problem behaviors, but there is less difference in their perception of the primary caregiver's coping with the stress of caregiving.

Caregiving (Type of Mentally Impaired Patient)

Researchers in Germany compared the burden on caregivers of recipients who had vascular dementia (that is, multi-infarct dementia; *see* Multi-Infarct Dementia) with the burden of caregivers of recipients who had Alzheimer's disease. They found that in the early stages of dementia, caring for a patient with vascular dementia created a greater burden than caring for a patient in the early stages of Alzheimer's disease. However, there was a reversal for patients who had reached severe stages of dementia. Here caregiving relatives of patients with Alzheimer's disease experience a greater burden than caregiving relatives of patients with vascular dementia. Recipients of caregiving seem to need different kinds of support that are dependent on the type of dementia they have.

Carrots

Carrots are an excellent source of antioxidants (*see* Antioxidants). Researchers at the University of Arkansas found that they have three times more antioxidants when they are cooked and pureed than when they are eaten raw. Keeping on the outer skin adds to the amount of antioxidants they contain.

Causes of Death

The leading causes of death for people age sixty-five and older are heart disease, malignant tumors, vascular disease, pulmonary diseases, pneumonia and flu, diabetes, accidents, and Alzheimer's disease.

Cautiousness

An impression held by many people is that older adults are more cautious in their behavior than are younger adults. A number of studies have revealed, however, that the greater cautiousness of older people is apparent for some behaviors but not for others.

There are two kinds of laboratory tasks for which elderly participants have consistently been found to be more cautious than younger participants. On learning tasks, elderly participants tend to wait until they are certain a response is correct before they give it. Until then, they are likely not to respond. Their errors are primarily errors of omission (that is, not responding at all). By contrast, younger participants are more willing to risk appearing foolish, and they often guess in regard to the correct response. Thus, they make many more errors of commission (responding but incorrectly) than do elderly participants (*see also* Verbal Learning).

A similar age difference is found when participants are asked to decide whether a weak sensory event (for example, a faint tone) is present or absent on each of many trials (with the tone present on half of the trials and absent on the other half). Elderly participants approach this task more cautiously than do younger participants. If elderly participants suspect the event may be present, but they are not certain, they are likely to avoid appearing foolish by responding "absent" (*see* Recognition Memory versus Recall Memory for a task in which elderly participants are likely to be less cautious than younger participants).

Age differences in cautiousness appear to be absent when the task involves a higher level of decision making. The standard procedure is to give participants a test describing lifelike situations in which they are to advise someone on the degree of risk he or she should take (for example, leaving a secure job with low pay to take a higher-paying job with a shaky company). Participants must choose among alternatives that are more desirable in some ways but more risky in others and among alternatives that are less desirable in some ways but less risky overall. In general, studies with this kind of task indicate little age difference in the willingness to take a risk. Of course, the task is only a simulation of everyday risks. Nevertheless, it does seem risky to conclude that there is some general characteristic of cautiousness—and that elderly people possess more of it than do younger people.

Centenarians

According to the 1990 census there were then about 36,000 centenarians (people one hundred years old or older) in the United States. In 1999 the number was estimated to be 70,000. By the year 2030 the estimated number is 324,000. Centenarians represent the most rapidly growing age range in the United States.

Their heredity apparently aids their resistance to cancer and other diseases that cause the deaths of most people well before they reach one hundred years of age. Studies of centenarians reveal that at least 20 percent have minor memory problems, but they function well anyway. About half of them do live in nursing homes. A number of community-dwelling centenarians have been studied by researchers at Iowa State University and the University of Georgia. About a third of their samples reported that their lives are exciting, and the vast majority reported that they maintained a social network.

However, they did report problems performing many of the instrumental activities of daily living (see Activities of Daily Living). For example, they were less likely to go to places alone or shop alone than when they were younger. Many did report feeling that their life satisfaction is only fair. Interestingly, centenarians in the University of Georgia study who scored high on extroversion also scored higher on subjective well-being than those who scored lower on extroversion. Dr. Leonard Poon is the head of the University of Georgia study. He describes the typical centenarian as being a woman with a grade school education who lives either alone or with an offspring. She has an annual income of four thousand to seven thousand dollars. She has vision or hearing problems, but she is generally satisfied with life.

Dr. Nir Barzilai of the Albert Einstein College of Medicine has found that centenarians tend to be optimistic and relaxed and do not necessarily live a healthy lifestyle. Their children tend to have a high level of HDL cholesterol (the good kind; see Cholesterol).

Do most Americans want to live to be one hundred years old? A recent survey suggests they do not. Only 27 percent said they did want to live that long. Reasons given for not wanting to live that long included suspected declining health with aging and a suspected declining supply of money. See also How Much Longer Do Seniors Want to Live?; Longevity (What Determines a Long Life?); Surgery Survival.

Cervical Cancer

The cervix is the lower part of the uterus where it opens into the vagina. There are more than thirteen thousand new cases of cervical cancer every year and about four thousand deaths from this cancer every year. The incidence of cervical cancer is higher among African American women than among white women.

Nearly 100 percent of the deaths from the cancer could have been pre-vented if the cancer had been detected early enough. Usually, there are no noticeable signs, other than possible bleeding and pelvic pain. However, it can be detected early if women have a yearly checkup that includes a test known as a *Pap smear* (the test is named after Dr. George Papanicolaou who introduced it in the early 1950s) in which the cervix's surface is scraped and the contents of the scraping are examined microscopically.

Women age sixty-five and older should have a Pap smear test every one to three years, more likely every year. In a study by Yale University researchers of nearly five hundred women (average age of sixty-four years) with advanced cervical cancer, nearly 29 percent had never had a Pap smear test. There is available a new, and more expensive, version of the Pap smear test known as a ThinPrep Pap smear test. The new test makes it easier to inter-pret Pap smears and to identify more abnormal cells by washing out blood and mucus that could hide abnormal cells.

When a Pap smear test is no longer needed is debated by the various cancer organizations and societies. The American Cancer Society recom-mends stopping at age seventy, and the American College of Obstetricians and Gynecologists believes that stopping should be decided individually. In general, you may be able to stop at age sixty-five if you have had three consecutive years of normal tests. Women should consult with their gyne-cologist for his or her recommendation about when to terminate the test.

Treatment in the early stage of the disease may involve medications called angiogenesis inhibitors. They are drugs that block the development of new blood vessels. The hope is that this will cut off the tumor's supply of oxygen and nutrients. The tumor may then stop growing and not spread to other organs.

There is a promise of preventing many cases of cervical cancer in the near future. Two types of the human papillomavirus cause 70 percent of all cervical cancers. There is a new vaccine called Gardasil that has been found in clinical trials to prevent infection from the two types of virus 100 percent of the time. The vaccine was approved by the Food and Drug Administra-tion in June 2006. The search is on for finding similar vaccines to prevent other forms of cancer.

Children View Aging Negatively

Try to remember what you thought about older adults when you were eleven years old. Were most older adults good, bad, or something in between? Your grandparents and older characters in the movies you saw (for instance, Gabby Hayes in cowboy movies) were probably the only older adults you knew enough about to form an opinion.

What about today's children? Their exposure to older adults has been increased considerably by watching television. They may be influenced negatively by the evil grandmother on *Malcolm in the Middle* or by the constantly bickering grandparents in *Everybody Loves Raymond.*

Not surprisingly, evidence gathered by researchers at the University of Texas Health Science Center at San Antonio indicates that most eleven- to thirteen-year-old children do have a negative view of seniors.

Nearly two thousand middle-school children completed such sentences as "Old is . . ." Most completions were negative in their tone, such as "when you can't remember anything." Many children by this age have already acquired a negative stereotype of aging and older people. The stereotype needs to be altered through education and by providing more positive models of seniors and fewer negative models in movies and television programs.

Chocolate

In a study of nearly eight thousand Harvard graduates, those that ate chocolate moderately were found to live almost a year longer than those who abstain. Researchers in the Netherlands found that older adults who eat the equivalent of one-third of a chocolate bar every day had lower blood pressure and a lower risk of death than other seniors who ate little chocolate. Especially beneficial is dark chocolate. But what about chocoholics? Note the word *moderately.*

Perhaps the reason for the apparent positive effect was discovered by researchers in the Netherlands. They found that the cocoa contained in dark chocolate contains four times the concentration of an antioxidant (catechins) contained in black tea, another substance known to have a positive effect on health. Cocoa beans also contain a substance that improves the functioning of blood vessels. The amount of cocoa in dark chocolate is much greater than that found in milk chocolate.

Cholesterol

The high risk of cardiovascular problems in late adulthood makes it especially important for older people to control the amount of cholesterol in their diets. Cholesterol is a waxy, fatlike substance that is found in all animal tissues and is needed in small amounts for many of the body's chemical processes.

The two most important forms of cholesterol are *low-density lipoprotein cholesterol (LDL)* and *high-density lipoprotein cholesterol (HDL)*. LDL is the "bad" cholesterol that increases the risk of heart disease, whereas HDL is the "good" cholesterol that may help to prevent heart disease. LDL collects on the walls of arteries, leaving less space for blood to flow through them. The consequence may be atherosclerosis and an eventual heart attack (*see* Cardiovascular Diseases). The body produces most of the cholesterol it needs for its chemical processes. To avoid harmful levels of LDL, elderly adults (and younger adults as well) should limit their intake of high LDL foods, such as butter, whole milk, cheese, egg yolks, and fatty meats, and replace them with such foods as cholesterol-free margarine, skim milk, egg whites, and lean meats.

Seniors should have their levels of HDL and LDL tested regularly. Their physician will inform them if their level of HDL is high enough and if their level of LDL is low enough. With a history of a prior heart attack or angina, it is especially important for seniors to maintain a level of LDL of 70 mg.dL or less, and the lower the level the better it is to help prevent future cardiovascular problems.

Limiting the intake of foods high in saturated fats (for example, red meat and poultry skin) is essential for maintaining a low level of LDL cholesterol and avoiding the risk of a heart attack or stroke. By contrast, polyunsaturated fats, found in such oils as safflower and soybean and in walnuts, are recommended because they tend to lower the level of LDL in the body (but they may also lower the level of HDL). Avoid trans fats found in hard margarine, baked goods, and imitation dairy products. They tend to raise the level of LDL cholesterol. There is some evidence that eating red grapefruit regularly may also reduce the level of LDL cholesterol. A diet containing whole grains, vegetables, and fruit raises the level of HDL cholesterol, as does wine with your evening meal and fish that contains omega-3 fatty acids (as in salmon and tuna).

Aerobic exercise, such as swimming, is often effective in raising the level of HDL cholesterol. You should check with your physician. Estrogen replacement therapy (hormone replacement therapy) tends to lower the level of LDL cholesterol and raise the level of HDL cholesterol. However, the therapy has a major disadvantage in that it increases the risk of various diseases (for instance, breast cancer; *see* Breast Cancer).

There is evidence indicating that statin drugs such as Crestor and Lipitor can be effective in lowering the level of LDL cholesterol. Especially intriguing is a study in 2006 by researchers at the Cleveland Clinic. It indicated that Crestor may actually shrink blockages in clogged arteries and reduce the risk of heart disease. Participants who took 40 milligrams daily for two years had an average reduction of 53 percent in the level of their LDL (from 130.4 to 60.8). In addition, there was a modest increase in their average level of HDL (14.7 percent). However, consumer advocates believe that the medication may cause more liver and muscle problems than other statin medications. *See also* Cardiovascular Diseases; Flaxseed; Grape Juice; Nutrition and Diet.

Chronic Respiratory Diseases

Chronic respiratory diseases that are especially prevalent in late adulthood are *chronic bronchitis, emphysema,* and *acute respiratory syndrome (ARDS).* In chronic bronchitis there is a continuous inflammation of the bronchial tubes (the air passages in the lungs). The inflammation produces a bronchitis cough that is an attempt to clear excess mucus caused by irritation of the air passages. In emphysema the air sacs become weakened and break. Elasticity of the lung's tissue diminishes, causing air to be trapped in the air sacs. The result is an impairment in the exchange of oxygen and carbon dioxide. Symptoms include shortness of breath, a cough, and little capacity for exercise. Chronic bronchitis and emphysema frequently occur together to create chronic obstructive lung disease. More than 3.1 million Americans have been diagnosed with emphysema. More than 90 percent are forty-five years of age or older. The disease rarely occurs in people under age forty-five. Men have a much higher incidence of the disease than women.

Both of these two respiratory disorders are rarely found in nonsmokers, suggesting the critical role of smoking in causing respiratory problems. Air-conditioning can help relieve the symptoms of emphysema. Treatment of emphysema consists of conditions to provide relief of the symptoms and steps to take to prevent more progression of the disease. These conditions and steps include prescription drugs that relax and open air passages of the lungs and breathing exercises to strengthen the muscles used in breathing. Above all, those with the disease must stop smoking, if they have not already done so. For more information, contact your area's local American Lung Association by calling 800-LUNGUSA.

ARDS consists of the air sacs being filled with fluid. The result is shortness of breath and depletion of oxygen in the blood. Among the causes are an infection, pneumonia, and smoke inhalation. Adults over age seventy-five have a 60 percent mortality rate from the disease. There is no one medicine that is widely recognized as a means of treating the disease. The usual treatment is mechanical ventilation.

Classical Conditioning

You are seated in a chair with your head firmly placed in front of a glass disk. Suddenly, the disk brightens, and shortly thereafter a puff of air is shot into your eye. Of course, you blink. Blinking your eye is an example of an *unconditioned response* to its natural stimulus (in this case, the puff of air). An unconditioned response is one that is automatically evoked when its appropriate stimulus occurs. Suppose the pairing of the brightening of the disk with the puff of air continues for many trials. Eventually, you will begin to blink when the disk brightens and before the puff of air is delivered.

Blinking to the brightness of the disk is an example of a *conditioned response.* A conditioned response is one that has been learned in the presence of what was originally a neutral stimulus or event (in this case, the brightness of the disk). The originally neutral stimulus is called a *conditioned stimulus;* the originally natural stimulus (in this case, the puff of air) is called an *unconditioned stimulus.*

The procedure described above is the most common one used to investigate age differences in classical conditioning. In classical conditioning, participants essentially learn to substitute one stimulus (the conditioned stimulus) for another stimulus (the unconditioned stimulus), such that the new stimulus takes over for the original stimulus in evoking a specific response. Classical conditioning is the simplest form of learning. It was introduced to psychology a century ago by Ivan Pavlov, the famous Russian scientist, in his research with dogs and other animals. Pavlov discovered, for example, that dogs could learn to salivate to such conditioned stimuli as a bell or a flashing light when the stimuli just preceded receiving meat powder in the mouth (the unconditioned stimulus).

There is much more to classical conditioning than simply training dogs to salivate or human beings to blink. Classical conditioning may be the simplest form of learning, but it is of great importance in shaping human behavior.

Some fears and phobias appear to be acquired through classical conditioning. Consider someone who has a painful fall while trying to avoid stepping on a spider. If the pain is great enough, there is the possibility that a component of the pain (an unconditioned response to the fall) will be conditioned to the sight of the spider (a conditioned stimulus). The conditioned response to future encounters with spiders is the anticipation of pain, an anticipation we call fear. In other words, this person has acquired via classical conditioning a fear or phobia of spiders. Psychologists believe that even some prejudices may be acquired by means of classical conditioning. In addition, classical conditioning serves as a form of therapy for eliminating some kinds of unwanted behaviors (*see* Psychotherapy). Given the importance of classical conditioning, age differences in the rate at which it occurs are of great interest.

Numerous investigators have found that elderly adults do acquire a conditioned eye-blink response with the procedure described above. However, the rate of acquisition is much slower than it is for younger adults. In fact, the slowing of acquisition is apparent by the midfifties. For example, researchers at Temple University gave participants in their twenties, forties, fifties, and sixties and older more than ninety pairings of the brightening disk and the puff of air. At the end of the pairings, participants in their twenties and forties were blinking to the disk alone about 80 percent of the time. By contrast, the older participants were blinking only about 40 percent of the time. Once an eye-blink is conditioned, its retention differs greatly among adults of various ages. Even after a five-year period young adults were found to be nearly 50 percent as proficient as they were five years earlier. By contrast, elderly adults had returned to the absence of the conditioned eye-blink response to the disk.

The eye-blink task may be far removed from conditioning as it occurs in the everyday world, but it does have the basic elements of classical conditioning. It is apparent that something happens with normal aging that inhibits the rate at which classical conditioning occurs. The slower rate of conditioning by older adults has both good and bad components. The good news is that older adults are less likely than younger adults to acquire new fears and prejudices by means of classical conditioning. The bad news is that older adults are less likely than younger adults to benefit from conditioning therapy.

Why is conditioning slower among older people? There is good reason to believe that it is one of the consequences of normal biological aging. Animal research has revealed that the cerebellum (a segment of the back portion of the brain; *see* Brain and Aging) is highly involved in acquiring a conditioned response. It is the loss of neural cells in the cerebellum that seems to result in slower conditioning by aging animals, including human beings.

Claudication

See Peripheral Arterial Disease and Claudication.

Clergy (What Do They Know about Aging?)

The emphasis older people place on religion (*see* Religion in Later Life) has important implications for members of the clergy. They usually have more contact with older people in their congregations than does anyone else other than seniors' closest family members. Members of the clergy are often the confidants older adults seek out for advice when they are confronted by a personal problem or crisis in their lives.

It is especially important therefore that clergy members have an understanding of what happens to people physically, mentally, and emotionally as they age. They need, above all, to reject the negative stereotype often associated with older people (that they are grumpy, rigid people) and discount the many myths about aging that place older people in an unfavorable light (that they are unable to learn anything new; *see* Myths about Aging).

Nevertheless, many clergy members do possess negative stereotypes of older people. They usually report that they were poorly prepared in their seminary training for working with seniors. Very few seminaries offer a course on the needs and concerns of older people. The number of older people in future congregations will be increasing greatly. It is important that seminaries find the means of better preparing their future graduates for interacting with older parishioners.

Clinical Dementia Rating Scale

Researchers at Washington University in St. Louis have designed a widely used rating procedure to measure the course of dementia (especially Alzheimer's disease) as it progresses in severity. The rating is based on an intensive clinical interview with the patient and with others close to the patient. The rating is on a scale ranging from 0 to 3. A score of 0 indicates the absence of dementia, a score of 0.5 indicates that the presence of dementia is questionable, and scores of 1, 2, and 3 indicate that the dementia is mild, moderate, and severe, respectively. Separate scores are given for six different categories of mental functioning that are affected by dementia: memory, orientation, judgment and problem solving, involvement in community affairs, involvement at home and in hobbies, and personal care. These category scores are then combined to give a single overall score.

Clinical Psychology

Clinical psychology is the component of psychology that deals with the diagnosis and treatment of emotional, adjustment, and behavioral problems. Clinical psychologists usually have a doctor of philosophy or doctor of psychology degree, and they are certified or licensed by the state where they practice in private practice or in hospitals or mental health clinics. They are well qualified to administer psychological tests of intelligence, memory functioning, personality, and depression and to supervise psychotherapy for patients. By contrast, psychiatrists are medically trained therapists who have a doctor of medicine degree and are able to prescribe drugs for the treatment of depression and psychosis and prescribe such treatments as electroconvulsive therapy.

Geriatric clinical psychologists are most likely to be involved in the diagnosis and treatment of depression and other emotional disorders in elderly people caused by stress or life crises. They may also be involved in the diagnosis and treatment of dementias, such as Alzheimer's disease. Unfortunately, clinical psychologists generally prefer to work with younger clients. Many clinical psychologists are active researchers into the causes of behavioral disorders, including those associated with aging, and in the discovery of better diagnostic tests and therapies of behavioral disorders.

Clock Drawing Test

The Clock Drawing Test is a screening test for dementia. A client is first asked to draw a circle, then add the numbers of a clock to the circle, and finally set the time at 8:20. Researchers at the University of Washington found the test to be nearly as sensitive as the Mini-Mental State Exam (*see*

Mini-Mental State Exam) in detecting probable dementia. Low scores on the test have been found to be a predictor of the need for twenty-four-hour home care for elderly residents in an independent living, continuing-care retirement community. It has also been found to be a better predictor of mortality than the Mini-Mental State Exam over several years for residents in a twenty-four-hour-care retirement community.

The minimal language required to take the Clock Drawing Test and the high acceptability of the test to patients make it especially valuable in screening poorly educated, non-English-speaking patients when interpreters are not available and time is limited.

Coffee

For years coffee was considered to be a nemesis for your health. The picture has changed in recent years, however. Two cups a day (caffeinated) probably affects your health positively. The apparent reason is that coffee is rich in antioxidants (*see* Antioxidants), even richer than blueberries and broccoli. Moreover, a report issued by the United States Institute of Medicine contained the information that coffee does quench thirst and does not deplete body fluids. *See also* Liver Cancer.

Cognitive Impairment (Incidence)

Has cognitive functioning been improving in recent decades? Improvements in instrumental activities of daily living (for instance, managing money) have been greater than those for physical activities of daily living (*see* Activities of Daily Living), indicating that cognitive functioning may be improving for more recent generations of older adults. There is evidence from surveys in 1993 and 1998 showing that the percentage of noninstitutionalized Americans aged seventy and older with severe cognitive impairment declined from 6.1 percent in 1993 to 3.6 percent in 1998. Especially impressive is the decline for those aged eighty-five and older, from 13.5 percent to 7.6 percent.

Cognitive (Mental) Stages of Development

In the 1920s Jean Piaget, the famous Swiss physician and psychologist, gave psychology one of its most influential theories. The theory postulated that all children go through the same progressive stages of cognitive or mental development, and in the same order. The earliest stage, the *sensorimotor stage,* occurs roughly from birth through two years. It is characterized by the child mastering such concepts as object permanence (that is, objects do not really disappear when they are out of sight).

The second stage, the *preoperational stage,* occurs from about age two to age seven. It is one in which children are influenced greatly by their senses. If given two rows with equal numbers of blocks but differences in the spacing between blocks, children in this stage of development are likely to say that the row with the greater length has more blocks in it.

The third stage, the *concrete operational stage*, begins at about age seven and ends at about age eleven. By now the child is able to say that the rows contain an equal number of blocks. This is accomplished by the child's ability to manipulate objects mentally and observe that it is only the spaces that distinguish the rows.

The final stage, the *formal operations stage*, occurs during adolescence. It is characterized by the development of reasoning abilities that enable individuals to think abstractly and to solve problems with which they have had no prior experience.

Piaget's stage theory has attracted interest in gerontology from two different perspectives. The first concerns the possibility of an age regression whereby some older adults return to a preformal stage of cognitive development. That is, their thinking processes are limited to those characteristics of the concrete operational stage or even the preoperational stage. Some researchers have found that some of their elderly participants are less capable than their younger participants in solving problems that should be solvable by the thinking processes characteristic of the concrete operational stage. However, it is quite possible that many elderly participants view simple problems, such as the rows of blocks problem, as being too childish. Moreover, when the elderly participants are carefully selected to ensure the inclusion of only those in good health and who are functioning well, there is no apparent difference from younger participants in the ability to solve such simple problems.

The second interest concerns the possibility of an additional stage of cognitive development, one beyond Piaget's final stage of formal operations. The fifth, or *postformal*, stage is one characterized by more diversified forms of thinking than found in individuals locked into the formal stage. Individuals in a postformal stage would have the capability of asking the right questions when appropriate and not just finding answers to questions. Individuals in this stage would also know that answers to questions often depend on the situations and conditions relevant to those questions. There is limited evidence to indicate that more older than younger individuals perform at this postformal level. The implication is that cognitive development may continue throughout adulthood, and does not end before early adulthood.

Cohort (Generational) Effect

People born in widely separated years necessarily come from different generations. Many conditions present during the childhood and adolescence of people born, say, in 1970 changed greatly from those present during the childhood and adolescence of people born, say, in 1920. For example, people from the 1920 cohort grew up without television and with the experience of living through a major economic depression. By contrast, people from the 1970 generation grew up with television and did not experience a major economic depression. In addition, child-rearing practices differed greatly between children born in 1920 and children born in 1970.

These differences in conditions in the home and in society are likely to have produced important behavioral differences overall between people born in 1920 and those born in 1970. If people born in those years had been tested on one of those behaviors affected by variation in home and societal conditions in 1990 when they were seventy and twenty years old, they would show a pronounced age difference. The age difference, however, would not be the result of a true age change in behavior. Instead, the age difference would be the result of a *cohort effect*.

This is the case, for example, for political and social attitudes. When tested in 1990, people who were seventy years old scored, on average, as being more conservative on attitude tests than people who were twenty years old (*see also* Attitudes [Political and Social]). However, this does not mean that people become more conservative with normal aging. People now age seventy were probably just as conservative when they were twenty years old. Moreover, people now age twenty are likely to remain as liberal when they reach age seventy. The present age difference in conservatism is the consequence of generational differences during the preadulthood period of development, and it therefore reflects a cohort effect rather than an age change.

In addition to political and social attitudes, there is evidence to indicate that age differences in scores on both personality tests and intelligence tests represent, at least in part, cohort effects. However, it is unlikely that age differences in performances on perceptual, learning, memory, and problem-solving tasks are greatly influenced by cohort effects. Age differences on these tasks are likely to be the consequence of normal aging. However, scores could be affected by the historical time in which the tasks are measured. *See* Longitudinal Method; Longitudinal Studies of Aging's Effects on Health and Cognition.

College Investments

A number of grandparents start a fund for their grandchildren's college education. A grandparent makes a contribution for a grandchild, and the state arranges for the money to be invested in stocks or bonds. The best-known plan is called the 529 Plan. Each state offers a savings plan, but the specifics generally vary among the states. However, each plan provides growth of the amount invested free of federal tax, provided the money is used for qualified educational expenses, such as college tuition, books, and room and board. A grandparent may invest in the 529 Plan of his own state or in the plan of another state. A grandparent should consult with a financial adviser to determine which plan is the most suitable one for him or her.

In addition, there are educational IRAs in which the grandparents can invest up to $500 a year for every grandchild under age eighteen. There is no annual tax deduction for the grandparent, but the profits are tax free if applied to higher education. To make the full contribution, a grandparent's income must be under $95,000 if single or $150,000 if married and filing jointly. For Series EE saving s bonds bought since January 1, 1990, the interest is partly or entirely tax free if applied to college tuition. However, the bonds must be owned by the child's parents, and the child cannot use EE bond money and education tax credit in the same year. For more information, contact http://www.collegesavings.org.

Colon Cancer

Colon cancer is the second leading cancer killer after lung cancer. The cancer is likely to involve the rectum as well as the colon. Both are parts of the large intestine. The incidence of colon cancer increases greatly between the ages of sixty-five and eighty-five.

Surgical removal of the tumor is the usual treatment, with about half of the cases of colon cancer cured by surgery. After surgery most relapses occur within five years, if at all, and they often spread to other organs of the body, causing death in many cases, especially if not treated by chemotherapy. Chemotherapy is usually with the drug 5-fluorouracil alone or in combination with the drug Oxaliplatin.

Most cases of colon cancer have no symptoms early in the disease. However, in some cases a persistent change in bowel habits, a weight loss with no known cause, and stools narrower than usual may be warning signs of colon cancer. Detection of either early colon cancer or relapses of the cancer may be made by a combination of diagnostic tests. Screening for the cancer should be part of routine physical examinations starting at age fifty. This is especially true for individuals with first-degree relatives who had the disease. Early signs of the cancer can often be detected (about 80 percent of the time) by a test for occult blood (blood that is not visible to the eye) in the stool. If the patient tests positive on the occult blood test, then the presence of cancer should be confirmed by colonoscopy or flexible sigmoidoscopy (in which an instrument is inserted into the colon) combined with a barium enema X-ray examination. A sigmoidoscopy is more commonly used, but it misses about half of precancerous polyps detected by the more expensive colonoscopy that probes the entire colon and not just the lower third.

Researchers in Minnesota have been following the health of forty-six thousand volunteers since 1976. They have found that participants who take the blood test every year have 33 percent fewer deaths from colon cancer than those who do not take the test. Nevertheless, the blood test does yield a fairly high rate of false negatives (the cancer is present but not detected) as well as false positives (cancer detected when it is not present). Modern technology is making considerable progress in improving both the diagnosis and the treatment of colon cancer.

Of great importance is the prevention of colon cancer by engaging in health-promoting behaviors and avoiding behaviors that are harmful to our health. Of primary importance in the prevention of colon cancer, of course, is to never smoke. The foods we eat are also of great importance. In a study involving half a million people in ten European countries, it was found that eating six ounces of red meat (beef, pork, or lamb) and processed meats (ham, sausage, bacon, and cold cuts) daily increased the risk of colon cancer by 35 percent compared to eating less than one ounce a day. Especially to be limited in your diet are red meats that were cooked well done and the excessive consumption of alcoholic drinks. Eating fatty foods does not seem to be associated with the risk of colon cancer (*see* Nutrition and Diet). On the other hand, eating about three ounces of fish daily was found to reduce the risk of colon cancer by about 31 percent compared to eating it less than once a week. In addition, frequent eating of cruciferous vegetables (such as cabbage, broccoli, and brussels sprouts) reduces the risk.

Taking a daily calcium supplement has been found to reduce the number of colon polyps that could become cancerous. Estrogen replacement therapy (hormone replacement therapy) consisting of estrogen along with progestin has been found to reduce by 37 percent the risk of colon cancer. However, this benefit must be considered in light of the adverse effects the therapy is likely to have on other diseases (for instance, breast cancer).

Consult your physician about additional sources of information on colon cancer.

Color Perception

Older studies on the ability of elderly people to discriminate among colors indicated that they are much less proficient in doing so than are young adults. These studies indicated that elderly adults, on average, are about 25 percent less accurate in identifying the colors of objects at age seventy than are young adults, and they are only about 50 percent as accurate at age ninety. However, more recent evidence suggests that the color weakness of elderly people may be apparent only when finer contour discriminations are needed, discriminations of the kind needed to distinguish among the colors in a tie that contains a complex, mutable pattern of shapes and colors. Regardless of the extent of the color weakness that occurs with aging, the difficulty in identifying colors is restricted largely to colors at the short wavelengths of the spectrum (that is, blue and violet). A major factor in producing color weakness is the yellowing of the lens of the eye that occurs with normal aging. The result is that less light reaches the retina or inner layer of the eye than in earlier adulthood.

Common Cold

Millions of older Americans annually join millions of younger Americans in suffering from a common cold caused by exposure to someone's germs. Seniors should avoid getting a chill from cold weather because it may reduce the number of white blood cells needed by their immune system to ward off a cold. If seniors feel a cold coming on, they should get plenty of rest, drink a lot of fluids, and gargle with warm saltwater (if a sore throat is threatening). To relieve the sore throat, use Tylenol or Advil and a lozenge. Decongestants ease breathing by shrinking blood vessels in the nose (do not use for more than three days). Antihistamines may relieve a runny nose, but older men with enlarged prostate glands should avoid antihistamines. Chicken soup should help because it contains antiviral substances.

There is some bad news for cold sufferers. A common symptom of a cold is a cough that irritates both the cougher and others near him or her. Billions of dollars are spent every year to get rid of the cough by an over-the-counter cough suppressant. However, most suppressants have been found to be ineffective in eliminating a cough. *See also* Diseases (Acute and Chronic).

Computerized Homes

"Be it ever so humble, there's no place like home" wrote John Howard Payne. For older adults, living alone in their own home gives them a feeling of independence and control over the events in their lives. This satisfaction can only be approximated by other living arrangements (for example, assisted living facilities). Fortunately, help is on the way for seniors who want to continue living in their own homes but have concerns about their physical and mental limitations. Several universities are developing computerized systems that will help these seniors "age in place."

For example, developers at the Georgia Institute of Technology are working on two different computerized systems. The first is an in-home monitoring system that informs family members living elsewhere about their relative's activities and health status and the problems he or she is having. The second system records recent actions of the older resident that may then serve as a substitute for memory when memory fails.

The developers estimate that it will not be expensive to computerize a senior's home. The price of equipment is decreasing rapidly, installation requires little, if any, structural changes to the home, and maintenance costs will be low.

Computers

According to a 1998 survey reported in *USA Today,* 40 percent of Americans over age fifty have a computer at home, and more than 25 percent of them have access to the Internet. In a later survey, 25 percent of Americans over age sixty-five reported using a personal computer, and 58 percent of those who do reported using the Internet. More older adults would surely use computers and the Internet if they could change their pessimistic attitude about their ability to use them. A study by researchers at the University of Florida reported that this attitude can be changed to a more optimistic one by providing older adults with the opportunity to perform several tasks successfully on a computer under supervision. AARP offers free computer and Internet demonstration sessions each month in a number of cities. For more information, call 800-240-5165 or visit the Web site at http://www. aarp.org.

There are a number of steps older users of computers may take to make them feel more comfortable while using a computer. To avoid eye fatigue, the top of the screen should be placed at or slightly below eye level. Users should look down at an angle of about ten to twenty degrees, and they should sit twenty to twenty-six inches from the screen. Lighting should be arranged to reduce glare. Reflection may be reduced by blinds or curtains. The screen should be kept free of dust and fingerprints. Reference material should be as close to the screen as possible to limit head and eye movements. Users should blink frequently to prevent their eyes from drying out. Most important, users should take frequent rest breaks (every fifteen to twenty minutes), looking away from the screen. *See also* Internet; Internet (Differences between Users and Nonusers); Motor Skill Learning.

Concept Learning

Big cars, little cars, blue cars, green cars, two-door cars, four-door cars—the list goes on and on. Despite the differences among them, they are all instances of the same category or concept, namely, an automobile. Members of the same concept are likely to differ in a number of ways. In the case of automobiles, they differ along several irrelevant dimensions, such as size, color, and number of doors. However, members of the same concept have characteristics in common along relevant dimensions. For an automobile, the relevant dimensions are source of power and number of wheels. For the power dimension, the common characteristic (or attribute) is being engine powered as opposed to animal powered (as in a carriage or stagecoach). For the wheel dimension, the common characteristic is four wheels as opposed to two wheels (as in a motorcycle). Thus, "automobile" is a concept that enables us to group together all variations of an automobile.

The concept in this case is called a *conjunctive concept* in that membership within the concept demands both something *and* something else. If either is missing, the object in question is not a member of that concept. There are also *disjunctive concepts;* here, membership is defined by a rule of "something *or* something else." Consider the concept of a strike in baseball. It occurs if a batter swings and misses a pitch or does not swing but the umpire says he should have—or if the batter swings and the ball goes foul and there are fewer than two strikes. Irrelevant dimensions include the location of the ball (inside corner, outside corner, or middle of the plate) and the direction of the ball hit foul. It is little wonder that people unfamiliar with baseball have difficulty understanding it when they see their first baseball game. Considerable concept learning must take place before they can understand the game. Another example of a disjunctive concept is a first down in football. It may be achieved by moving ten or more yards either in the air or on the ground.

Much of our concept learning takes place during childhood. We learn concepts like that of "a puppy" (a conjunctive concept—a member of the puppy concept must be both a dog and not fully grown) and "a daddy" (a conjunctive concept—male and a parent).

Concept learning does not stop in childhood, however. In recent decades, adults have learned such new concepts as "a black hole," "AIDS," "a space station," and even variations on old concepts, such as "gas guzzler" and "compact" for "an automobile."

To study age differences in concept learning, participants are given such tasks as the poisoned food task. Here, patients in a hospital are described as receiving a meal consisting of three components (for instance, rice, corn, and beef), with the patient either dying or living after eating the meal. The task is to discover what the poisoned meals have in common and thus identify what defines the concept of "a poisoned meal." Elderly participants have greater difficulty, on average, in learning the concept in question than do younger participants. However, as with other forms of learning, learning does take place, albeit somewhat more slowly, in general, than it does for younger adults. The implication is that normally aging elderly people are perfectly capable of learning new concepts as they occur in our world; they simply are likely to need more time to do so.

Conformity

Conformity means yielding to group pressure. Suppose you are a member of a club consisting of ten people. You have gathered to vote on whether Mr. Smith should be admitted to your club. You have studied Mr. Smith's credentials, and you have decided he would make an excellent addition. The voting is done openly and in alphabetical order. Your name makes you last in the voting order. One by one the other members of your club vote "no" to admit Mr. Smith. Now it is your turn to vote. Would you conform to group pressure and also vote "no"—or would you stay with your original conviction and vote "yes"?

A standard laboratory task is used to study conformity of the kind present in our club voting situation. Members of a group are shown pairs of lines differing in length. They are asked which member of each pair is longer. One member of the group is the true participant whose conformity is being observed. The other members are all stooges of the investigator. As in the fictitious club voting situation, members of the group respond one by one with which line in a pair appears longer. The real participant is the last one to respond. For some of the pairs, the stooges unanimously pick the wrong line. Surely, to the real participant, it is the other line that appears to be longer. Research with this task has revealed that a larger percentage of elderly adults than younger adults conform to group pressure in this situation. The research suggests that current elderly people, in general, may be more conforming to group pressure than are younger people.

However, little is known about age differences in conformity in other situations, especially those likely to be encountered in everyday life. Making judgments about lengths of lines is a task in which most elderly adults are likely to feel they have no expertise. Given a situation where most elderly people do believe they have expertise, elderly adults may well show less conformity than younger adults. That this may be the case was demonstrated in a study at Stanford University. Here, both stooges and real participants made judgments about emotions expressed on faces. Elderly adults do have considerable expertise in regulating their own emotions (see Emotions). Judgments were made individually with the participant being the last to respond. For some of the faces the stooges gave an atypical response to the emotional expressions. In these cases, the elderly participants were found to conform less to group pressure than did younger adults who were also participants.

There is evidence indicating that elderly people in a nursing home who are rated high in conformity to the staff's regulations are also rated higher in adjustment by the staff than are elderly residents who do not conform. This outcome should not be surprising. Conforming residents in a nursing home are the ones who behave in a manner that pleases staff members. They therefore could be rated high in adjustment for this reason alone.

Constancies of Perception

As you are walking down the street, a stranger approaches you from the opposite direction. When first spotted, the stranger is about fifty feet from you. Eventually, the stranger is within a few feet of you. The stranger appeared to be about six feet tall whether fifty feet from you or five feet. This is true even though the image of the stranger does become larger on the retinas of your eyes as the distance separating the two of you decreases.

This is an example of the important principle of *size constancy* in perception. Your eyes provide information that enables your brain to tell you that size is remaining constant. For example, as an object changes distance from you, so does the degree of convergence of your eyes. That is, your eyes converge more and more as the object keeps coming closer to you. This helps to inform you that the distance of the object from you is changing, and therefore the size of the object's image on the retina must also be changing.

This is obviously not the only source of information fed to your brain. We know that people with one eye do have size constancy. Accommodation of the lens (flattening or thickening of its shape) occurs as distance changes, thus providing additional information to the brain for size constancy. This is a monocular cue (that is, present separately in each eye), and it is therefore present for people with only one functioning eye. We also know that size constancy is retained well with normal aging. Elderly adults are no more likely than younger adults to be deceived by changes in the size of objects on the retina when those objects are perceived at different distances.

Age changes are also likely to be slight, if any, for the other basic perceptual constancies. One of these is *brightness constancy*. Consider the appearance of a piece of white paper in a room you occupy. Initially, the paper appears bright in illumination. Then the lights in the room begin to dim. As they do, you perceive no change in the whiteness of the paper. Similarly, a white duck swimming in a lake on a bright sunny day continues to look white when a cloud dims the sunlight. This is because the ratio of the illumination from the object in question to the illumination from the background stays constant as the background illumination decreases. This constant ratio provides information that the brightness of the object has not changed.

Another basic constancy is that of *shape constancy*. As you look at an opening door, the shape of the moving door projected on the retina of your eyes keeps changing, but your perception of the door's shape does not change. Similarly, a coin tossed in the air continues to be perceived as circular even though the images on the retina are unlikely to be circular. These are familiar examples of shape constancy. Our past experiences with these objects provide the information needed to know that they are not changing shapes, even though what is seen by the eyes is changing. Fortunately, shape constancy is as true for elderly adults as it is for younger adults. Otherwise, we would be living in a chaotic perceptual world as we grow older.

Consumer-Directive Care for Disabled Seniors

Physically disabled seniors who live in their own homes and need help to perform the physical activities of daily living (bathing and toileting) traditionally receive that help from governmental or charitable agencies that recruit, train, and supervise the home-care providers. However, in recent years consumer-directive health care has become an available alternative.

Physically disabled seniors receive money from some program, usually Medicaid, to hire and train their own home-care providers (usually family members or friends). This gives them some control over their daily activities of living. In general, seniors who have selected consumer-directive care have been receiving caregiving services that are either similar or more positive than agency-based services. A problem with consumer-directive care is that many disabled seniors do not want to have family members or friends perform such demanding activities.

Consumer Fraud

Telephone interviews with a nationally representative sample of nearly one thousand consumers revealed that consumer fraud and deceptive sales practices cost consumers an estimated one hundred billion dollars a year—much of it from older people. Tips for avoiding consumer fraud include not paying anything for a so-called free prize and refusing to be rushed into buying something or sending money to some uncertain firm or enterprise. Check any offers or so-called bargains with your local Better Business Bureau or your state attorney general's office, or call the National Fraud Information Center at 800-876-7070. *See also* Scams.

Consumers of Merchandise in Stores

It is estimated that people age fifty and older spend about 48 percent of consumer dollars. They buy about 48 percent of all luxury cars, and they are responsible for about 80 percent of luxury travel. They even buy about 25 percent of all toys annually (there are about fifty-five million grandparents age fifty years and older in the United States). Nevertheless, marketing and merchandising programs commonly treat these customers as if they are much older. For example, there is the myth that older consumers are fixed on certain products and are unwilling to try new alternative products. Therefore, why should advertising of a new product be directed at older consumers? In fact, a survey of five hundred people over age fifty in shopping malls revealed that about 80 percent of them were quite willing to try new products.

Merchants can do more to appeal to older consumers. For example, they could advertise merchandise of interest to older people at nontraditional times on television, such as during the noon news when the proportion of older people viewing the programs is likely to be greater than the proportion of younger adults. They should also have a number of older salespeople or age-sensitive younger salespeople. Above all, they should not have rock music playing in the background when they have sales of special interest to older people.

Continuity versus Discontinuity in Adult Development

Do elderly adults behave in the same ways they did when they were younger? If they were shy as young adults, do they continue to be shy through middle age and late adulthood? Do those elderly adults who were good problem solvers as young adults continue to be so as elderly adults, at least relative to other elderly adults who were not good problem solvers earlier in life?

In general, the answers to those questions are yes. We know that many personality traits and characteristics change little from early to late adulthood (*see* Personality Traits). Shy persons may become more or less shy as they grow older, but they are likely to remain more shy than most other people their own age. Similarly, there may be some modest decline in problem-solving ability with normal aging (*see* Problem Solving), but people who were proficient early in life are likely to retain their advantage later in life. These are examples of continuity in adult development. Continuity does not mean the absence of changes in behavior with aging, but it does mean that the changes are primarily quantitative in nature. That is, people may possess more or less of a behavior than they did earlier, but the basic pattern of behavior remains unaltered. In many mental processes and activities, only quantitative changes are observed with normal aging. People who are good readers early in life continue to be good readers later in life, but they read more slowly than they did earlier. Memory processes are basically unaltered, but they do occur more slowly than they did earlier in life (and therefore are somewhat less proficient). Older people have memory spans slightly shorter than they did as young adults, but they are nevertheless still able to hold considerable material in short-term memory (*see* Memory Span). These are all examples of quantitative, but not qualitative, changes that take place in adult development.

At the same time, there is some discontinuity in adult development. Some behavior and mental process changes are qualitative in nature rather than merely quantitative. In effect, elderly adults are presumed to be quite different with respect to those behaviors and processes than they were earlier in life.

For example, the stresses and crises confronting elderly adults are usually quite different from the stresses and crises they faced as younger adults. The ways in which they must cope with these stresses and crises are likely to be quite different from the coping strategies they used to solve earlier crises in their lives (*see* Stress and Coping with Stress).

Some memory processes may change qualitatively from early to late adulthood. When given stories to read and remember, younger adults typically try to recall the ideas of the story. By contrast, many elderly adults will focus less on the specific content and more on the moral of the story and implications of the story's content for their own lives (*see* Discourse Memory).

Control over Life's Events

"It's up to me to keep my mental faculties from deteriorating." "No matter what I do, if I am going to get sick, I will get sick." Responses to such statements are used to measure the personality characteristic known as *locus of control*. The characteristic is anchored by two extremes labeled "external" and "internal." People who score at the external end of the dimension of locus of control seemingly believe that many of the events in their lives are determined or controlled by forces external to themselves (chance or fate). Such persons are likely to respond false to the first statement, one dealing with the belief about control over one's intellectual functioning, and true to the second statement, one dealing with the belief about lack of control over one's health. People who score at the internal end of the dimension are likely to respond true to the first statement and false to the second statement. They believe that they have the capacity to control many of the major events of their lives.

A number of studies, both cross-sectional and longitudinal, have indicated that people tend to become more external in their beliefs as they age normally. They tend to lessen in their belief that they have considerable control of many of life's events. This is somewhat unfortunate, since there is evidence to indicate that, with normal aging, older people who score as being internal express greater satisfaction with their lives than do people who score as being external. The same evidence suggests that this difference in life satisfaction between "internals" and "externals" is especially pronounced for elderly women.

Moreover, there is also evidence indicating that those older people who appear to be "internals" in regard to their intellectual functioning score higher on intelligence tests than do those older people who appear to be "externals." Other evidence indicates that there are increases in control with age from twenty-five to seventy-five over work, finances, and marriage, but decreases in control over relationships with their children and their sex life.

"Externals" tend to rely more heavily on assistance from other people than do "internals" when confronted by mentally demanding tasks. The reliance on others for such tasks is likely to be especially true for women and for less educated older people. For most older people, the decline in mental ability is likely to be so moderate (if it exists at all) that they have little reason to fear facing mentally demanding tasks.

Similarly, those older people who appear to be "internals" in regard to their health make fewer visits per year to a physician than those who appear to be "externals." People over age eighty who feel they have control over their own health have lower rates of hospitalization than others of that age who believe they have little control over their own health. In addition, Canadian researchers found that elderly people with arthritis who had low levels of belief in control of their own health used more health services and had more visits to physicians than elderly people with arthritis who believed in their own health control.

Researchers at the University of Michigan determined for participants age sixty-five and older what were the three most important roles they played in their lives (for example, spouse, grandparent, provider). They found that feelings of control over the single most important role significantly reduced the odds of death in the near future. However, control over the second and third most important roles was not related to mortality.

Seniors with physical impairments who feel they have control or mastery over their environment have a lower level of depression than other impaired seniors with less feelings of mastery. Mastery enables a senior to prevent or manage health-related problems and, in turn, results in effective strategies for coping with impairment.

Residents of nursing homes live in an environment where there is little opportunity to control the events in their lives. There has been research revealing that when these individuals are given an opportunity to control a major event of their lives (such as the timing and duration of visits from family members and friends), their well-being, both physically and mentally, may improve considerably.

Conversation Memory

"What was it you said about her?" "Oh, I just don't remember." Such frequent conversational exchanges are testimony to the fact that our memories of past conversations with other people are often imperfect. Our interest rests in the possibility that the imperfection may increase from early to late adulthood.

As with memory for the content of television programs (*see* Memory for Television Programs), memory for the content of conversations in the everyday world would seem to occur incidentally. That is, we neither have the intent to commit conversational content to memory, nor do we even try to rehearse it in an attempt to increase its memorability. The very act of attending to and comprehending what is being said to you is sufficient to ensure the automatic registration of at least part of the content in memory, but not always accurately.

Memory for conversational content is an important component of our everyday memory. Failure to remember important parts of a conversation can on occasion have serious implications. This is the case, for example, in our memory of a conversation with our physician. Inability to recall correctly parts of that conversation can result in the misapplication of a treatment for an injury or a disease. We seem to be especially vulnerable to errors in memory when the content is in terms of instructions on how to reach a specific locale or how to assemble a particular piece of equipment.

Despite the importance of conversational memory in everyday functioning, there has been little research on age differences in the proficiency of conversational memory. Researchers at the University of Missouri at Columbia did bring conversational memory into the laboratory by having young adults and elderly participants engage in a series of conversations with the investigator. Each conversation centered around a specific topic, such as the presidency of the United States. For each topic, the participants were asked several questions, and after each question they were asked to explain the reason for their answers (for example, "Should presidents be limited to one six-year term in office?"). They were later asked to recall the topics discussed and the specific questions asked.

Interestingly, memory was almost as proficient for participants, young and elderly, who did not know in advance that their memory for the contents would be tested (that is, incidental memory) as it was for participants who did know (intentional memory). The recall of both topics and questions was far from perfect for the young adults, and it was even more imperfect for the elderly adults (about 20 percent less proficient).

However, when tested for the recognition of the topics discussed and the questions asked, both young and elderly participants had essentially perfect scores. The imperfection of conversational memory seems to be largely in the retrieval stage (that is, getting information out of memory storage) rather than in the encoding stage (getting information into memory storage). Older adults have moderately greater retrieval problems than younger adults (*see* Recognition Memory versus Recall Memory).

When dealing with important conversational content, such as that of the instructions of a physician or the advice of an attorney, people of all ages should not rely on their own memories. The information should be written down and read back to the person delivering the message. This is especially true for elderly people.

Coping with Frailty

Many frail elders have relatively low levels of psychological well-being (*see* Well-Being [Psychological]). However, some frail elders adjust to their condition and report relatively high levels of psychological well-being. One reason is that many of these elders have strong spiritual or religious beliefs that help them cope with their poor health. The positive effect of a high level of spirituality has been found to have a much greater effect on well-being for elders who have a relatively high level of frailty than for elders who have a relatively low level of frailty.

Cornell Medical Index

The Cornell Medical Index (CMI) is a checklist on which people report various physical and psychological symptoms they are experiencing. The

CMI includes sections for both physical and psychological symptoms. Twelve different categories of symptoms are included in the physical section (for instance, cardiovascular or respiratory) and six different categories in the psychological section (including anxiety and depression).

The CMI has been widely used in studies comparing adults of different ages regarding the frequencies with which they report different symptoms, both physical and psychological. The most comprehensive of these studies are those conducted with participants in the Baltimore Longitudinal Study (National Institute on Aging) and participants in the Normative Aging Study (*see* Longitudinal Studies of Aging's Effects on Health and Cognition). These studies revealed only a modest increase in physical symptoms with increasing age for men ranging in age from seventeen to ninety-seven in the Baltimore Longitudinal Study and from twenty-one to eighty in the Normative Aging Study, and an even smaller increase in psychological symptoms. By contrast, the personality trait of neuroticism is strongly related to the number of symptoms reported quite independently of age.

Creativity

Galileo was only twenty when he discovered the law of the pendulum. Isaac Newton was only twenty-three when he began his discoveries of gravitation, and Albert Einstein only twenty-six when he advanced the theory of relativity. Remarkable achievements by individuals so young—sufficiently so that these individuals were labeled as "geniuses."

Are youthful achievements of this magnitude limited to physicists? Certainly not. Chemistry has had its share of young superstars, such as Antoine-Laurent Lavoisier who, at the age of thirty-four, unraveled the mystery of combustion as the combination of a burning substance with oxygen. Ernest Hemingway was only twenty-seven when *The Sun Also Rises* was published and thirty when *A Farewell to Arms* was published. David Hume, the philosopher, was only twenty-eight when his major work, *A Treatise of Human Nature,* was completed. Nor has psychology been void of its youthful masters. B. F. Skinner was in his early thirties when he discovered the principles of reinforcement and operant learning that were to make him internationally famous, as was Sigmund Freud when he published his major work on the interpretation of dreams.

Creativity involves originality, or the discovery of a unique solution to a problem (*see* Originality). However, creativity involves much more than just originality. It also means that the solutions or contributions have significance for society, and through them important advances are made in mathematics, science, philosophy, literature, and, yes, even psychology.

Is creativity possessed only by young adults? Or, at least, are important discoveries by older individuals more the exception than the rule? Those who follow the awarding of Nobel Prizes each year may be misled to conclude that many older individuals have made great discoveries in their fields. However, in most of the cases of awards to older scientists, the discoveries of those scientists were made when they were much younger. It simply took the test of time for their discoveries to be recognized.

The classic analyses of the relationship between age and creativity conducted by H. C. Lehman provide partial answers to our questions. Beginning in the early 1940s and continuing through the early 1960s, Lehman reported analyses of highly creative contributions made by individuals at various age levels in several different academic disciplines. A "highly creative contribution" was one that was widely cited in introductory textbooks of a given discipline. Of interest to Lehman was the age of the contributor at the time his or her most cited contribution was produced. Overall, Lehman found that the peak age range was between thirty and thirty-nine. Beyond that age range there was a pronounced and progressive decline in the percentage of contributions that he ranked as being truly creative, so much so that the percentage of contributions made by individuals in their seventies was close to zero.

Lehman's classic analyses did not go unchallenged. However, the challenge rested largely on the issue of productivity and not creativity. Later researchers found that productivity in various academic and artistic endeavors shows only a modest decline after ages thirty to thirty-nine. At stake, however, is the quality of the products of one's creative activity. True creativity, as defined by Lehman, ends with a startling, perhaps even world-shaking, discovery that changes the course of a discipline's future.

Many older scholars, researchers, inventors, and artists certainly contribute effectively to their disciplines, but it does seem usually that the contributions are at the level of a modest increase to knowledge in their discipline and to their own careers. It should be noted further that a massive longitudinal study (that is, following the same individuals over a period of years) of research psychologists indicated that researchers who were the most productive when they were young continued to hold their advantage over less productive researchers during the later stages of their careers.

Of course, we know that artists like Claude Monet and Pablo Picasso created some of their greatest pictures near the end of their lives. Many creative artists, composers, and writers may simply develop new creative styles in late adulthood. Dr. Dean Simonton of the University of California at Davis found that creativity does not decline with age, but it may change form. For example, Igor Stravinsky composed music differently late in his life than he did earlier in his life.

There are probably many reasons that creativity appears to decline with age. One contributing factor has nothing to do with aging as a biological process. Potentially creative individuals are often "rewarded" for their earlier achievements by being made executives of an industrial company or administrators of their universities at a relatively early age. Consequently, the opportunity to pursue further their research or artistic careers is denied them.

It has also been argued that creativity is adversely related to certain personality characteristics that are more pronounced in older than in younger individuals (for example, intolerance of ambiguity). However, given the generally stable nature of personality over the adult life span (*see* Personality Traits), age differences in personality seem unlikely to be a major determinant of age differences in creativity.

Another possibility is that there is some underlying mental ability that declines with aging. We do know that there are modest age differences in originality, an ability many have suspected to be a determinant of creativity. However, the extent of these age differences does not seem to be great enough to account for the pronounced age differences in creativity reported by Lehman. What remains is the possibility that we have yet to discover further mental abilities that affect creativity, abilities that do decline significantly in proficiency with aging. Considerable progress in identifying these abilities should occur in the near future because new theories of creativity and new methods of studying it are appearing at a rapid pace.

Cremation

The number of cremations in the United States has been increasing steadily in recent years. In 1970 they accounted for less than 5 percent of the disposal of human bodies after death. By the year 2000 they had accounted for more than 25 percent. By the year 2025 the percentage is expected to be greater than 50 percent. One reason is that a cremation is less expensive than a burial. Cremation may even avoid the expense of embalming, and it is not necessary to have all of the arrangements needed with a funeral home for a burial. Most seniors simply cannot afford the cost of a funeral and burial. *See also* Funerals.

Crime Prevention

There are a number of ways crimes against older people (and younger people too) may be prevented. For example, at home, keep outdoor lighting on all night, do not display your name on your mailbox (burglars could look up your phone number and call to see if you are home), keep doors locked, and change locks when you move into a new residence. While driving, keep your windows up and your valuables out of sight. If you feel threatened driving in a strange area, leave that area as quickly as possible. While traveling, shield your luggage identification tags (so a thief will not know you are away from home); leave a record of your travelers' checks, your itinerary, and your tickets with a friend; and when leaving your hotel, store your valuables in the hotel's safe-deposit vault.

A number of communities have established what is called a triad. It is a cooperative effort that combines the local sheriff, the police chief, and older individuals and organizations to combat crime and help police serve the needs of older people. For information about triads, write to Triad, 1450 Duke Street, Alexandria, VA 22314-3490.

Crime (Victim of and Fear of)

Are you afraid to leave your home for fear of being mugged? Do you have difficulty falling asleep because you fear your home will be robbed? In some cases, of course, such fears may be realistic and serve to help an individual avoid being the victim of a crime. In other cases, however, the fear of being a victim of a crime may be irrational and may interfere with normal every-day functioning.

Are such fears especially prevalent among elderly adults? If so, they would provide evidence to support what is called the victimization/fear paradox. Crime statistics reveal that it is teenagers and young adults, not elderly adults, who are most likely to be the victims of crime. People age sixty-five and older are less likely to be victims of violent crimes than are younger people.

The United States Justice Department reported that there were 5.3 violent crimes each year for every 1,000 older people from 1992 through 1997 compared to 56 violent crimes per 1,000 people age twelve through sixty-four. Elderly people are less likely to go out at night (when most violent crimes are committed) than are younger people, and they are less likely to fight back when attacked than are younger people. In a survey of elderly victims of a violent crime, only 49 percent reported arguing with the attacker, running away, calling for help, or fighting the attacker, compared to 70 percent of those under age fifty.

For some years it was believed that fear of crime was much more prevalent among older adults than among younger adults. Thus the paradox—greater incidence of fear despite the lower incidence of victimization among elderly adults. However, a recent study indicates that the paradox does not really exist. It is younger persons, not elderly persons, who are most afraid of most types of crime. In the same study it was found that at every age women are more likely than men to fear being the victim of a crime.

Cross-Sectional Method

Are there adult age differences in the rate of solving anagrams (scrambled words), in scores on intelligence tests, in performances on various kinds of memory tasks? Do younger and older adults differ in their performances on such tasks and many other tasks? To answer this question, gerontological researchers most often use the cross-sectional method.

This method requires the selection of a different group of people for each age level being compared, and comparison of the scores among the age groups for the task being evaluated. Consider the simplest kind of cross-sectional study in which young adults (say, twenty to twenty-nine years of age) are to be compared with elderly adults (sixty-five to seventy-four years of age) on a learning task. A group or sample of young adults is selected along with a group of elderly adults. The two groups are then given the same learning task at approximately the same time. Suppose we discover that the young group averages eight trials to learn the task and the elderly group averages ten trials. Thus, the cross-sectional age difference reveals an age difference in which the elderly group averaged 25 percent below the level of performance of the young group.

What can we conclude about this age difference? Is the age difference in proficiency really the result of a decline in learning ability with normal aging? This conclusion depends on how the groups were selected.

Suppose our participants at each age level had been selected randomly from the total populations of people in the age ranges of twenty to twenty-nine and sixty-five to seventy-four. If so, then the young participants would be representative of all adults in the twenty-to-twenty-nine-year age range with respect to the proportions of men and women in the total population, proportions of different races in the total population, socioeconomic backgrounds, educational backgrounds, and so on. Similarly, the elderly participants would be representative of all adults in the sixty-five-to-seventy-four-year age range. If such representation is truly satisfied, then the age difference for our two groups should be generalizable to the entire populations of millions of people in the two age ranges used in this study. We would be able to conclude that learning on this particular task occurs at a rate for all adults age sixty-five to seventy-four that is about 25 percent slower than the rate for all adults age twenty to twenty-nine. It is through the use of the cross-sectional method with groups that are representative of their total populations that age norms are developed (*see* Norms).

Our hypothetical study with representative groups at different age levels clearly describes the existence of an age difference in learning. But does it permit us to conclude that it is aging itself that caused the age difference? Not necessarily.

By selecting representative groups of young and elderly adults we had two groups that undoubtedly differed in a number of ways besides their ages. These differences arise because people of different ages who are tested at the same time must come from different cohorts or generations (*see* Cohort [Generational] Effect). The two groups in our study probably differ on such characteristics as their years of formal education. That is, the young adults will have had, on average, more education than the elderly adults. This creates a definite problem in concluding whether the age difference is the consequence of normal aging. We know that amount of education does correlate with learning proficiency (*see* Educational Level). Consequently, it may be the difference in educational level that is responsible for our observed age difference, with aging itself having little effect on the difference in scores earned by the two groups.

To determine the role of aging on the observed age difference in learning, we would have to make certain that our age groups are matched in educational level. This could be done, for example, by selecting only college graduates as participants. We may then discover that the young college graduates and older college graduates average five and six trials, respectively, to learn the task. We are now better able to view the age difference of 20 percent as resulting from a moderate decline in learning proficiency with normal aging. At the same time, we are likely to underestimate the magnitude of the age difference that exists in the total populations of younger and older adults. Remember that our hypothetical study with representative age groups estimated that difference to be about 25 percent.

The matching of age groups on such important characteristics as educational level is a common practice in research with the cross-sectional method when the objective is to determine whether aging itself is the reason for an observed age difference in task performance. However, there is the risk of failing to match the age groups on some other characteristics that could affect performance on a given task.

For example, age groups matched only for education may differ in their degree of introversion. However, this would present a problem only if degree of introversion is known to relate to performance on the task in question. If it is, then the age groups would have to be matched on introversion as well as on education. For many tasks, introversion is unlikely to be related to performance. Consequently, matching the age groups in scores on a test of introversion would not be needed. Age groups are also likely to differ in many other respects, such as their average heights, their amounts of gray hair, and so on. These are usually age differences that should not affect performances on most of the tasks used in gerontological research.

Cultural Differences in Memory

Cultures vary in their views of normal aging. Of interest is the extent to which negative views of aging contribute to the age-related differences found in memory studies conducted in societies holding this view. There is evidence to indicate that age-related differences in memory performances do not differ between cultures with positive and negative views of aging.

However, other components of cognition seem to differ between Americans and Asians. They tend to differ in how they perceive objects. Americans focus on objects in a scene, whereas Asians focus more on the context in which objects appear. Categorization also seems to differ. Americans are likely to group objects by type (for example, dogs and human beings are

both animals), whereas Asians are more likely to group them by relationships (dogs and human beings both eat meat).

Curiosity

Curiosity is rumored to have killed the cat—but what does it do to human
beings? Wouldn't life be dull if we were not curious about the world and
universe in which we live? How much of your time is spent seeking information about that world? Children are well known to be very curious individuals. But what about adults of different ages? One of the beliefs about aging
is that curiosity decreases from early to late adulthood. However, there is
considerable evidence to indicate that this is simply another myth of aging
(*see* Myths about Aging).

Recent evidence was provided by researchers at the National Institute on
Aging. They tested a large sample of individuals of various ages over the adult
life span. The participants responded to a number of statements related to
both interpersonal curiosity and impersonal-mechanical curiosity. Interpersonal curiosity refers to the desire to know more about other people.
Examples of the statements for this form of curiosity were "I like to read
about the personal lives of people of public prominence" and "I have little
interest in the private lives of my schoolmates or fellow workers." Impersonal-
mechanical curiosity refers to wanting to know more about things and science in general. Examples of the statements for this form of curiosity were "I
like to read about new scientific findings" and "I do not like to visit factories
and manufacturing plants." The participants' responses to these statements
indicated the extent to which the statement applied to them.

The researchers found the degree of curiosity to be about the same for
young, middle-aged, and elderly adults. Curiosity may be considered a trait
of personality, and like other traits, it is affected little by aging (*see* Personality Traits).

Interestingly, elderly adults who score higher on the trait of curiosity
seem to live longer than those who are low on the trait. Evidence in support
of this possibility was provided by researchers in California who measured
curiosity by responses to the kinds of statements included in the study at the
National Institute on Aging.

D

Daily Help

Many disabled seniors receive either no help (paid or unpaid) to fulfill all of their daily needs or some help, but it is not enough. They have the risk of encountering serious consequences. For example, the absence of assistance in transferring from bed to chair increases the risk of falling (*see* Falls).

Researchers have found that those seniors who receive no care are characterized by less severity of disability, lower levels of insurance coverage, and less informal support from family and friends than those seniors who receive some but an inadequate amount of care.

Dancing

Researchers at the Albert Einstein College of Medicine in New York City demonstrated the benefits of dancing for avoiding dementia. The participants in their study were 469 community-dwelling adults over age seventy-five. They were all free of dementia at the beginning of their study. The participants reported the frequency with which they engaged in such physical activities as swimming, bicycling, and dancing. They were then followed closely for five years.

Over that period 124 participants developed dementia (mostly Alzheimer's disease and vascular dementia). Dancing was the only physical activity associated with lowering the risk of dementia. Participants who danced three or four times a week had an incidence of dementia that was 78 percent less than that of participants who danced either once a week or not at all.

Why dancing? The researchers believe it's because dancing, unlike most other physical activities, combines physical and mental activities. It also involves emotional activity, namely, joy. So put on your dancing shoes!

Dark Adaptation

Most people have experienced what happens when they enter a dimly lit movie theater. It takes some time before they can see well enough to find an unoccupied seat. They are experiencing the important visual phenomenon of dark adaptation. The receptor cells in the retina are adapting to the change in illumination. This process takes a number of minutes before complete adaptation occurs. The time needed for complete adaptation may be several minutes longer for elderly adults than for younger adults, although the evidence in this area is somewhat ambiguous. However, it has been well established that the vision of elderly adults in dim illumination is impaired to a much greater degree than it is for younger adults. This is a major contributing factor to the reluctance of many elderly people to drive a car at night or at twilight.

Partial dark adaptation is a related visual phenomenon that has important implications for aging. It occurs when the eyes are exposed to intermittent changes in brightness. A familiar example occurs when driving at night and the headlights of occasional cars moving in the opposite direction are encountered. Frequent shifts from bright-light vision to dim-light vision are needed to maintain control of the car being driven. Elderly adults find these shifts more difficult to accomplish than do younger adults. This is another reason many elderly adults, especially those age seventy-five years and older, should avoid driving at night as much as possible.

Daydreaming

One of the myths about aging is that elderly people daydream more than younger people. This myth probably had its origin in the belief that many older people spend much of their time reminiscing. These reminiscences are thoughts that interrupt the ongoing task in which the elderly person is engaged, whether it is listening to a lecture, raking the leaves, or washing the dishes.

A daydream need not be reminiscing about the past. A daydream is any thought that intrudes while we are doing something else. For example, a college student listening to a professor's lecture may find himself or herself suddenly thinking about a party to be held that coming weekend. Daydreams are typically spontaneous. They seem to just "pop" into the mind without the individual's intent to have those intruding thoughts. In addition, daydreams need not be erotic, romantic, or bizarre. In fact, they are often routine or commonplace in content (for example, thoughts about what in the world we are going to serve our guests for dinner tomorrow night).

Does daydreaming actually increase from early to late adulthood? Evidence gathered by Dr. Leonard Giambra of the National Institute on Aging's Gerontology Research Center indicates that the opposite is actually true. Dr. Giambra's research has involved two different methods. The first consists simply of interviewing adults of all ages about their daydreaming and answering a questionnaire. These answers reveal that both men and women report less frequent daydreaming as aging increases. That is, the older the individual, the less frequent the daydreaming.

The other method consists of studying daydreaming under controlled laboratory conditions. Adults of varying ages are given a boring laboratory task to perform for an extended period of time. They are also trained to report each time they have an intruding thought or "mindwandering." The results of this laboratory research confirm's Dr. Giambra's interview data: the oldest individuals reported far fewer "mindwanderings" than the youngest individuals. A researcher at Furman University failed to find less "mindwandering" by elderly adults than by young adults but, nevertheless, found that elderly participants did not exhibit more "mindwandering" than young adults.

The content of the daydreams reported is of further interest. Dr. Giambra discovered that for all but the youngest adults in his studies (ages seventeen to twenty-three), the most frequent daydreams involved problem solving of some kind. That is, the content was concerned with some problem currently facing the individual.

For the youngest adults, the most frequent daydreams were, not surprisingly, sexually oriented (but problem-solving daydreams ranked second even for them). Daydreams do seem to play an important role in our everyday lives by helping us to cope with our problems. It is as if our subconscious mind is struggling with a problem even as our conscious mind is occupied with other things, perhaps leading to a solution to that problem (for instance, "Hey, let's have stroganoff" for the guests at dinner).

Even the daydreams of the most famous dreamer of all time, Walter Mitty in James Thurber's *Secret Life of Walter Mitty,* may be viewed as a form of problem solving. Mitty frequently engaged in exotic and adventurous daydreams in which he played the heroic role. Remember that he engaged in these daydreams when he was subjected to nagging by his wife. The daydreams represented a form of coping with a problem.

Death and Dying

Thousands of elderly people die every year. Contrary to popular belief, most of them do not die of "old age." "Old age" is not a disease. Most elderly people who do not die as a result of an accident, murder, or suicide die of a life-threatening disease that is more prevalent in late adulthood than in earlier adulthood (such as heart disease; *see* Cardiovascular Diseases).

One of the myths about aging is that people become increasingly more fearful of death and more anxious about death as they grow older. However, this does not appear to be true. In a survey of more than eighteen hundred Americans age forty-five and older, younger adults expressed more fear of dying (about 30 percent for those in the forty-five to forty-nine age range) than seniors (about 15 percent for those aged seventy-five and older).

Women overall are more afraid of dying (24 percent) than men (18 percent) and more afraid of being in pain at the end of life than men (52 percent versus 40 percent).

The intensity of fear of dying does vary greatly among older adults. In general, religious older people have less fear of dying than less religious people. However, some religions might increase the fear of dying by involving the belief of possible punishment in the afterlife. Seniors with greater feelings of self-efficacy (feeling mastery of events in one's life) tend to have less fear of the unknown following death than seniors with less of this feeling. This seems to be true for both men and women. Seniors who face old age with the feeling of integrity in their lives (their lives were worth living) have less fear of dying than seniors who are confronted by despair that their lives were not worth living.

Is there any consistent pattern to how people face death when they know they have a terminal illness and will die fairly soon? This question is of particular interest in gerontology because a large proportion of the terminally ill population consists of elderly people. In the early 1960s, Dr. Elizabeth Kubler-Ross provided evidence to suggest that many terminally ill people progress through a series of emotional stages. Her stage theory was based on interviews with two hundred terminally ill individuals.

According to Dr. Kubler-Ross, the first stage is one of shock and disbelief in which the individual feels a diagnostic mistake must have been made and denies the reality of the diagnosis. However, most terminally ill individuals eventually accept the diagnosis and move into a stage characterized by the expression of anger and hostility directed toward healthy people. They seem to be expressing their frustration and feeling of unfairness as to why they rather than other people are dying. This stage is followed by a bargaining stage in which they may appeal to a higher being that they will be better persons if they are allowed to live. Eventually, they realize that the bargaining is ineffective, and they enter a stage in which they experience depression, guilt, and shame about their lives. Discussing these experiences with others helps them enter the final stage in which they accept the inevitability of their own deaths.

Thus, the five stages are disbelief and denial, anger and hostility, bargaining, depression, and acceptance. Dr. Kubler-Ross recognized that not all terminally ill people progress through all of these stages, and that even those who do move through them do so at different rates.

Although the stage theory has attracted considerable attention, it has also encountered considerable criticism. Several later studies have revealed that many terminally ill people remain basically the same throughout their illness, rather than progressing through stages. It was found that some terminally ill people simply continue to live their daily lives as they did before their illness was diagnosed, whereas others withdraw from further social interactions.

Most important, a number of patients were found to cling to the denial of the severity of their illness until the end, rather than accepting it fairly early after diagnosis. In addition, the presence of depression in terminally ill people may be the consequence of their medications, rather than a stage of their adjustment to their impending deaths. As the end of life nears, many terminally ill people vacillate between feelings of contentment and feelings of hopelessness, rather than being continuously depressed.

Dr. Victor Cicirelli of Purdue University presented hundreds of alert community-dwelling adults ranging in age from sixty to one hundred with a number of different end-of-life situations. About half of the participants favored continuing life even if they had a terminal illness that would greatly lower the quality of their lives (for instance, dependence on others). Only about 10 percent favored ending their lives under such conditions. About a third expressed the need to have a family member, close friend, or their physician make the decision for them.

Decision Making

When making decisions based on written material (such as a brochure containing information about a health insurance policy), elderly adults do not utilize as much information from the material as do younger adults. Elderly adults base their decisions largely on their own experiences. However, middle-aged adults tend to utilize both their experience and information from the material in making a decision regarding what that material is presenting. *See also* Accidents (Automobile); Advance Directives; Cancer (General Information); Cautiousness; Delayed Rewards; Stress and Coping with Stress.

Defibrillators

A fibrillating heart is beating randomly and needs to restore normal rhythm. Especially life threatening is ventricular fibrillation (that is, fibrillation in the ventricle chambers of the heart). A defibrillator is a machine that assesses if the heart needs an electric shock to restore that rhythm and then provides that shock if needed. Heart attack survival decreases by between 7 percent and 10 percent for every minute between fibrillation and the application of a defibrillator.

Technology has made it possible to have defibrillators that are easier to apply than are those in a hospital. They may be placed in schools, libraries, offices, malls, and other places where people gather. They are therefore readily available for use if an emergency occurs.

Delayed Rewards

Consider this situation: A decision needs to be made between buying a

stock that will make a quick profit or buying another stock with little immediate reward but with a large reward in the future. At stake in making your
decision is what is called temporal discounting. It refers to decreases in the
subjective value of a delayed reward as the duration of the delay increases.
Researchers at Washington University in St. Louis gave younger and older
participants hypothetical situations involving immediate versus delayed
rewards (for example, one involving stocks). Older adults (mean age of
seventy-one) with lower income had a greater temporal discounting than
did either higher-income older people or younger adults (mean age of
thirty-three). Older adults with a reduced income seem to prefer short-term
rewards, even when they are less in amount than later rewards.

Delirium

Delirium is a mental condition brought about by physiological brain dysfunctioning. It is characterized by mental confusion and incoherence that
may include hallucinations and delusions. The symptoms may also include
disturbances in sleep-wake cycles. It is unfortunately a fairly common condition for hospitalized elderly patients. Its incidence has been found to vary
between 10 percent and 39 percent, but may often be labeled as depression
rather than delirium. Patients who display delirium tend to have longer
hospital stays and greater risk of death in the hospital than patients who do
not display delirium.

   Behaviors in the hospital that are predictive of delirium are restlessness,
difficulty in thinking clearly, enhanced sensitivity to visual and auditory
stimuli, insomnia, and nightmares. Relatives of elderly hospitalized patients
should be aware of these forewarnings and inform the hospital staff of their
occurrence. Once forewarned, there may be ways of preventing delirium or,
at least, reducing its duration and intensity. Unfortunately, physicians fail to
diagnose 30 percent to 50 percent of delirium patients. They are often
likely to view the patient's delirium behavior as being caused by dementia
or depression.

Dementia

See Senile Dementia.

Demography of Aging

The population of elderly people in the United States has increased steadily
over the years. The trend toward an increasing population of elderly people is expected to continue through the first few decades of the twenty-first
century. The United States is not alone in the population boom of older
people. Similar trends have occurred in most developed countries of the

world, but not in many of the underdeveloped countries where life expectancy falls well below that found for developed countries.

The United Nations classifies a country as being *old* if more than 7 percent of its population is age sixty-five or older. The United States and such countries as Canada, England, Germany, Japan, Poland, and Spain fall into this category. Countries with 4 percent to 7 percent of the population in the age sixty-five and older range are classified as mature countries. Included here are such countries as Brazil, Panama, South Africa, and Turkey. Countries with less than 4 percent of the population age sixty-five or older are classified as young. Among these countries are Burma, Colombia, Egypt, India, Iran, Kuwait, and Mexico. However, even developing countries are showing signs of becoming older. In the period 1991–1994 their annual growth rate of people age sixty-five or older was 3.2 percent compared to 2.3 percent for more developed countries.

In 2005 it was estimated that there were 35 million Americans who were age 65 and older (about 13 percent of the total population), 59 percent of them women. In 1900 there were slightly more than 3 million people age 65 and older in the United States and about 25 million in 1980. By the year 2030 it is estimated that the number of people age 65 years and older will be 65 to 70 million. By the year 2030 the percentage of the total U.S. population age 65 or older is expected to reach 20 percent.

Especially striking is the increase in individuals in the more advanced age ranges. The number of people age 76 to 84 in 1990 exceeded 10 million, which is a gain of more than 30 percent of the number in 1980. The number of people age 85 or older in 1988 was more than 3 million, which is 23 times larger than in 1900 and a gain of 38 percent over the number in 1980. By the year 2000 the number reached 4.5 million. With further increases in longevity, the number of the "old" in the total U.S. population is expected to show further dramatic increases in the twenty-first century.

The gain in the number of elderly people in the United States over the years is reflected further in the dramatic increase in the median age of the country's population. In 1900 it was 22.9 years; in 1990 it was estimated to be 32.9 years and in 2000 35.3 years. The increase in the number of elderly people has been greater for females than for males, as might be expected given the longer life expectancy of women (*see* Life Expectancy). For women age 65 and older the percentage in the total population was 8.5 percent in 1950 and 14.7 percent in 1996.

Just as countries may be classified as "old" or "young" depending on the percentage of the population age 65 or older, so may the states of the United States. "Old" states are those in which the percentage of their population of elderly people exceeds the 13 percent of elderly people in the total population of the United States. The state with the highest percentage in 2005 was Florida (17.6 percent). Second was Pennsylvania (15.6 percent). Other old states are Arkansas, Missouri, Iowa, Kansas, Nebraska, and South

Dakota in the Midwest and Massachusetts and Maine in the East. "Young" states are those with less than 10 percent of their population made up of people age 65 or older. Included here are Texas, New Mexico, Colorado, Utah, Wyoming, and Nevada in the Southwest and West; Louisiana and Georgia in the South; and West Virginia in the East.

The increase in the elderly population of the United States has been accompanied by a change in their locations within states. By the late 1970s the majority of elderly people lived in metropolitan areas, rather than in small towns or rural areas, as was true for earlier periods. By the late 1980s only about one-fourth of elderly people lived in nonmetropolitan areas. Especially dense is the current population of elderly people in the suburbs of metropolitan areas, especially the older (established) suburbs. This means that suburban areas now carry the major burden of providing services and care for disadvantaged and needy elderly people, a responsibility once carried largely by inner cities.

Depression (Diagnostic Tests)

There are several widely used tests in which those taking the test give self-reports of the symptoms of depression. The Beck Depression Inventory is one in which the test taker rates on a four-point scale the intensity of various psychological and physical symptoms of depression. On the Zung Self-Rating Scale, people respond to such statements as "I am more irritable than usual" and "I feel downhearted, blue, and sad." The Center for Epidemiological Studies Depression Scale (CES-D) has twenty items representing various symptoms of depression (such as "I felt sad") in which the respondent rates the frequency of a particular symptom during the week before the test. Various problems arise in the use of these tests with elderly people. Perhaps the greatest problem is the likelihood that they will often yield high scores indicative of severe depression, largely through the presence of physical symptoms of depression on the tests (for instance, "My sleep was restless" on the CES-D scale and similar questions on the other tests). Such physical symptoms may be indicative of depression for younger adults, but they may simply be physical problems encountered by elderly people as part of normal aging.

In addition, the format of these tests in terms of forced choices or estimating frequencies of occurrence is one that discourages a number of elderly adults from completing the test. Some of the tests state some items positively and others negatively, a procedure that causes confusion for some elderly respondents. A recently published test, the Geriatric Depression Scale, was designed to avoid these problems. It has thirty yes/no items dealing only with psychological symptoms. Respondents answer questions about how they felt during the past week. There is evidence to indicate that elderly adults who take the test find it easy to complete.

Depression may also be diagnosed by means of clinical interviews by trained psychiatrists and psychologists. There are standard forms for the nature of the interview (such as the Hamilton Rating Scale for Depression).

Depression (Incidence, Symptoms, Causes)

Many adults at all age levels feel depressed at times. They feel depressed in the sense of having negative feelings (sadness, melancholy, or self-disparagement), often accompanied by apathy, difficulty in concentrating, difficulty in sleeping, and some loss of appetite. The duration of their depression, however, is usually fairly brief, and they return to a more normal state in which they have positive feelings about life and themselves. Clinical depression is another matter. Intense negative feelings persist for a long time, while the physical symptoms, such as loss of appetite, intensify. Some cognitive functions may also be adversely affected. Adaptation to the hassles of daily living becomes difficult, if not impossible.

A common belief is that the incidence of clinical depression is much greater for elderly adults than for younger adults. This belief received support from early studies revealing that as many as 65 percent of elderly adults report an excessively large number of depressive symptoms on self-report tests of depression (*see* Depression [Diagnostic Tests]). The problem with these early studies is that emotional symptoms (such as "I feel sad") were combined with physical symptoms ("I have difficulty sleeping") to yield a total symptom score. Physical symptoms such as difficulty in sleeping and loss of appetite may be symptoms of depression when present in younger adults. However, when present in elderly adults, they may simply be manifestations of normal aging.

More recent studies have revealed that the incidence of elderly adults who report excessively high nonphysical symptoms of depression is far less than 65 percent. For example, the percentage of elderly adults in their sixties who report depressive symptoms is usually found to be only from 15 percent to 20 percent (but it is somewhat higher for people age seventy-five or older). High scores on self-report tests do not necessarily indicate the presence of clinical depression. More intensive evaluations with psychiatric interviews of people of various ages generally indicate that the incidence of clinical depression among elderly adults may be quite low (perhaps no more than 5 percent). However, the percentage may be as high as 50 percent for those elderly people who are physically ill and 70 percent for those elderly people in nursing homes.

There is the danger that the incidence of clinical depression among elderly adults, especially those age seventy-five or older, may be underestimated. A diagnosis of dementia may be made in some elderly adults when their memory problems and lowered mental functioning may actually be caused by depression. The mental dysfunction may be confused with symptoms found in patients with Alzheimer's disease. An error in diagnosis could have disastrous consequences. Depression is a reversible disorder; Alzheimer's disease is not. Contemporary psychiatrists and clinical psychologists have found very effective treatments of clinical depression in late adulthood (*see* Depression [Treatment]). However, a major problem is that depression may go untreated in as many as 60 percent of the elderly people with depression. Much of the problem stems from the fact that Medicare pays reduced amounts for psychiatric and psychological treatment of emotional disorders, thus making this service unavailable to many depressed older people.

Melancholy and self-disparagement are the major emotional symptoms commonly associated with depression. However, there is evidence indicating that these symptoms are more likely to be present in depressed younger adults than in depressed elderly adults. For elderly adults, the emotional symptoms are more often those of apathy, a feeling of worthlessness, and a general sense of hopelessness with their lives. Dr. Margaret Gatz of the University of Southern California, an expert in the clinical psychology of aging, has speculated that elderly adults may have a form of depression that differs from what is commonly considered to be clinical depression. One possibility she proposes is what she calls a depletion syndrome, characterized by uninterest in life and a sense of hopelessness, but not the self-blame and guilt often found in younger clinically depressed adults.

The reasons for depression among elderly adults are many. Reduced income, for example, can be sufficiently stressful to produce depression. Elderly adults who are experiencing severe financial strain have been found to have more depressive symptoms than those elderly adults who are more financially secure. Loss of spouse and the occurrence of a physical disability are other possible causes that are more likely to be present in late adulthood than earlier in adulthood. Depression is likely to persist longer with the occurrence of a severely restricting physical disability than with the death of a spouse. Researchers at Duke University found that chronic physical disability is highly related to both physical and emotional symptoms for depressed elderly adults. However, disease does not seem to be a significant predictor of depression in elderly adults. Another common cause of depression among elderly adults is a major change in their social support system as a result of the deaths of friends, reduced physical mobility, and so on.

Depression is common among elderly adults with dementia. As many as 30 percent of patients with Alzheimer's disease have severe depression, and an even larger percentage is likely to have at least some depressive symptoms. Depression limits further the ability of such individuals to function well mentally. Older adults with depression before the onset of Alzheimer's disease are more likely to develop the disease than those without earlier depression. Some patients with mild degrees of dementia may be treated effectively for their depression (*see* Depression [Treatment]; Psychotherapy with Nursing Home Residents).

Depression (Performances with)

An important issue concerning depression among elderly adults is the extent to which it may impair their performances on a variety of mental and cognitive tasks. For most memory tasks, the evidence rather convincingly shows that the performance of depressed elderly adults does not differ greatly, if at all, from that of nondepressed elderly adults. For example, researchers at the University of Florida found that scores of depressed elderly participants on a depression test did not predict performance on tasks designed to simulate everyday memory tasks (memory for telephone numbers, memory for names, and so on). Researchers in Sweden even found that depression in very late adulthood (age ninety and older) did not affect performance on several memory tests.

Nevertheless, complaints about memory proficiency are more common among depressed than nondepressed elderly adults (37 percent depressed complainers and 22 percent nondepressed complainers in a study conducted in the Netherlands). Researchers at Pennsylvania State University have found that mnemonic training (*see* Memory Training) reduces the memory concerns of depressed elderly adults and may even reduce the degree of their depression as well.

On the other hand, there are some tasks on which depressed elderly adults may perform more poorly than the nondepressed, such as tasks that combine visual scanning with motor performance (for instance, the Trail Making Test; *see* Trail Making Test) and tasks that require spatial ability. Researchers in England also found that older adults who had nonclinical depression (that is, not overly severe) performed more poorly on tests of both crystallized and fluid intelligence (*see* Intelligence) than did nondepressed older adults.

Depression (Prognosis)

Once depression is treated, and presumably recovered from, the question remains, "Will the elderly patients stay free of depressive symptoms in the future?" That is, what is their prognosis? An Australian researcher found that 41 percent of older (age sixty and older) depressed patients remained recovered after four years following treatment. Another researcher in New York followed 127 patients who were age sixty and older for a year. Recovery was defined as eight continuous weeks with no evidence of symptoms or only minimal symptoms. Only 19 percent of the patients relapsed during the year. Patients who did not recover were those who were likely to have a spouse or adult children with psychiatric symptoms or who were in poor physical health.

Depression (Treatment)

Mild forms of depression are usually temporary and spontaneously disappear. By contrast, severe or clinical depression is likely to be a long-term disorder that requires treatment to remove the symptoms. The most effective treatment of clinical depression in young and middle-aged patients is by the administration of antidepressant drugs, such as heterocyclic antidepressants and Nardil, Norpramin, and Serzone. At one time Prozac was the most widely prescribed antidepressant drug, but there is currently little use for it in treating depression, especially for elderly adults.

Many elderly clinically depressed adults are required to take other drugs and medications that prevent the use of antidepressant drugs. In addition, antidepressants often have adverse side effects for many elderly people, especially when they receive improper dosages. A new antidepressant drug called SAMe is comparable to the other antidepressant drugs in its positive effects on depression, and it seems to have no side effects. In 2006 the U.S. Food and Drug Administration approved a selegiline transdermal patch to treat depression. The patch had previously been used in only the treatment of Parkinson's disease. When antidepressants are given to elderly patients, they have been found to reverse the symptoms of depression in more than 70 percent of cases.

An alternative to antidepressant drugs is the administration of electroconvulsive (ECT) or electroshock therapy. ECT therapy often results in some immediate symptom relief. When it is effective with elderly patients, it usually requires only a few administrations. ECT therapy is no longer considered to be as risky with elderly patients as it was once thought. However, patients with severe cardiovascular problems may be advised against its use because of the transient increase in blood pressure that often occurs with ETC therapy. In addition, ECT therapy often creates some memory problems that may add to those produced by aging.

Psychotherapy, particularly cognitive therapy, is the major alternative for those elderly patients who are at risk with either drug therapy or ECT therapy (see Psychotherapy). In addition, cognitive therapy has also been found to relieve depressive symptoms for some patients with mild dementia or mental impairment as well as depression (see Psychotherapy with Nursing Home Residents). Psychotherapy is also often used in conjunction with either drug or ECT therapy to accelerate the treatment effects. In a study by researchers at the University of Pittsburgh Medical School, groups of depressed older patients (age sixty and older) received either a combination of an antidepressant drug and psychotherapy, the drug alone, psychotherapy alone, or a placebo only. The combination of drug and psychotherapy prevented a recurrence of depression in nearly 80 percent of the combination group, compared to 57 percent in the drug-only group, 36 percent in the psychotherapy-only group, and 19 percent in the placebo group.

Drug therapy and psychotherapy have also been used to treat a milder form of depression. Seniors receiving the drug seem to show greater decrease in the symptoms than those receiving psychotherapy.

Dr. Dolores Gallagher-Thompson of the Older Adult and Family Center at the Palo Alto, California, Veterans Administration Medical Center has developed a behavioral intervention that teaches depressed elderly patients practical coping skills, such as cognitive reframing (getting rid of unproductive thinking patterns), assertiveness, and relaxation. There is a manual for therapists and a workbook for patients. Interestingly, exposing depressed patients to a bright light periodically was found by researchers at Cornell Medical School to improve the benefits of antidepressant drugs.

There is evidence that moderate exercise may reduce depressive symptoms. For example, in a Canadian study a group of moderately depressed elderly women participated in a walking exercise program for six weeks. Three sessions were held each week; the duration of the early sessions was twenty minutes, and the duration of later sessions was forty minutes. After six weeks a significant decrease in depressive symptoms, both physical and psychological, was found, on average, for the participants. In addition, Australian researchers have found that high-intensity progressive-resistance exercise training is an effective way of treating older clinically depressed patients. There is also evidence indicating that combining mild exercise with listening to music and imagining pleasant things further reduces symptoms of depression in elderly adults.

Researchers at St. Louis University have discovered a biological alternative to medication in the treatment of severe depression. They invented a device that delivers electrical stimulation to the brain via stimulation of the vagus nerve. The stimulation appears to activate several parts of the brain involved in depression, including the prefrontal cortex. The device was approved by the FDA for adults who have tried at least four antidepressant drugs without improvement.

Depth Perception

When you look at an object you are able, usually immediately, to identify three attributes of it: its height, its width, and its depth. What makes the perception of depth truly remarkable is the fact that you are seeing a third dimension even though the image of the object on the retina (inner layer of the eye) is cast in only two dimensions. You perceive depth because of several cues provided by the eye that provide you with the necessary information to "see" a third dimension. For example, your two eyes are separated by several inches; therefore, the image of an object on the retina of the left eye is slightly different from the image of the same object on the retina of the right eye. This slight difference provides important information that your brain knows how to interpret. Even people with only one functional eye have depth perception to some degree. This is because other kinds of cues from either eye alone provide further information of depth that is interpreted by the brain.

The proficiency of depth perception varies among individuals. This may be seen by measuring depth-perception proficiency through the use of a device similar to the one used to test vision to obtain a driver's license. You look at three vertical bars projected on an illuminated screen and are asked to make decisions about these bars in a number of test trials. For example, is bar X in front of or behind the other two bars? Research with this device has revealed that age differences make up a major portion of the individual differences in depth perception.

Young adults, in general, are quite proficient. This proficiency shows little decline for people until they reach their fifties. At this age the decline is rather large. However, further decline with aging, at least through the seventies, seems to be modest. Distance perception is closely related to depth perception. Perceiving an object in depth, of course, means that you are aware that some parts of the object are at a greater distance from you than other parts. Older people are likely to have some difficulty in judging distances of objects. Certain problems in everyday living are the likely consequence. For example, parallel parking becomes more difficult because it requires judging distances between nearby cars and the car being parked. Diminished depth perception is also a likely contributor to the increased incidence of falls among elderly people.

Deteriorating Neighborhoods

If littering, vandalism, crime, and drug use are increasing in a neighborhood, the stress experienced by its residents is likely to increase. The decline of a neighborhood affects senior residents the most. The problems occurring in the neighborhood may prevent them from leaving their homes, and they are likely to feel vulnerable and isolated. This can lead to anger, depression, and anxiety, as well as various physical symptoms.

Surprisingly, the amount of support received from friends and relatives does little to reduce these symptoms. Other conditions need to be discovered—conditions that are more effective in reducing the stress produced by living in a deteriorating neighborhood.

Diabetes

Type 1 diabetes develops when the body's immune system destroys pancreatic cells that are the only cells that make the hormone insulin. Insulin regulates the body's blood glucose level. Children and young adults are the ones who usually have the disease, although its onset can occur at any age. It accounts for 5 percent to 10 percent of the diagnosed cases of diabetes.

Type 2 diabetes was once called non-insulin-dependent diabetes mellitus or adult-onset diabetes. It accounts for 90 percent to 95 percent of all cases of diabetes. It is especially prevalent for seniors, African Americans, and Hispanics. Type 2 diabetes is a lifelong disease that develops when the pancreas cannot produce enough insulin or when the body's tissues become resistant to insulin. Consequently, the blood sugar level rises above the safe level.

Signs of diabetes may include extreme thirst, frequent urination, unusual tiredness, and an unexpected weight loss. Diabetes may lead to blindness, heart attack, stroke, kidney failure, and amputation. Unfortunately, detection of Type 2 diabetes in elderly people may be difficult unless they have regular physical examinations that include tests for diabetes. Often the disease is not detected until elderly people experience conditions such as blurred vision caused by their diabetic condition. Less than half of older diabetics are given a test to check for degeneration in the retina of the eyes.

Diet and exercise (for instance, moderate levels of strength training) enable many Type 2 diabetics to keep their condition under control. They may also reduce the risk of healthy seniors developing the disease. However, about one-third of seniors with the disease require either drugs or insulin to maintain control of their blood sugar levels.

Considerable progress is being made in the diagnosis and treatment of diabetes, including the use of inhaled insulin devices to replace injections. For more information about diabetes, visit the Web site of the American Diabetes Association (http://www.diabetes.org) or the division of the National Institutes of Health that deals with diabetes (http://diabetes. niddk. nih.gov).

Diary Keeping

Keeping a daily diary has been a tradition for centuries. Seniors who keep one seem to cope better with stress than those who do not. In effect, it is a form of self-therapy in which the keepers work out daily hassles on paper. Writing about yourself also gives you confidence in knowing that you have something that is important enough to be on paper.

Diary Studies of Memory Failures

Asking people of various ages to keep a daily diary in which they record each day's memory failures is one means of studying age differences in memory performances. Of interest is the extent of the probable increase in the number of everyday memory failures from early to late adulthood. Critics of laboratory studies of age differences in memory performances have argued that the memory tasks encountered in the laboratory, such as memorizing lists of words, are too artificial to indicate how memory operates in the everyday world. They believe that studies conducted with these tasks tend to overestimate the extent to which memory proficiency (especially episodic memory proficiency; *see* Episodic Memory) declines with normal aging. Diary studies offer an alternative to laboratory studies in determining the extent to which memory is affected by normal aging.

Several diary studies of age differences in memory have been conducted. In the most comprehensive of these studies, the participants ranged in age from twenty to seventy-six. For an extended period of time participants recorded in their diaries each day's failures to remember such things as an item they forgot to purchase at the supermarket. The older participants reported themselves to be more upset about their memory failures than did the younger ones (younger adults are likely to take the imperfections of memory in stride). The number of memory failures actually recorded was only moderately greater for the older than for the younger participants.

This difference must be interpreted cautiously, however. Diary recordings may underestimate the magnitude of memory problems facing elderly adults. If people older than age seventy-six had been included in the study, the age difference may have been much greater. Moreover, older adults may forget their own memory failures more frequently than younger adults, and therefore fail to record all of them. It seems reasonable to conclude that laboratory studies do provide fairly realistic estimates of age differences in episodic memory performances. Diary studies reflect the fact that many normally aging elderly people are concerned about their memory problems, perhaps much more than necessary (*see* Memory Complaints).

Disability (Adaptation)

Researchers at the University of Toronto studied nearly three hundred women age fifty-five and older who were disabled from osteoarthritis or osteoporosis. They found that the women used a wide range of adaptations to their disability. They were not helpless. Instead, they employed many self-care efforts to manage their condition. The form of adaptation varied with the type of activity. For example, for discretionary activities, they often limited their participation. By contrast, for personal care and mobility, they turned to forms of compensation, such as using gadgets or assistive devices. *See also* Disability (Assistance with Activities of Daily Living).

Disability (Assistance with Activities of Daily Living)

Some people with a disability receive no help for performing the activities of daily living (for instance, dressing or toileting), and some receive not enough help. Researchers at Brown University discovered that women in the eighteen-to-forty-four-year age range were more likely to have inadequate help than older women or men. For those receiving no help, neither age nor sex was a factor. However, those divorced, separated, or never married were more likely to have no help. African Americans were more likely than whites to have no help.

Disability (Educational Level)

Researchers at the National Institute on Aging provided evidence showing that disability is greater for adults age sixty-five to eighty-four who have less education than for adults of the same age range with more education. However, recovery from disability was not found to be related to educational level.

Disability (Effect of Social Support)

More than four thousand people in North Carolina who were age sixty-five and older were followed for seven years to determine if social networks and support from friends affect the incidence of disability. Social interactions with friends were associated with a reduced risk of disability. However, social interaction with relatives was not associated with the reduced risk of disability.

Disability (Incidence and Assistance)

There are two ways to define disability, both of which may be used to estimate the number of older people who have a disability. The first is based on the presence of an illness that produces long-term physical impairments. The second way is in terms of an individual's ability to perform critical physical activities of daily living. These activities include feeding oneself and dressing oneself (*see* Activities of Daily Living).

Researchers at Miami University used the latter method to estimate the percentage of elderly people affected by a disability. They further classified disability into severe disability and moderate disability. Severe disability occurs when an individual has impairments of two or more important physical activities of daily living, and moderate disability when only one such activity is impaired. Information from 1986 census figures enabled the researchers to estimate separately the percentages of people in the sixty-five-to-seventy-four-year age range, people in the seventy-five-to-eighty-four-year age range, and people age eighty-five and older having disabilities. The percentages of people with severe disability were 4.4 percent in the sixty-five-to-seventy-four-year age range, 9.9 percent in the seventy-five-to-eighty-four-year age range, and 28.9 percent in those eighty-five and older. Comparable percentages for moderate disability were 5.8 percent, 11 percent, and 21.3 percent. With one exception, the percentage of women with a disability was only modestly greater than that of men. The exception was for severe disability in the eighty-five-and-older age range; the percentage was 21.7 percent for men and 31.7 percent for women.

Elderly women are more likely to receive assistance from other people than are elderly men. Elderly women and elderly men, however, do not seem to differ in the extent to which they receive assistance from devices, such as walkers and raised toilet seats. For people age sixty-five and older, the probability of developing a disability is estimated to be 35 percent higher for those without private non-Medicare insurance than for those with it.

According to the National Long Term Care Survey there was a decline in disability from 1982 to 1994. The decline presumably resulted from reductions in various health problems, such as circulatory diseases, and from better knowledge about health in the total population.

Researchers in New York investigated the hours of assistance received by disabled elderly people. Compared to those who are helped only by non-relatives, those with a network of assistance from a spouse and children have forty additional hours of help per week. Those with a network of children received only twenty-nine additional hours of help per week if the disabled individual resided with other adults and ten hours if not. *See also* Obesity (Effects on Longevity and Disability); Sarcopenia.

Disability (Psychological and Social Consequences)

Disability caused by illness or an accident is a major source of stress for those elderly people who experience it. They are likely to experience considerable distress, low self-esteem, and low life satisfaction. These negative consequences of disability appear to have a longer duration than those found with other sources of stress for elderly people, such as bereavement. Researchers at Arizona State University found that depression was less pronounced for bereaved elderly persons than for disabled elderly persons.

Adjustment to a disability typically progresses through four phases or stages. The first consists of shock, in which disabled individuals are likely to have diminished mental functioning to the point that they may even be unaware of their condition and are likely to be dependent on others to care for them. The second phase is called defensive retreat. At this point, disabled individuals realize that they have a disability, and they are likely to be frightened greatly by it. They are also likely to begin coping with and adjusting to their disability. During this period they often deny the permanence and severity of the disability. To maintain this denial they may avoid any behavior that may call attention to their disability. This may even include avoiding social interactions with family members and friends and avoiding appearances in public for fear of embarrassment. After a while, denial becomes ineffective in eliminating stress, and a phase called acknowledgment begins. It is during this phase that anxiety, grief, and depression are most pronounced. The final phase is called adaptation—one that will last for the remainder of the disability. Disabled individuals usually learn to cope with their disabilities and to live satisfactory lives, including renewing old friendships, finding new friends, increasing social interactions, and participating in volunteer and community services (for instance, helping other people who recently became disabled to cope with their disabilities). It is during the early period of this phase that various forms of psychotherapy are especially useful to disabled older people.

Researchers at the University of Pittsburgh have discovered that the amount of social support and social contact of disabled elderly people is strongly related to their well-being and their ability to function in the community. Depression among disabled elderly people was found to be lowest for those who were optimistic about the future and believed that they could control important events in their lives (*see* Control over Life's Events). Other researchers have reported that lower feelings of well-being for elderly disabled men are associated with greater reliance both on others and on devices for aiding their activities. By contrast, lower feelings of well-being for elderly disabled women were found to be associated with reliance on devices but not with reliance on other people.

Self-care coping strategies tend to increase as the severity of disability increases, except for the most severely disabled. These strategies include the use of devices and appropriate risk-avoiding behaviors. Increase in the use of these strategies has also been found to be related positively to the amount of assistance received from other people.

Discourse Memory

You have just finished reading an interesting novel. The plot centers on a man living in a medium-size town who, because of a strange genetic mutation, has become a vampire. His affliction is eventually cured by the love he feels for a small child living nearby. The child's widowed mother falls in love with the vampire, and they eventually marry.

How much of the story are you likely to remember? Even some time later you will probably recall the central theme of the story ("A vampire is cured by his love for a child"). You may even remember major subplots ("The vampire marries the child's widowed mother"). However, you probably will not remember much of the more detailed information, even after you just finished reading the story.

The summary statements you have in your memory are called *propositions* by memory researchers. A proposition is an abstraction of information that summarizes content. Propositions differ in *levels*. The highest-level proposition is one that summarizes the central theme of the story ("A vampire is cured by his love of a child"). Intermediate-level propositions are those that summarize more important subplots ("The vampire marries the child's widowed mother"). Low-level propositions are those that deal with more trivial information ("The action takes place in the city of Aorta, Texas"). Propositions are encoded and transmitted to your memory store by the very nature of your comprehension of what you read. This is usually accomplished incidentally. We have memory for content without the intent to remember it or to rehearse the content actively.

The later retrieval of these stored propositions enables you to describe the story to someone else. Propositions are also the content in memory of informative articles we read in a newspaper, magazine, or encyclopedia. For example, after reading an article about a new treatment for arthritis, you may remember the general nature of the treatment, but have difficulty recalling a number of the details.

Memory researchers refer to the memory of stories and articles as *discourse memory*. Age differences in discourse memory are studied by having younger and older participants read an unfamiliar story or article (usually several hundred words in length) and then having them paraphrase the content.

In general, the results of many studies have indicated little age difference in memory for high-level propositions, a moderate age difference favoring younger participants for intermediate propositions, and a more pronounced age difference favoring younger participants for low-level propositions. This is usually the case whether the content read is narrative (a story) or expository (an article). The inability to recall more trivial details should not concern older people. Such details are usually unimportant. One could always reread the story or article if there is a need to recover the information. In addition, older adults often go beyond the specific content of a story or article and find moral implications and lessons to be learned from what they have read that younger adults do not find (*see* Continuity versus Discontinuity in Adult Development). *See also* Longitudinal Studies of Aging's Effects on Physical Health and Cognition.

Diseases (Acute and Chronic)

Diseases may be classified into two broad categories: acute and chronic. *Acute diseases* are those that have a rapid onset and a short duration, usually from a few days to a few weeks. They include the common cold as well as influenza and pneumonia (*see* Influenza; Pneumonia).

A myth about aging is that people age sixty-five or older have the highest incidence rates of acute diseases. In reality, young adults have the highest rates for most acute diseases, including the common cold. Even such conditions as sprains and muscle strains have a higher yearly incidence rate among young adults than among elderly adults. Diseases such as sinusitis and hay fever are usually not disabling. Sinusitis is an inflammation of a sinus (an air cavity in one of the cranial bones). Hay fever is an intense nasal catarrh (inflammation of a mucous membrane brought about by an allergic reaction to a foreign substance, such as a particular pollen). Both sinusitis and hay fever are more prevalent in the forty-five-to-seventy-four-year age range than any other age range, and especially for women.

Chronic diseases have a slower onset and a longer duration than acute diseases. They include many various forms of cancer, different kinds of cardiovascular disease, arthritis, emphysema, and diabetes. The chronic diseases that are especially prevalent in late adulthood are discussed in separate entries (for example, *see* Breast Cancer; Diabetes). Chronic diseases account for nearly all deaths that do not result from an accident, suicide, or murder. Cardiovascular diseases are the leading cause of death among people age sixty-five or older, followed by cancer, stroke, and influenza/pneumonia. Although it is true that if all diseases were to be eliminated today, many more people would live to old age, it is also true that the average length of life would probably increase by no more than ten to fifteen years.

Disengagement Theory

During the 1950s an extensive survey of elderly people living in Kansas City was conducted. One of the major products of that survey was the development of what became known as disengagement theory. The investigators found that elderly adults commonly withdraw to some degree from their earlier social roles and activities, including their involvements with other people. In effect, their increased self-preoccupation produces social "disengagement." It was theorized at the time that society *expects* elderly adults to show such individual disengagement and demonstrates this expectancy by withdrawing its interest in elderly people. Elderly adults who succeeded in conforming to the disengagement expected of them by society were viewed as being more satisfied with their lives than elderly adults who continued to strive for social engagement.

Disengagement theory is clearly contrary to the notion that keeping active is the most effective way of combating the adverse effects of aging. Not surprisingly, the theory stimulated considerable research, most of which has refuted the theory. Disengagement may have been common in the 1950s when there was little concern about the welfare, both financial and psychological, of elderly people. More recent years have seen dramatic changes in society's treatment of older people, most of which have been beneficial to them. Disengagement is no longer the route elderly people are encouraged by society to follow, and conditions likely to enhance life satisfaction have changed greatly. The need for elderly adults to remain socially active is now emphasized (*see* Activity Theory).

Disuse Principle

A familiar theme in gerontology is that mental skills and abilities become "rusty" if they are not used regularly, and therefore a decline in proficiency occurs. Elderly adults, in general, are commonly believed to use these skills less often than do younger adults, presumably because elderly adults are faced with fewer demands to use them than are younger adults (for instance, in job performances). Consequently, elderly adults are affected more by the negative effects of disuse than are younger adults. Conceivably, the remedy for overcoming the negative effects of disuse is prolonged practice of a given task. It is hoped that, with such practice, elderly adults will eventually recover their earlier skill and begin to perform as well as most younger adults. This would be true if the actual skill or ability to perform the task had not declined with aging—it had simply become "rusty" for lack of use, an impairment that could be remedied by the practice needed to restore its original state.

Several researchers have discovered that elderly adults do indeed greatly improve their performances on various kinds of tasks with practice. One of these tasks is the digit symbol substitution task. Participants receive rows of boxes in which different digits, such as 1 and 2, are placed in the tops of the boxes. The participants are given a code, such as 1 = * and 2 = <, and they are asked to write in the bottom of each box the symbol that codes the digit it contains. After one hundred trials on this task, researchers at the University of Wisconsin at Milwaukee found that their elderly participants had increased the number of substitutions they could complete by more than 30 percent. However, they also found that their young adult participants also increased their number completed by more than 30 percent. As a result, the age difference in number of substitutions completed favoring the young participants was as great after one hundred trials as it was on the first trial.

It seems likely that the age difference in performance on this task is the result of a moderate decline in ability with aging and is not simply the result of the lack of recent use of that ability by elderly adults. Researchers at the University of Missouri at Columbia reported similar outcomes for several other tasks in which the participants received hundreds of practice trials. Practice improves performance regardless of age, but usually no more for elderly adults than for younger adults.

However, there is one other important result of these practice studies. At the end of a lengthy practice period, elderly participants have consistently been found to perform at a level characteristic of young adult participants at the beginning of practice. Practice may not make performance perfect, but it does have the potential for making the performances of elderly adults equivalent to those of young adults who have not had the benefit of similar amounts of practice.

Disuse has also been used in a more general sense to refer to the possibility of diminished mental activity in late adulthood and the negative effects in performance such disuse may have on a wide variety of mental tasks—that is, the "rustiness" may affect performance on virtually any demanding mental task. In question is the benefit of "mental exercise" in overcoming such "rustiness" (*see* Activity [Mental] and Mental Performance).

Diverticulitis

Diverticulitis refers to the bulging of pouches (called diverticula) in the outer wall of the colon. About half of people age sixty and older have it. It is caused by the lack of dietary fiber that would add moisture in undigested food. If the diverticula become inflamed, you are likely to experience severe stomach pain, nausea, and vomiting and should consult your physician. *See also* Flaxseed.

Divided Attention

Many times during an ordinary day you are in situations that require you to divide your attention between two or more ongoing events. While driving, you are listening to the car radio (or, dangerously, answering your ringing cell phone) while watching the traffic around you. When introduced to someone at a party, you may be trying to attend not only to that person's name but also to the conversation behind you. Is dividing attention (or, more likely, alternating rapidly between simultaneous events) more difficult for elderly people than for younger people? Is there an age difference in the ability to "program" attention so that it may be divided between two events in such a way that attention to either event is not greatly diminished?

Research on age differences in divided attention began in the early 1960s with the *dichotic listening task*. Participants hear successive pairs of digits, with one member delivered to the left ear and the other member delivered at the same time to the right ear. For example, they hear 3 (left ear) and 6 (right ear), followed by 7 (left ear) and 4 (right ear), and then 1 (left ear) and 8 (right ear). Note that as each pair is presented, the participants must divide their attention between the left ear and the right ear. After the last pair is presented, the participants attempt to recall the digits, one ear at a time. For some sequences of pairs they may be asked to recall first what was heard in the left ear, and then recall what was heard in the right ear. For other sequences, the order is reversed (that is, the right ear first).

In general, digits delivered to the right ear tend to be recalled better than digits delivered to the left ear. This is an example of what is called the *right-ear advantage*, an advantage found for adults of all ages. The right-ear advantage results from the fact that messages delivered to the right ear are transmitted directly to the left cerebral hemisphere of the brain where language centers are located for most people. By contrast, messages delivered to the left ear are transmitted directly to the right cerebral hemisphere and must then be relayed to the language centers in the left hemisphere.

Elderly adults perform more poorly on the dichotic listening task than do younger adults. However, their poorer performance is found mainly for the left ear, with little age difference in memory for what was heard in the right ear. This complicates any conclusion that can be reached about a declining ability in dividing attention with normal aging. The age difference in performance on this task could be the result of greater degeneration of the right hemisphere than the left hemisphere with normal aging (*see* Brain and Aging). In addition, the age difference in dichotic listening performance could be largely the result of memory deficits that accompany aging rather than divided attention deficits.

Not surprisingly, more recent research has turned to other kinds of tasks to determine whether there are indeed age differences in the ability to divide attention. For example, in a recent study participants were given a visual and an auditory task to perform. Two different versions of the tasks were constructed, one easy, the other difficult. On some trials, one task was performed alone—sometimes the easy visual task, other times the difficult visual task, or the easy or difficult auditory task. Two tasks had to be performed on other trials. Sometimes the two tasks consisted of the easy visual task and the easy auditory task. At other times the easy visual task was performed along with the difficult auditory task (or the easy auditory task with the difficult visual task). Finally, on some trials the two difficult tasks were performed together.

Evidence from this study, and other recent studies using related procedures, indicates that elderly participants, like young participants, experience little difficulty when two easy tasks are performed together. Both tasks are performed nearly as well when combined as when they are performed alone. However, the more difficult the combined tasks, the greater the advantage favoring young adults. Thus, performance of the two difficult tasks when performed together, relative to their performance singly, is especially difficult for elderly participants. Provided the two tasks are relatively easy, little difficulty in performing them together would be expected with aging. This would be the case, for example, in dividing attention between the car radio and watching the traffic flow when traffic is very light.

As one or both tasks become more difficult, elderly adults, on average, would be expected to have greater difficulty than younger adults in dividing attention between the two. This would be the case when the traffic flow is heavy. At this point, it would probably be a greater advantage for the older driver than for the younger driver to turn off the radio (or tell a passenger to be quiet) and concentrate on the traffic alone. *See also* Attention and Stroke Recovery; Attention (Overview); Bingo.

Divorce

Divorce occurs most frequently for people in the age range of thirty to forty-five. The incidence of divorce is higher for those people who marry before the age of twenty than for those who marry after age twenty. Although divorce is less common for elderly adults than for younger adults, its incidence is, nevertheless, fairly high. It is estimated that more than half a million people age sixty-five or older are divorced, and that about an additional ten thousand elderly people join the ranks of the divorced annually.

Divorce is usually a stressful event for elderly people—more so, on average, than it is for younger people. Divorce is less a normative (or expected) event in late adulthood than in earlier adulthood. In general, divorce is likely to be more stressful to elderly people than is widowhood or widowerhood (which is a normative event in late adulthood; *see* Widowhood and Widowerhood). Surveys of divorced people of various ages indicate that, immediately after separation, older people tend to show greater negative emotions and unhappiness and fewer positive emotional experiences than younger people do.

Negative life events are usually followed by a decline in life satisfaction. However, the decline for most such events is only temporary. Those affected tend to rebound to the level of life satisfaction they had before the event. Divorce seems to be the exception for older people. The decline in life satisfaction does show a rebound for most divorced seniors, but the rebound is not sufficient to raise life satisfaction to the level it was before the divorce.

In general, people age fifty and older show the most maladaptive behavior after separation. People in their forties more closely approximate the functioning level of young adults after separation. Elderly men tend to show greater unhappiness after divorce and greater change in their perceived health status than do elderly women. However, older women tend to have more psychological symptoms and appear to be more disorganized after divorce than elderly men. Elderly women also tend to express greater dissatisfaction with their lives for more years before the divorce than do elderly men.

In general, elderly women tend to show improvement in physical health status after divorce, seemingly reflecting their release from what they may perceive to have been confining lives. However, there is also evidence that, over the long term, elderly women may experience more problems in their postdivorce lives than do elderly divorced men. Part of the problem facing many elderly divorced women is their poor financial status. A 1989 survey revealed that more than a fourth of divorcées age sixty-two and older had incomes below the official poverty level. Only 4 percent of elderly divorcées received any alimony payments, and only 23 percent had an income from both Social Security and an employer pension plan.

Divorce is usually a crisis situation for elderly people. Both spouses would profit greatly from psychological counseling at least as much as, if not more than, younger divorced people. Of course, divorce is an alternative to what is usually an unhappy marriage. Researchers in California have found that there is a relationship between marital satisfaction and health, one that is stronger for women than for men. In unhappy marriages, elderly wives tend to report more mental health and physical health problems than do their husbands.

There is another aspect of divorce that has important implications for elderly people. Of concern is the effect of divorce in early adulthood on relationships years later with the now adult children. In general, these adult children have less contact with both elderly parents, and their relationships with both parents are more negative, than is the case for adult children whose parents stayed together while they were growing up. Negative relationships are likely to be more pronounced with fathers than with mothers. In addition, adult children are likely to feel less loved by divorced fathers than by divorced mothers. *See also* Stress and Coping with Stress.

Dizziness

Dizziness is a problem for many elderly adults in which they feel light-headedness. The light-headedness is caused by insufficient blood reaching the brain, a condition brought about by a sudden drop in blood pressure or from dehydration. It is estimated that dizziness results in eight million outpatient visits per year in the United States. It occurs more often among the old than among the young and more among women than among men. It is often associated with anxiety or depression. Dizziness can become a long-lasting condition that may be associated with disability. Researchers in Chicago interviewed more than six thousand adults age sixty-five and older. Dizziness in their study was defined as an episode of light-headedness at least once a month. The incidence increased from 6.6 percent in the sixty-five-to-seventy-four age range to 18.4 percent in the eighty-five-and-older age range.

Dizziness may also result from a problem in the inner ear's vestibular system that helps to maintain the body's balance. The number of nerve hair cells in the vestibular system decreases with aging, beginning at about age fifty-five. The decrease in the number of cells increases in severity as aging progresses, and it is accompanied by other changes in the vestibular system. Several different forms of dizziness known as vertigo may be the result of these changes. Vertigo, in general, is characterized by feelings of spinning and being in motion.

A common form of vertigo is labyrinthitis, a condition that may occur after influenza or a severe ear infection caused by irritation of the hair cells that are in the labyrinths (fluid-filled canals of the vestibular system). Another common form of vertigo is benign paroxysmal positional vertigo that is caused by small loose particles floating in the fluid. Ménière's disease is a less common form of vertigo associated with ringing in the ears and progressive hearing loss.

Vertigo is treatable by vestibular therapy and various medications. Consult your physician if you are experiencing frequent light-headedness or vertigo. *See also* Falls; Postural Change and Orthostasis; Syncope.

Domestic Violence

See Elder Abuse.

Drivers (Having Passengers)

The presence of passengers in an automobile may have either a positive or a negative effect on senior drivers. The positive effect may come when a passenger alerts an older driver about a dangerous driving condition that could cause an accident. The negative effect may result when a passenger distracts an older driver and directs his or her attention away from road conditions. This could result in a serious accident.

Researchers at Lakehead University in Ontario, Canada, analyzed data from the United States Fatality Analysis Reporting System. They discovered that the presence of a passenger reduced the number of unsafe actions by older drivers relative to driving with no passengers by 11 percent for drivers age eighty and older. This reduction could be even greater if passengers avoid distractions that cause an older driver to miss road signs and other warnings. *See also* Accidents (Automobile); Divided Attention.

Drivers (Improving Their Skills)

AARP has a training program, called AARP 55 Alive, for drivers age fifty and older to help them improve their driving skills and perhaps recapture some lost skills, especially for elderly drivers. The program has had more than six million participants since its inception in 1979. There are eight hours of classroom instruction that stress physical changes with aging that affect driving skills and ways of compensating for those changes. For more information, call 888-227-7669 or visit the program's Web site at http://www.aarp.org/55alive.

Driver's License Renewal

You recently turned seventy-nine. On your birthday you received notice that you need to renew your driver's license. "What, already?" you thought. "I just did this three years ago. My sister who is sixty-nine doesn't have to renew for six years." You are one of many older people caught in what is called accelerated renewal for older people. Sixteen states require older adults to renew their license after fewer years than younger drivers. The age when this begins is usually seventy years, but in some states it is older. Also, in some states it is less than every three years.

Is accelerated renewal for older drivers a form of age discrimination? Probably not, given the fact that older drivers do have a higher probability of an automobile accident than drivers of all other ages except teenage drivers (*see* Accidents [Automobile]). But what is accomplished by having more frequent renewals unless there are procedures employed to identify which older drivers have the greatest risk of an accident? One such procedure is to require a visual test. Declining visual ability is a contributing factor to the greater accident rate of older drivers. But is it age discrimination when drivers of all ages are required to take the visual test on each renewal? Only five states require the visual test for older drivers only.

Why not require older drivers to take a road test? Two states do have this requirement—but only for drivers age seventy-five and older. Is a road test for only older drivers a form of age discrimination? Perhaps not. However, it is not very practical. Should it be given only in fair weather or only in foul weather? Should it be given only in busy traffic or only in minimal traffic? A better procedure would be the use of a driving simulator in which driving proficiency could be tested in a wide variety of conditions.

Driving (Activity after Cessation or Reduction)

Some older drivers voluntarily cease driving. Does this affect their out-of-home activities? Researchers have found that it presents a handicap for many former drivers. Activities such as shopping, going to a restaurant, attending religious services, and playing bridge may be greatly restricted. Alternative means of transportation need to be found before they give up driving. However, even with alternatives, the quality of their lives may never be the same as it was when they were driving.

Researchers have found that the cessation of driving, or even a major reduction in the amount of driving, is a sufficiently negative event to cause symptoms of depression for many former drivers. Even having a spouse serve as their driver had little effect on relieving the depression. The loss of independence is very difficult to tolerate for many older former drivers.

If retraining of driving skills does not restore driving, then friends and relatives of former drivers need to offer positive support in the form of reminding the former drivers of the benefits they have gained by no longer driving. These include the saving of considerable money for gasoline, mechanical service, and insurance and the avoidance of future fender benders. If depression continues to worsen anyway, the former drivers should be encouraged to seek professional counseling.

Driving (Identifying Cognitively Unqualified Drivers)

It is very important to have ways of identifying those individuals whose cognitive abilities have declined to a level that they present a sufficient safety risk to prohibit further driving. Accomplishing this objective is not easy, however.

The most obvious way is to give a road test to see how their abilities operate under actual driving conditions. The tester accompanying the driver should then be in the position of evaluating the skills of the driver, sufficiently so to recommend whether they should continue driving.

This method does have problems. Evaluating a driver's skills is somewhat subjective and dependent on the tester's evaluation skills and perhaps even his or her mood that day.

A more effective method is to use a driving simulator in which various driving conditions may be introduced. This procedure offers a more objective means of evaluating driving skills.

There are a number of neuropsychological tests that might further test the kinds of skills needed for driving. Many of these tests have been used in a number of studies with drivers who have Alzheimer's disease. They include tests of attention, memory, and visuospatial ability. Scores on these tests have been correlated with scores earned by drivers on road tests and simulated driving tests.

Researchers at the Veterans Affairs Puget Sound Health Care System in Tacoma, Washington, recently reviewed twenty-seven of these studies. They concluded that of all of the tests tried in these studies, tests of visuospatial ability correlated the highest with both kinds of driving tests. Visuospatial ability is the ability to integrate disparate visual information into a meaningful whole. It affects driving by determining a driver's judgment of distances and maneuvering of an automobile's position. One of these tests is the Clock Drawing Test (*see* Clock Drawing Test). It has been found to correlate significantly with driving proficiency. *See also* Driver's License Renewal.

Driving (Why Many Seniors Limit or Quit Driving)

Older women are more likely to reduce their driving or to stop driving completely than are older men. Why would any senior, woman or man, want to reduce or quit driving? Driving is very important for most seniors in order to maintain their independence. What physical, social, and psychological factors lead to the decline in driving?

Researchers at the University of California at Berkeley asked several thousand adults age fifty-five and older who had limited or quit driving to identify from a list of twenty-one reasons (fourteen medical and seven non-medical) one or more reasons for their decision. A problem with eyesight was the most frequent medical reason given by both women and men.

Nearly 49 percent of the women age seventy-five and older reported it. No other medical reason had a frequency greater than 7 percent.

Two nonmedical reasons were identified by both women and men. One was the fear of being in an accident (27 percent of the women and 17 percent of the men age seventy-five and older). The other was having no reason to drive (18 percent of the women and 17 percent of the men age seventy-five and older). Women, but not men, frequently reported concern about crime (17 percent of the women and 4 percent of the men age seventy-five and older).

Drug Abuse

Researchers of drug abuse generally agree that, relative to younger people, the use of illegal drugs (for instance, marijuana) by older people is rare. The main problem for community-dwelling elderly people is the misuse of legal drugs, both those prescribed by physicians and those bought over the counter. However, the problem is more likely to be the underuse of prescribed drugs than the overuse. By contrast, elderly people in nursing homes are often the victims of overuse as a result of physicians' instructions to "administer as needed" and by error in the administration of drugs.

Researchers at the University of California at Berkeley have compared normally aging misusers and nonmisusers of drugs on a number of psychological characteristics. In general, misusers did not differ from nonmisusers on most characteristics, including the number of "hassles" or stresses they had experienced. However, misusers reported that they experienced their hassles more intensely than nonmisusers, and they also reported greater dissatisfaction with their ability to cope with stressors than did nonmisusers.

Drug Tests (Clinical Trials)

New drugs that may aid patients in combating a physical or a mental disorder are constantly being discovered. Before these drugs are made available to the general public by the U.S. Food and Drug Administration, they must pass a series of rigorous clinical tests to determine whether they are actually beneficial and whether they may have harmful side effects.

Testing usually starts with animals. If these tests are successful, the next step is likely to be tests with healthy volunteers who are free of the disorder for which the drug is intended. If no harmful side effects are found, the next step is usually the testing of a small group of volunteer patients with the disorder. If these patients show some improvement in their clinical condition and the absence of serious side effects, then the final step is extensive clinical trials with larger numbers of volunteer patients at many locations across the country. These tests are carefully controlled and include treating other patients with a placebo (a neutral substance) in place of the new drug.

Neither the patient nor the physician knows whether the patient is receiving the drug or the placebo. A careful evaluation is then made of the drug's effect on the disorder before it is available for physicians to prescribe to their patients.

This is the procedure used to determine the effectiveness of a new drug in treating, for example, memory problems in patients with Alzheimer's disease. A number of drugs have been so tested in recent years, and clinical trials are planned for other drugs (see Alzheimer's Disease). Elderly adults interested in finding a clinical trial suited for their needs should contact the Web site http://www.clinicaltrials.gov.

Unfortunately, the number of elderly people who participate in clinical trials is not very large. Although nearly 65 percent of cancer patients are age sixty-five and older, they make up only 25 percent of the trials of new cancer treatments. One reason is that Medicare does not reimburse the cost of experimental trials (if there are any). A second is that people of these ages are often too sickly to tolerate aggressive new treatments.

E

Ecological Validity

Ecological validity in aging research refers to the generalizability to the everyday world of the results obtained in a laboratory study on age differences for some mental task. For example, substantial age differences favoring younger adults may be found in the acquisition of face-name pairs studied in the laboratory with a number of such pairs. Are elderly adults likely to be this different from younger adults in acquiring names to pair with faces in their everyday encounters with new people? That is, to what extent does the laboratory age difference in acquisition apply to real-life acquisition?

The less the result can be generalized, the lower the ecological validity of the study from which the generalization could be made. The nature of the laboratory task may be such that the results exaggerate the extent of the age difference outside the laboratory (*see* Everyday Memory). Nevertheless, the study may have some degree of ecological validity in terms of the determination that there is a likely difference of some kind between younger and older adults in performance on the task investigated in the laboratory. Researchers must then determine the reason for that age difference, no matter how large it may be.

Educational Level

For some years elderly adults have averaged fewer years of formal education than have younger adults. The age difference in educational level in the 1950s may be readily seen from the nature of the large sample used by David Wechsler in the standardization of his revised intelligence test (*see* Wechsler Intelligence Tests). At each age level a major, and largely successful, attempt was made to make the tested sample representative of the total population in the United States at that age level.

More than 43 percent of the sample in the age range of twenty-five to thirty-four had attended college for 1 or more years. By contrast, only 16 percent of the sample in the age range of seventy to seventy-four had attended college for 1 or more years. In 1960 it was estimated that fewer than 20 percent of the elderly population of the United States had graduated from high school. Even in the 1980s a substantial "educational gap" separated elderly and younger adults. In the mid-1980s it was estimated that nearly 72 percent of those adults age twenty-five to fifty-five had completed high school, but only 34 percent of adults age seventy-five and older.

Nevertheless, there has been a definite trend toward a better-educated older population. Between 1970 and 1985 the median number of years of formal education for elderly people increased from 8.7 to 11.7, with about 50 percent of elderly white persons completing high school. Unfortunately, the educational level of older members of minority groups has lagged well behind that of older white people. In the mid-1980s fewer than 20 percent of older minority group members had completed high school. In the near future it is estimated that two-thirds of the elderly population will have at least graduated from high school. However, to increase this trend even more for future generations as they age, it is clear that greater educational opportunity must be given to members of minority groups.

The age difference in educational level is important in evaluating the effects of aging on mental functioning. At all ages educational level is known to correlate positively and moderately with scores achieved on an intelligence test. When younger and older participants are carefully equated in educational level, much of the age difference in scores disappears. In most cross-sectional aging studies on learning, memory, problem solving, reasoning, and so on, the investigators are very careful to ensure that their younger and older age groups are equal in terms of educational level. An age difference in performance that persists with this condition is likely to be related to aging itself rather than to a generational difference in education.

Interestingly, the number of years of formal education also correlates positively with longevity. Of course, this does not mean that more education causes people to live longer. It suggests that people with higher levels of education find better-paying occupations. With better pay they can afford better nutrition and better health care—factors that do affect longevity.

Life expectancy tables estimate how much longer people are expected to live when they have attained any given age. The years a person is expected to live are increased by such factors as nonsmoking and regular exercising—and amount of education. For example, it is not unusual to see instructions telling you to add 3 years to your life expectancy if you have 4 or more years of college, 2 years if you have 1 to 3 years of college, and so on. Researchers in California found the decline in cognitive functioning with normal aging to be slower in women with a college education than without. Researchers in New York also found the incidence of Alzheimer's disease to be less for adults age sixty and older with higher levels of educational attainment than for those with lower levels.

African Americans show a faster rate of decline with aging than whites in functional health (ability to perform normal activities of daily living, such as bathing and dressing). Even when African American and white participants are equated for health status at the beginning of a study, the African Americans, nevertheless, show a faster rate of decline in functional health than the whites. Why this persistent racial difference? African Americans, in general, have less education and less income than most whites in late adulthood. When this difference is controlled, there seems to be no difference between the races in the rate of decline for functional health. The more the education and the greater the income, the greater the likelihood of exhibiting health-promoting behaviors and taking advantage of available professional health services.

Elder Abuse

There is no generally acceptable definition of elder abuse. Should it include both verbal and physical abuse? Should neglect be considered a form of abuse? Some statutes regarding elderly abuse are broad in what is to be considered abuse, but the implementation of those statutes is usually rather limited and often restricted to physical abuse. Moreover, various authorities are likely to have different views of what constitutes abuse. For example, police officers are likely to consider only physically aggressive acts as forms of abuse, whereas social workers are likely to consider verbally aggressive acts as being as abusive as physical acts.

There are, however, at least four generally accepted categories of elder abuse: physical (physical assault), psychosocial (verbal assault, verbal threats, and emotional abuse, such as lack of affection), financial and material (money or property mismanagement), and neglect (deprivation of basic needs). In an Illinois survey of more than five hundred substantiated cases of elder abuse it was found that the most frequent forms of abuse were financial exploitation and neglect. However, when the abuser had a substance-abuse problem, the most frequent forms of elder abuse were physical and emotional.

Elder abuse has undoubtedly existed for many years. However, concern about elder abuse did not receive national attention until the 1970s. In part, society's awakening to elder abuse resulted from surveys of small samples of older people that indicated more than a million elderly people were abused annually. Such surveys received considerable attention in newspapers, and terms such as *granny bashing* became widely used. This was a period in which general concern about elderly people had been aroused, and the existence of elder abuse became a major part of that concern.

How many elderly people are the victims of abuse? As noted above, estimates in the 1970s were based on small samples of elderly people. The results of a much larger survey were published in 1988. More than two thousand community-dwelling elderly people in the Boston metropolitan area were surveyed. The percentage of elderly people who reported abuse in one form or another was 3.2 percent (thirty-two per one thousand elderly people). A more recent survey of nearly three thousand community-dwelling elderly adults over a nine-year period reported the frequency of well-corroborated abuse was somewhat less than that found in the Boston survey (1.6 percent). This may be a conservative estimate because in many cases abuse is never reported.

Two-thirds of the victims of elder abuse are women. Abuse may be either intentional, that is, the abuser intends to cause pain or injury, or unintentional, that is, the abuser lacks appropriate coping skills to take care of an elderly person harmlessly. Abusers are more frequently men than women, and they are often children of the victims.

The potential for abusing demented elderly patients by caregivers is high, and it may take place often without the caregiver realizing it. Researchers at the Benjamin Ross Institute have developed a handbook for caregivers to help them identify their potential risk of abuse and how to seek appropriate interventions to prevent it.

Domestic violence is a form of abuse that usually takes the form of physical assault against one's spouse (85 percent of the victims are wives). Most people are likely to consider domestic violence to involve only younger adults. However, older adults may also be the victims of domestic violence. Surveys in the late 1990s indicated that about 5 percent of older adults (age fifty and older) suffered from domestic violence. Unfortunately, the percentage is probably higher because many older victims do not report the abuse.

Of further concern is the extent of abuse toward residents of nursing homes. In a survey conducted several years ago, nearly six hundred nurses and nursing aides working in nursing homes were asked how often they had observed incidents of abuse by staff members at their institutions in the past year. The most frequently observed physical abuse was the excessive use of restraints; 6 percent of those surveyed reported its occurrence ten or more times in the previous year, and 79 percent reported never having observed it. Such acts as pushing and shoving residents were observed to occur even less frequently. Only 1 percent of those surveyed reported observing its occurrence ten or more times in the previous year, and 83 percent reported never having observed it.

By contrast, verbal abuse appears to occur much more frequently in a nursing home. Of those surveyed, only 30 percent reported never observing residents being yelled at in anger, 15 percent reported observing its occurrence ten or more times, and 11 percent reported residents being insulted or sworn at ten or more times during the past year. In another survey, 10 percent of nursing assistants reported committing at least one act of physical abuse toward residents, and 40 percent reported committing at least one act of psychological abuse.

Fortunately, the incidence of abuse among residents of nursing homes may be reduced greatly by providing appropriate training for nursing assistants. This has been demonstrated by the application of a training program developed by the Coalition of Advocates for the Rights of the Infirm. The objectives of this program are to increase staff awareness of potentially abusive situations and to teach strategies for the effective resolution of conflicts that arise with residents and lead to abusive actions.

Suspected elder abuse should be reported to the Adult Abuse and Neglect Hotline (800-392-0210) or to the social service office in the victim's state. For victims of domestic violence, there is also the National Domestic Violence Hotline (800-799-SAFE). They may also receive advice about actions they could take by contacting the National Coalition against Domestic Violence (303-839-1852). The American Psychological Association has a booklet on elder abuse. To obtain a copy, call 202-336-6046 or send an e-mail to http://www.publicinterest@apa.org.

Elderhostel

Elderhostel programs offer continuing education programs of many kinds for older adults. The concept, introduced in 1975, was patterned after the youth hostels that were popular with young people traveling in Europe. Many of the programs are given on college and university campuses both in the United States and in Canada and in seventy other countries as well. More than two thousand institutions offer educational programs for those people who are age fifty-five and older.

In the United States programs usually include five days of lessons with many field trips and usually six nights of accommodations in dormitories or in hotels, motels, or retreat centers. The cost varies from program to program, and it includes the registration fee, housing, food, and instruction. The typical program offers three courses, each usually meeting for one and a half hours each day. The objective is to present older adults with courses that are relevant to their everyday lives and are enjoyable. For example, one such course is on microcomputers. The students receive hands-on experience in word processing and the use of various software programs. There are no examinations and no homework. In addition, the students are given the opportunity to participate in a variety of extracurricular activities.

Elderhostel programs are not limited to academic subject matter. For example, AARP initiated in the year 2000 a series of courses that are far removed from traditional academic subjects. Among these courses are learning to sail on Alabama's coastal waters and helping to restore a World War II aircraft carrier. Courses dealing with participation in voluntary organizations are also becoming increasingly popular.

For more information about elderhostels, write to Elderhostel, 75 Federal Street, Boston, MA 02110-1941. Alternatively, call 877-426-8056 or visit the Web site at http://www.elderhostel.org. For information about

AARP's courses, call AARP at 800-294-8056 or visit its Web site at http://www.aarp.org/elderhostel.

Emotions

Fear, anger, disgust, joy, sadness—these are all emotions experienced by adults of all ages. However, are they experienced in the same way during the course of the adult life span? A familiar theme in aging is that they are not. One of the popular beliefs has been that there is both a blunting or flattening of emotion (that is, becoming less intense) in late adulthood and a preponderance of negative emotions (for example, sadness) as opposed to positive emotions (such as joy) relative to earlier stages of adulthood.

However, research by Dr. Carol Zender Malatesta and her associates has demonstrated that these beliefs are really among the myths of aging (*see* Myths about Aging). The researchers extensively interviewed a large sample of people of various ages about their emotional experiences. The results indicated that there is no reason to believe that emotions are either less intense in late adulthood than in early adulthood or more negative than in early adulthood. If anything, the frequency of experiencing negative emotions is less in late adulthood than in early adulthood, and the frequency of experiencing positive emotions is greater in late than in early adulthood. Psychologists at Stanford University have proposed that people become increasingly aware that "time is running out" and that they should not waste dwindling time on trivial negative emotions. In addition, researchers at Fordham University found that the most happy emotions are experienced by older men who are married and extroverted.

Another important finding emerged from Dr. Malatesta's interviews. Children in our society are generally taught, as much as possible, not to display their emotions. By the time young adulthood has been reached, control of the facial muscles has largely succeeded in hiding emotional expression. By contrast, elderly adults are much less concerned with the need to conceal their inner feelings. This is especially true for elderly women. Paradoxically, elderly women seem more likely than elderly men to mask their true feelings by controlling their outer expressions of emotion. Conversely, when asked to relive a past emotional experience, older women report feeling a more intense emotion than do older men.

On many occasions we are unable to control our emotional expression. We do hear such remarks as "You look sad today" or "Something good must have happened. You sure look happy." The implication is that our nonverbal language is communicating our emotional inner feeling to other people. Especially important in this nonverbal communication is our facial expression. Even with the emphasis during childhood to mask our expression of emotion, we often find it difficult to control our facial expression while experiencing an emotion.

Of further interest is the extent to which our nonverbal communication becomes less reliable as an indicator of a specific emotional state for elderly people relative to younger people. Dr. Malatesta has provided some intriguing evidence with regard to this point. People of various ages were asked to recall particular experiences in their lives during which they felt sad, other experiences when they felt happy or angry, and so on. The goal of this task was to recapture to some degree the experience felt originally (a procedure known as mood induction). Participants were videotaped as they relived these experiences. The videotapes were then shown to other participants of differing ages, who were asked to evaluate each tape in terms of the intensity of emotion displayed and the specific nature of the emotion.

In general, young adults were found to judge emotions most accurately when the tapes were of fellow young adults. Middle-aged and older adults were also most accurate when they judged the expressions of others their own age. Overall, the facial expressions of elderly adults were most difficult to judge accurately.

Largely unresolved is the possibility that the importance of emotions to people's lives changes from early to late adulthood. Gerontologists have debated for some years whether emotions are of greatest importance in the lives of young or elderly adults. Evidence provided by researchers at Stanford University suggests that salience may actually be greater for elderly adults. Participants in their study read and then recalled a story that contained both emotional and nonemotional content. The amount of emotional content recalled was found to increase progressively from the twenties through the early eighties, thus implying increasing importance of emotions from early to late adulthood.

The researchers at Stanford made another important discovery: elderly adults were found to be better than younger adults in regulating their emotions and controlling their negative emotions. That is, older adults seem to have more of what psychologists call emotional intelligence than do younger adults. Emotional intelligence consists of the ability to monitor your own feelings and those of other people as well, and use your emotional knowledge to help guide your thinking and behavior. Older adults seem more likely than younger adults to control their anger when confronted by relatively minor irritations—and therefore are less likely to express anger of the kind called road rage and other unproductive forms of anger.

Some evidence indicates that a high level of emotional intelligence may be as important, if not more so, than traditional IQ-type intelligence in order to excel in life. Your degree of emotional intelligence is measured by a paper-and-pencil or computer test that contains a forty-minute test battery (Mayer-Salovey-Caruso Emotional Intelligence Test) with such questions as "What mood(s) might be helpful to feel when meeting in-laws for the very first time?" Adults who score high on the test have been found to have greater success in personal and work relationships than adults who score low on the test.

Of further importance is the nature of emotions expressed by residents in nursing homes who have Alzheimer's disease or other dementias. An immediate question is how to measure their emotions when verbal expressions are unreliable. Psychologists at the Philadelphia Geriatric Center have found the answer to this question. They developed the Philadelphia Geriatric Center Affect Rating Scale. Emotional experiences are evaluated by observation of a resident's facial expressions, body movements, and other clues that are independent of verbal expressions. With the use of this scale, researchers have found that positive affect is the highest for residents without depression and least for residents with major depression. Conversely, they found negative affect to be lowest in nondepressed residents and highest in depressed residents. The hope is that better understanding of the emotional life of cognitively impaired elderly adults will lead to ways of improving the quality of their lives.

Emotions and Memory

Older adults tend to experience more positive emotions and fewer negative emotions than younger adults. This suggests that older adults' memory for positive emotional information may be better than their memory for negative emotional information. By contrast, young adults may not differ in memory for positive and negative information.

This hypothesis was tested by researchers at Stanford University. Young adult and older adult participants were presented with a series of images on a screen. Some evoked positive emotions (images of babies and animals), while others evoked negative emotions (mutilations and bugs). The participants recalled as many of the images as they could.

Older adults, but not younger adults, recalled many more positive than negative images. Consequently, the age difference favoring the young adults was much smaller for the positive images than for the negative images. However, a similar difference in memory by elders for positively and negatively toned words was not found by German researchers. Words are less likely to evoke positive or negative images of what they represent by elders than by younger adults (*see* Imagery; Verbal Learning). Activation of images seems to be needed for elders' greater memory of positively toned words than negatively toned words to be manifested.

End-State Renal Disease

The incidence of end-state renal disease (ESRD) is very high for older adults. Hypertension and diabetes are responsible for about 65 percent of all cases of ESRD. ESRD occurs when a patient's kidneys fail to the degree that there is insufficient excretion of water, salt, and other substances from the body. As a result, the volume of water contained in the body increases and tissues swell. Among the signs of kidney failure are swelling (especially in the ankles), lower back pain, puffiness around the eyes, and often painful urination. Treatment consists of dialysis or a kidney transplant. Dialysis is expensive, about fifty thousand dollars per year, with medications adding five thousand to ten thousand dollars.

Entitlements

An entitlement in the federal budget is a mandatory expenditure. Individuals included in some entitlement program in the federal budget are not affected by their income levels. That is, they are entitled to payments regardless of the level of their income. Social Security and Medicare are among these non-means-tested entitlements (that is, there is no test to pass in terms of a specified income level). They account for about 21 percent and 10 percent, respectively, of federal spending. Other entitlements, such as Medicaid, are means tested in the sense that only individuals who pass the test of low income qualify to receive them.

A belief held by many younger people is that Social Security and Medicare benefits go largely to elderly people with incomes high enough that they do not need the benefits. In fact, however, less than 2 percent of the benefits go to those whose family income is more than one hundred thousand dollars, and more than 67 percent go to those whose family income is less than thirty thousand dollars. In 2002 there were nearly seven million beneficiaries of Social Security who received nearly thirty-four billion dollars that year.

Social Security receives its funds from employees' payroll tax and from their employers' contribution to the fund. Full benefits are now available for those persons who retire at age sixty-five, and reduced benefits are available for those who retire between the ages of sixty-two and sixty-five. The age-sixty-five benefit will be raised gradually to age sixty-seven by the year 2007.

Social Security benefits represent 83 percent of the total income for seniors in the lowest 25 percent of annual income and 20 percent of seniors in the highest 25 percent of annual income. For nearly 44 percent of older women and 29 percent of older men, Social Security benefits represent 90 percent to 100 percent of their retirement income. Approximately 10 percent fell below the official federal poverty income level in 2003. African American and Hispanic seniors are more than twice as likely as whites and Asian Americans to live in poverty (*see also* Income of Elderly People).

If you retire early and are still below the full retirement age, your benefits will be reduced slightly if you earn a certain amount per year. However, after you reach full retirement age, you are able to collect retirement benefits and still continue working without any reduction in your benefits. If you plan to continue working past your full retirement age, you can choose to delay your retirement benefits; delayed retirement credits may increase your eventual benefits.

Social Security payments may be made by electronic direct deposits in a recipient's bank account. More than thirty million beneficiaries do have their checks deposited electronically, but more than seven million beneficiaries who have bank accounts, nevertheless, receive their check by mail anyway. Direct bank deposit does benefit beneficiaries by eliminating theft of checks from mailboxes or fees charged by check-cashing services. For more information, contact http://www.socialsecurity.gov.

Environmental Press

Our environment places various demands or pressures on us. These demands may consist of various combinations of physical, mental, interpersonal, and social demands. If these demands exceed our capacities to cope with them, then we are likely to experience distress. For most people of all ages, their capacity exceeds or equals these environmental demands. However, some elderly adults do not have the capacity to meet these environmental demands or presses.

For example, physical demands are more likely to be a problem for elderly adults than they are for younger adults. Consider, for example, an individual living on a third (or even second) floor of an apartment house without an elevator. The need to climb the stairs is surely likely to be a greater environmental press for an elderly resident than for a younger resident. The less the physical competence of the elderly resident, the greater will be the impact on him or her created by the environmental press.

Distance from a shopping center is also likely to have a greater impact on an elderly person who must walk to shop, relative to a younger person who is more likely to drive. Fortunately, designers of residential centers and retirement communities have become increasingly aware of the need to plan physical facilities that consider the physical capabilities of their elderly residents. Similarly, manufacturers of drugs and medicines prescribed for elderly individuals are increasingly packaging them in forms that are less taxing on the memory abilities of their clientele.

Interpersonal demands involving unhappy relationships with family members or friends may exceed our capacities to deal with them. Social demands may become excessive when, for example, new social customs conflict with those firmly established from one's earlier life. According to environmental-press theory, stresses created by excessive demands may be treated either by increasing the capacities of the persons involved or decreasing the extent of the environmental demands.

Episodic Memory

Do you remember the first spill you had on a bicycle? Where did it take place? What was the name of your date at your high school prom? What did you eat for dinner last night? How many times have you seen a beer commercial on television during the past week? When was the last time you balanced your checkbook? What was it your spouse said to you when you left the house? Do you remember where you parked your car at the shopping mall?

These are all examples of what memory researchers call episodic memory, or memory for personally experienced events. Episodic memory and semantic memory are the main broad components of the human memory system. Episodic memory refers to memory for personally experienced events or episodes in your life (for instance, the memory of your first spill on your bicycle). Such memories are stored in reference to the context in which they occurred. Context refers to the when and where of an episode, that is, the time and place that it occurred (it was your sixth birthday, and it happened on the sidewalk in front of your house). In this respect, episodic memory differs from semantic memory, which contains general knowledge information that is ordinarily stored without reference to the context in which it was acquired (*see* Semantic Memory).

When elderly people complain about their memory problems, they are usually referring to their episodic memory. The study of age differences in episodic memory, including the reasons for their occurrence, is complicated, however, by the complexity of episodic memory. Episodic memory is both short-term and long-term in nature. Short-term episodic memory (also called *primary memory*) is for information held briefly in consciousness. Age-related declines in short-term memory proficiency are, in general, modest (*see* Short-Term Memory). Long-term episodic memory is either for newly acquired episodic information (called *secondary memory*) or for information acquired some time ago (very long-term memory, or *tertiary memory; see* Autobiographical Memory; Very Long-Term Memory).

Most laboratory research on age differences in memory has centered on secondary memory. Age-related declines in secondary-memory proficiency usually range from moderate to fairly substantial, depending on the form of secondary memory involved. These deficits may occur in either the encoding of episodic information (that is, transforming it into a memory record or trace) or the retrieval of the resulting memory traces from the long-term store of episodic-memory traces. The encoding of episodic information may be, in turn, either effortful or automatic.

Effortful encoding means that there is the intent to commit information to memory, and mental effort is exerted to transform the information into a memory trace. Effortful secondary memory is commonly studied with words as the to-be-remembered events. After studying a lengthy list of words, participants are asked either to recall the words or to recognize them among destructors or new words. Note that the participants are not really "learning" the words—they are already present in the participants' semantic memories. Instead, they are asked to remember which of the many words they know were encountered at a particular time and place (the where and when of episodic memory).

On average, elderly participants recall fewer words than do younger participants. Part of the problem lies in the generally less proficient encoding of the episodic events by older adults relative to younger adults. Younger adults tend to make greater use of what is called *elaborative encoding* than do older adults, presumably because the former have a greater capacity of what is called *working memory*, the place in the memory system where encoding takes place (*see* Working Memory).

Elaborative encoding makes the resulting memory trace more distinctive and more accessible for later recall or recognition than does simply saying a word to yourself. One form of elaboration is to construct an image of a word serving as an episodic event. Another form is the use of an organizational strategy whereby a connection or relationship is found between the words in the list. For example, four different animals may be named in the list, but they are widely separated. By making use of the animal relatedness, you may be able to recall their names together. Memory training programs for elderly adults usually stress the use of elaboration to improve the encoding of episodic events (*see* Memory Training). Part of the older adult's problem in episodic memory results from the greater difficulty in retrieving information from the episodic-memory store. This may be seen from the results of research studies in which recognition memory has been contrasted with recall of the same information (*see* Recognition Memory versus Recall Memory).

Automatic encoding refers to forms of episodic memory in which memory occurs without the intent to commit information to memory and without a conscious effort to encode that information. This is the case for the memory people have of their own actions, the memory of conversational contents, the memory of television programs they watched, and the memory of stories they have read. In general, younger adults are more proficient in these forms of memory than are older adults, but the extent of the age difference is less pronounced than it is for effortfully encoded material.

Another important distinction in regard to episodic memory is that between *retrospective memory* and *prospective memory*. Retrospective memory, or remembrance of things past, refers to the forms of memory just discussed. That is, it consists of memory for previously encoded episodic events that have been registered in either a short-term store or a long-term store. By contrast, prospective memory refers to memory for performing some future action, such as remembering to mail a letter or to stop at the store on the way home from work to purchase some needed item (*see* Prospective Memory). Interestingly, recent research has indicated that prospective memory may be largely resistant to any pronounced declines in proficiency from early to late adulthood.

The complexity of retrospective memory is increased further when we realize that it refers not only to memory for the content of episodic events but also to other attributes of events. You may remember playing bridge with the Smiths, but you do not remember when. In this instance it is the temporal (time) attribute of the event and not its content that is at stake. Or you may remember how many times you played bridge during the past month. This is the frequency-of-occurrence attribute of the event and not its content that is at stake. You may remember that the last time you played bridge with the Smiths was at their house and not your house. Here it is the spatial attribute of the event and not the content that is at stake. Or you may remember that it was George Smith and not Nancy Smith who said you are a great bridge player. Here it is the source attribute of the episodic event and not its content that is at stake.

Age differences in each of these attributes have been widely studied in the laboratory by the use of procedures that vary these attributes in much the same way that they are varied in the everyday world (*see* separate entries for the attributes, such as Frequency-of-Occurrence Memory).

Esophageal Cancer

The incidence of esophageal cancer is relatively rare compared to lung cancer, colon cancer, and prostate cancer. The American Cancer Society reported that there were 13,900 new cases of the cancer in 2003. Its incidence is greatest for men and women in the age range of forty-five to seventy. Other risk factors include race (African Americans have three times the risk of the cancer than whites), tobacco use, excessive alcohol use, and, especially, a history of acid reflux over a long period of time. Symptoms may include trouble swallowing, unexplained weight loss, and a frequent pain in the chest that feels like heartburn.

Estate Taxes

Prior to 2006 people did not have to pay a federal tax on the first $625,000 of their estate. This amount was increased to $1 million in 2006. The amount includes life insurance, bank accounts, jointly owned property, retirement accounts, and property in revocable trusts. In addition, you may make a yearly tax-free gift of up to $10,000 to children, grandchildren, or other relatives. The maximum is increased annually to adjust for the rate of inflation.

Estrogen Replacement Therapy (Hormone Replacement Therapy)

Between 15 percent to 40 percent of postmenopausal women are on estrogen replacement therapy (or hormone replacement therapy). The therapy may be with estrogen alone or with estrogen combined with progestin. Estrogen is a female sex hormone produced by the ovaries that decreases in its level with menopause. Progestin is also a female hormone that prepares the uterus for the reception of a fertilized ovum.

Estrogen replacement therapy has been commonly used to reduce the risk or treatment of symptoms of various diseases. Included are Alzheimer's disease, blood clots, breast cancer, colon cancer, heart disease, gallbladder diseases, osteoporosis, stroke, and uterine cancer. However, most studies have indicated that the therapy may have more harmful effects than beneficial effects for most of these diseases. There are new products called designer estrogens that may reduce these risks. *See also* Alzheimer's Disease; Breast Cancer; Cardiovascular Diseases; Cholesterol; Colon Cancer; Facial Appearance; Gallbladder Diseases; Osteoporosis; Ovarian Cancer; Stroke; Uterine Cancer.

Euthanasia

One of the greatest ethical debates in contemporary society is in regard to the practice of euthanasia, the killing of someone with a seemingly incurable and mentally devastating disease or disorder. The debate is likely to intensify in the coming years as the elderly population increases and the number of individuals with Alzheimer's disease increases accordingly.

There are two forms of euthanasia. The first is *active euthanasia,* in which a person's life is deliberately cut short by some action that terminates life immediately to avoid further suffering. This form of euthanasia has received considerable attention in recent years with the advent of so-called death machines that aid the person to commit suicide. Suicide assisted by a physician is against the law in thirty-eight states, and several other state legislatures have been considering laws to make it illegal. Only in Oregon is physician-assisted suicide legal as determined by a state law passed in 1997. Oregon's law has been challenged by various groups, including the present administration of the United States. These challenges eventually reached the United States Supreme Court to determine the legality of the law. In January 2006 the Court upheld the legality of Oregon's law. As a result, we are now likely to have other states passing a law similar to that of Oregon.

The other form of euthanasia is *passive euthanasia,* in which efforts are no longer made to sustain the life of the person through the use of lifesaving medical equipment and procedures. This form of euthanasia has been the center of recent court cases in which the right to withdraw lifesaving equipment has been debated. It is hoped that many of the ethical concerns about euthanasia will be reduced by the existence of advance directives in which people make known their desire not to have their lives sustained by artificial means when there is no apparent hope for their recovery (*see* Advance Directives). In some states, administrators of nursing homes are required to ask about residents' wishes and to keep these documents on file. However, the extent to which these documents are legally binding and will dictate the treatment received from a medical team is debatable.

Everyday Memory

"Did I mail that letter?" "I must remember to stop at the supermarket on my way home from work today." "What is that new neighbor's name?" "When was it that we last played bridge together?" "I know the name of that movie, but I just can't think of it now." These are examples of everyday memory experiences. One of the most frequent complaints expressed by older people is that their everyday memory is not as proficient as when they were younger. When elderly people rate their own memory proficiency, they characteristically rate it lower than do younger adults (*see* Metamemory; Metamemory in Adulthood [MIA] Questionnaire and Metamemory Functioning Questionnaire [MFQ]). The implication is that the imperfections of memory found at all ages are greater in late adulthood than in earlier adulthood.

How accurate are elderly people in their complaints about their memory proficiency? Ideally, it would be best to study memory as it operates in everyday life, and then compare people of different ages in its proficiency. This is difficult to accomplish. The very presence of an investigator watching you throughout the day could alter your memory performance (the Heisenberg principle—the mere act of observing an event is likely to change the nature of that event). There is the possibility that you could be your own observer by keeping a diary in which each day you record your memory failures and imperfections. There have been several diary studies of this kind (*see* Diary Studies of Memory Failures). However, the procedure is not very satisfying. How can you rely on reports of memory failures from people who may have memory problems and are unable to remember their own memory failures?

Given the problem of observing memory as it functions in everyday life, memory researchers concerned about age differences in memory proficiency have turned largely to bringing everyday-like memory into the laboratory where it may be studied under controlled conditions. They give participants of various ages memory tasks that they believe approximate those encountered in everyday living. Thus, to study age differences in learning to associate names with faces, a task elderly people claim is very difficult for them in the everyday world, participants learn a list in which ten faces of strangers are paired with surnames. In general, elderly participants take much longer to learn such a list than do younger participants.

What do such results reveal about the difficulty of elderly people in learning names to go with faces in the everyday world? How often does an elderly person need to learn ten new face-name pairings at essentially the same time? We usually meet new people one at a time or perhaps two at a time. In general, elderly people may have a bit more trouble in mastering the names than younger people, especially when they fail to pay attention to the name(s) in the first place. The laboratory results on face-name acquisition do indicate a decline in proficiency with normal aging (*see* Verbal Learning). However, it is likely that the extent of that decline as evidenced in everyday face-name acquisition is exaggerated by declines observed in the laboratory (that is, the results of the research may have limited ecological validity; *see* Ecological Validity).

Similarly, many studies of age differences in memory for words in a lengthy series of words reveal a fairly substantial difference in the average number of words recalled between younger and older participants. Such results do suggest that older people are somewhat less proficient than younger people in both encoding and retrieving episodic information. The results seem to exaggerate the extent of the deficiency in everyday memory proficiency.

How often does an elderly person attempt to memorize a lengthy series of events? The memory of older adults for a short shopping list is probably nearly as good as most younger adults. If it is a much longer shopping list, why not write the items down and take the list with you when you go shopping?

There have been important trends toward research on adult age differences for laboratory tasks that more closely approximate those of everyday memory and therefore seem to have greater ecological validity (that is, generalizability from the laboratory to the everyday world). With verbal material, research on age differences in memory for the contents of stories, articles, conversations, and television programs has become a popular area of aging memory research (*see* Conversation Memory; Memory for Television Programs). Our everyday memory functioning surely includes frequently encountering contents of these kinds. Similarly, an important new area of laboratory research on aging consists of memory for actions and activities (*see* Action Memory). The objective of such studies is to approximate the kinds of memories we have for our everyday actions, such as turning off the gas on a stove and locking a door. This is a component of everyday memory about which elderly people often complain.

Exercise Capacity

Researchers at Stanford University and the Veterans Administration Medical Center in Palo Alto, California, studied more than six thousand men who had been referred for treadmill testing. Each participant had a health problem that suggested the need for the test. The participants were then followed over the next six or seven years. Exercise capacity (measured in metabolic equivalence) was found to be the predictor of survival or death for both those with a cardiovascular disease and those without the disease.

Exercise (Relationship to Physical/Mental Performances)

Some elderly people have been regular exercisers for many years, whereas others have lived more sedentary lives. Long-term exercisers have been found to be physically healthier and to be faster in responding on a variety of tasks than nonexercisers. For example, older runners who had been running for an average of twelve years at the start of the study were compared with older nonrunners in a study at Stanford University. The two groups were studied over a period of eight years. At the beginning of the study the runners had fewer medical problems, fewer joint symptoms, and less disability than the nonrunners. Over the eight years the incidence of disability and mortality increased at a much slower rate for the runners than for the nonrunners.

There is also evidence to indicate that regular long-term exercisers perform at a higher level on a variety of mental tasks (such as reasoning tasks) than nonexercisers. Given the high proportion of currently young adults who are regular exercisers, there is good reason to believe that future generations of elderly people will show less mental decline than current and past generations of elderly people who were less likely to be regular exercisers. This depends, of course, on current younger exercisers continuing to exercise through late adulthood.

A related question concerns what happens to those sedentary elderly people who become exercisers late in life. Researchers at Duke University Medical Center have been active in their attempt to answer this question. In their studies, elderly participants engage in intensive aerobic exercises for several months. They are then evaluated in terms of how they compare at the end of the exercise program both with their initial findings and with other elderly people who were engaged in no vigorous activities during the same period. The results have shown that exercise late in life does have some physical health benefits. There is evidence indicating that seniors who delayed participating in an exercise program until late in life have the same low incidence of physical disability as other seniors who have been long-term exercisers.

There have been a number of other studies that demonstrated the positive physical benefits of a relatively short-term exercise program. For example, Canadian researchers found that adults ranging in age from sixty to eighty who were given two years of twice-a-week weight training (for instance, leg presses) exhibited increased endurance in cycling, walking, and stair climbing. Similarly, older adults (sixty to eighty-eight years) given one year of twice-a-week low-intensity exercise maintained or improved their strength, balance, and mobility after one year. Another study with fifteen hundred National Aeronautics and Space Administration workers showed that even moderate exercise, such as a brisk thirty-minute walk three times a week, helps older adults to avoid the ill effects of aging.

In the Duke University study the exercisers reported at the end of the program that they were sleeping better than at the beginning, and they reported that their social life had improved. They also believed that their concentration had improved after completion of the program, as had their mental functioning. Unfortunately, laboratory performances failed to show any significant improvement in scores on either memory tests or intelligence tests. The implication is that initiating regular exercise late in life does not seem to be a cure-all for moderate mental declines that may occur with normal aging.

However, in a later study, researchers at the University of Illinois at Urbana found that mental functioning, including memory, improved significantly for older adults who had aerobic exercise consisting of vigorous walking. They had not previously been regular exercisers. On the other hand, anaerobic exercise, such as weight lifting, did not affect mental functioning. This is an important topic that obviously needs much more research before we know if regular physical exercise initiated late in life really improves mental functioning. Of course, we realize that it surely cannot hurt mental functioning, and it carries with it many physical benefits.

Although the many benefits of physical exercise are obvious, what is not clear is the extent to which elderly patients are encouraged by their physicians to be regular exercisers. Unfortunately, such encouragement does not happen often enough. In a study conducted in 1990 only 50 percent of older men and 45 percent of older women with high blood pressure reported being advised by their physicians to exercise as a way of lowering their blood pressure. In a more recent survey, only 48 percent of older adults reported ever receiving a recommendation from their physician to exercise. Most alarming is the fact that older adults who do receive a recommendation to exercise are about 60 percent more likely to enroll in an exercise program than those older people who do not receive a recommendation.

The physical benefits of an exercise training program are not limited to community-dwelling older adults. Researchers at Tufts University have demonstrated that benefits occur for many frail residents of nursing homes as well. Many participants in their study had illnesses such as lung disease, arthritis, and high blood pressure, and many had some degree of dementia. They worked out vigorously for forty-five minutes a day for three days a week for several weeks. The participants used exercise machines to strengthen their thighs and knees, and they lifted weights to strengthen other muscles. At the end of the program the participants averaged an increased walking speed of

12 percent and an increased stair climbing ability of 28 percent. They appeared to be less depressed than they were at the start of the program. Most important, they walked around their rooms on their own much more than they did before the program.

This is important because many residents of nursing homes have such poor leg strength that they are confined to chairs and unable to walk to the bathroom on their own. They would benefit greatly from this kind of exercise program. *See also* Walking.

Exercise Types

One popular myth about aging is that exercise is dangerous for many elderly people. In truth, exercise in the right form and the right amount is likely to improve the health, strength, flexibility, and stamina of many older people. However, before beginning any exercise program, elderly people should be checked out thoroughly by their physician, and they should consult with exercise experts. The three main kinds of exercise are *low-intensity* or *anaerobic, aerobic,* and *resistance.*

Light walking, golfing, bowling, and some calisthenics are example of low-intensity exercises. Low-intensity exercise has some effect on improving cardiovascular and pulmonary functioning, and it does help in weight control and increasing muscle strength (*see* Walking).

Aerobic exercise is vigorous and raises the heart rate by more than 40 percent from the resting rate to the maximum rate. Examples of aerobic exercising are jogging at a moderate or fast pace, walking at a brisk pace, swimming, and riding a bicycle. When used in the right form and duration, aerobic exercise should help to improve cardiovascular and pulmonary functioning for many older people.

A major study of elderly male exercisers indicated that participants who exercised moderately had more than a 20 percent lower risk of mortality, whereas elderly men who exercised more strenuously had a 50 percent lower risk of mortality. Among the health benefits of regular exercise is that it is likely to increase your level of HDL cholesterol (the good cholesterol; *see* Cholesterol), thus reducing your risk of a heart attack or stroke. Aerobic exercise is also likely to improve agility and balance. Researchers in Vermont found that even postcoronary patients (for example, myocardial infarct) may benefit in peak oxygen consumption from aerobic exercise. Caution is important, however. An exercise regimen that is too strenuous can lead to an increased risk of mortality.

Leg presses, tricep presses, and weight lifting are examples of resistance exercise. Researchers in California demonstrated that resistance exercise is not just for the young. Their more than sixty participants in a yearlong training program showed significant increases in muscle strength, with the increases occurring primarily during the first three months of training.

In addition, researchers at Tufts University found that a twice-weekly weight-lifting program increased bone density of the hips and spine for their older women participants, all of whom had a prior sedentary lifestyle. Increases in bone density help to reduce the risk of osteoporosis (*see* Osteoporosis). In general, the participants in this training program also improved balance and muscle strength, therefore reducing the risk of falls (*see* Falls). Canadian researchers found that a weight-lifting program for elderly people served to improve treadmill-walking endurance and stair-climbing ability. Experts in weight lifting recommend that trainees warm up and stretch their muscles before they begin to lift weights and that they lift weights only every other day.

There is also a special kind of exercise called tai chi, a traditional form of Chinese fitness exercise. It combines deep breathing with the diaphragm and relaxation with slow, gentle movements, both isometric and isotonic. The exercise is performed while the mind is tranquil but alert. Researchers at Emory University found that participants age seventy and older given fifteen weeks of tai chi reported their lives to be positively improved. A form of exercise especially valuable for older adults with physical limitations is the ROM Dance Program. It includes instruction in both exercise and relaxation. The dance takes about seven minutes to complete and can be performed sitting or standing. It includes a special hand exercise, and it is accompanied by soft music and a poem. It is especially recommended for patients with rheumatoid arthritis, fibromyalgia, Parkinson's disease, or lupus.

Unfortunately, many elderly people ignore the benefits of exercise, either because they believe they do not need it or because they have accepted the myth of exercise's dangers. It is estimated that about 22 percent of all instances of heart disease, colon cancer, and bones broken because of osteoporosis are caused by lack of exercise. Inactivity also increases the risk of developing high blood pressure, breast cancer, and stroke. Physicians and health experts need to increase their efforts of informing elderly people of the many benefits derived from regular exercise.

Staying with an exercise program once it is started is also a problem for many elderly people. Adherence to a program depends in part on physical factors, such as few new medical problems, but even more on psychological factors, such as a positive attitude and a low level of depression. The use of certain medications may also create a problem in adhering to an exercise program.

To find more information about exercise and health and other health-related topics, you should consult the booklet *Healthy Aging*. To obtain a copy, write to ETNET, P.O. Box 7536, Department P, Wilton, CT 06897; you must enclose a check or money order for $1.50 and a self-addressed envelope.

Expertise

The United States has recently had two presidents who may be considered "old," at least in terms of their chronological ages. Numerous studies have demonstrated age-related declines on many mental abilities, including those of memory and reasoning. However, our older presidents seem to have functioned quite well in office (although one did admit to having memory problems). Older business executives have been found to perform well below the levels of younger executives on many laboratory tasks and clinical tests of mental abilities, yet the older executives were known to have performed their jobs very well, despite their apparent decline in what may be considered basic mental abilities.

The same outcome has been found for university professors. Older professors who are well known for their continuing excellence in teaching and research have scored well below the levels of younger professors on tests of many basic abilities. However, it is a different matter when older professors are required to comprehend new textual material and integrate that new information with their existing knowledge. These are skills that college professors have used repeatedly throughout their careers. Not surprisingly, researchers at the University of California at Berkeley discovered that professors in their sixties performed as well as professors in their thirties on laboratory tasks requiring these comprehension and integration skills. These are skills that give the professors expertise in their profession, skills that continue well into late adulthood.

Computer programmers are no exception to the continuation of expertise into later adulthood. Older experienced programmers have been found to function at a level comparable to that of younger and well-trained programmers. Most bridge players are likely to know elderly players who are exceptionally skilled in bridge and are regular participants in duplicate bridge tournaments. Their skill in playing the mentally challenging game of bridge seemingly denies their likely declines in many basic mental abilities. In each of these cases, expertise in a particular endeavor or field is the issue. Many people who are experts in a particular endeavor, whether it be in politics, business, or a skilled game, tend to retain their high level of performance in that endeavor, despite whatever declines they may experience in various mental abilities. They apparently compensate in some way that enables them to continue their expertise.

In the case noted above, and in most other cases, compensation is likely to be in the way of the added knowledge gained with experience in their vocation or avocation. Thus, the older expert has a broader knowledge base or background for aiding in the making of decisions (for instance, what response to give to your partner's opening bid for a hand of bridge). This kind of knowledge has been well documented for older chess players. Older master chess players have the ability to scan for several seconds a chess board containing as many as twenty-five pieces and then reproduce the pieces in their exact locations on the board. This is true, however, only when the pieces are arranged in accordance with standard and acceptable chess moves. Less experienced players lack the knowledge of chess plays that older masters have, and they are unable to match this remarkable memory feat. The older expert's knowledge of chess enables him or her to "chunk" the information on the board so that it circumvents the ordinary limits of short-term memory (*see* Short-Term Memory).

Retaining expertise in later life is also possible in some occupations by the development of a special skill that compensates in some way for a decline in other skills that are ordinarily essential for a high level of job performance. This kind of compensation may be seen for older skilled typists. Rapid movements of the fingers are seemingly essential for fast typing. Such movement does slow down with normal aging, thus apparently placing the older typists at a considerable disadvantage relative to younger typists. However, expert older typists have been found to type at a rate that is about the same as that of younger experts. The older typists have also been found to read several characters farther ahead in the text being typed than younger typists. This skill in reading farther ahead comes with experience and seemingly compensates for the overall slowing of the finger movements of the older expert typist.

One area of mental performances in which everyone should seemingly become an expert as a result of years of practice is memory. If true, one would expect to find few age-related declines in memory performances. For several components of memory this does seem to be the case. Semantic memory involving our general knowledge of words shows relatively little decline with normal aging (*see* Lexicon; Semantic Memory). Our expertise in using this knowledge seems to ensure its automatic retrieval well into late adulthood. Prospective memory (remembering to perform some future planned action; *see* Prospective Memory) also seems to be largely immune to the negative effects caused by aging, as is short-term episodic memory.

Age-related deficits in proficiency are most likely to occur for long-term (secondary) episodic memory (*see* Episodic Memory). One reason for this failure is that much of our everyday memory takes place automatically and incidentally (for example, memory of our own actions). Consequently, there is little opportunity for people to acquire with experience compensatory strategies that may offset age-related declines. With effortful forms of long-term memory, adults are frequently unaware of the kinds of strategies that could enhance their proficiencies, thus making it unlikely that they could develop compensatory strategies to offset age-related declines in proficiency. In fact, it is the purpose of memory training programs to make elderly adults aware of such strategies and to encourage them to use them (*see* Memory Training).

Eyewitness Testimony

Witnessing a criminal commit a crime usually occurs under incidental memory conditions (that is, there is no intent to memorize) and with little opportunity to study carefully the criminal's face. Nevertheless, eyewitnesses may later be asked to identify the suspected criminal in a police lineup. Accurate identification, of course, will aid the justice system in convicting the criminal. However, a false identification could lead to the prosecution of an innocent person.

Psychologists have been very active in investigating the accuracy with which people make such identifications. Of particular interest is the age of the eyewitnesses. In the laboratory setting older people have been shown to be less accurate than younger people in their memory of faces (*see* Face Memory). Especially disturbing is the high false-alarm rate (that is, falsely identifying a new face as one previously seen) of elderly participants. This is especially true when the faces seen are those of young adults. Criminals are more likely to be young adults than older adults. The likely problem of many older people as eyewitnesses is demonstrated further by having elderly participants observe a crime that is simulated in the laboratory. In such situations they are much less accurate than younger observers and have a much higher false-identification rate. However, a researcher at Mississippi State University found that elderly adults are as accurate as younger adults in recalling the details of a crime (the actions and objects involved in a crime) simulated on a videotape.

F

Face Memory

"I remember your face, but not your name." Such a statement implies that memory for faces is quite good. But is it, regardless of age? Face memory is tested in the laboratory by presenting a series of pictures of faces (usually from a college yearbook) to participants and then testing their memory with a list consisting of a mixture of old faces and new faces (that is, ones not included in the prior series).

Research with this procedure has demonstrated that even young adults have far less than perfect memory for faces. It has also been demonstrated that elderly participants are much less accurate than younger participants in recognizing old faces as being truly old. This is true even when participants are required to study each face thoroughly and to make a decision about it (how friendly does it look?). Moreover, elderly participants misidentify new faces as being old ("false alarms") considerably more often than do younger participants. Face memory does seem to decline in proficiency from early to late adulthood. This decline has implications for a probable age difference in the accuracy of eyewitness testimony (*see* Eyewitness Testimony).

Facial Appearance

We are all well aware of the changes that occur in our faces from early to late adulthood. One of the first changes is the presence of lines in the forehead that usually appear by age thirty. Other lines then appear in the face between the ages of thirty and fifty. Many of these lines are the result of years of squinting and frowning, and these lines may be largely prevented by wearing appropriate glasses and avoiding frowning as much as possible.

After age fifty more pronounced changes in the face, such as wrinkles, usually begin to appear. Water inside the facial skin decreases in amount, as does collagen, a fiber that gives the skin resilience (*see also* Body Build and Body Characteristics). The facial skin tends to become stiffer, leading to more pronounced lines and sometimes to bags under the eyes and sagging skin on the cheeks. Puffiness below the eyes may result from blood seeping into loose skin below the eyes. This usually occurs at night, and it may be reduced by propping your head on two pillows. During late adulthood, cartilage accumulates in the nose, and it may increase both the width and the length of the nose. The earlobes tend to become slightly fatter and longer, and the circumference of the head increases slightly. Fat may accumulate in the chin of some elderly men.

The rate at which changes in the skin occur is determined in part by heredity. Slower rates of change are possible by avoiding ultraviolet rays as much as possible. Facial cosmetic surgery is available for prolonging more youthful skin, as are cosmetics for covering up blemishes in the skin. In 1996 the U.S. Food and Drug Administration approved retinoic acid (a cream known as Renova) as a treatment for wrinkles caused by aging. It takes months, however, for it to smooth the skin, if it works at all. Changes in the face are often more noticeable in older women than in older men. This is largely because the production of skin oil declines in women after menopause.

Thinning of the hair occurs, especially after age sixty-five, as the rate of growth of hair decreases and the diameters of the strands of hair decrease in size. Although many aging men retain much of their hair, some have a hereditary form of baldness known as male pattern baldness in which the top of the head eventually becomes completely bald. A substantial percentage of elderly women also experience some degree of hair thinning to the point that they may wear a wig.

Hair on the top of the head begins to turn gray between the ages of twenty-five and forty-three for whites, slightly later for African Americans, and slightly earlier for Asians. Elderly men tend to experience growth of hair in the ears, nostrils, and eyebrows, whereas many elderly women experience excessive growth of hair over the lips and on the chin. The growth of facial hair on elderly women is the result of an imbalance of sex hormones after menopause because estrogen (female sex hormone) production decreases and testosterone (male sex hormone) tends not to decrease. Unwanted hair may be removed by electrolysis, shaving, application of wax, or laser therapy. There are also some medications that negate the effect of testosterone on hair follicles.

There is some good news for senior citizens. Researchers in Denmark found no relationship between longevity and the extent of grayness, baldness, or facial wrinkles. There is other good news as well. The incidence of acne in late adulthood is very low.

Facts of Aging Quiz

This is a well-known test to appraise the knowledge that laypersons have about aging. It consists of twenty-five true-false statements about the physical, economic, psychological, and social characteristics of elderly people. The average American answers about half of the statements correctly (which, of course, is chance). It is hoped that readers of this book will do much better than that on this quiz.

Falls

Falls vary in terms of their type. The three main types are same-level falls, falls from one level to another level, and falls from stairs and steps. Same-level falls from slipping, tripping, or stumbling account for the majority of falls by older adults.

Elderly people fall frequently. About one-third of community-dwelling elderly adults fall annually, and in 2003 more than 421,000 seniors were hospitalized for fall-related injuries. However, it is estimated that only 5 percent to 15 percent of their falls result in injuries that seriously restrict their mobility. Nevertheless, there is good reason to be concerned about falls during late adulthood. Nearly two-thirds of the more than 10,000 fatal accidents each year among elderly people result from falls, making falls the most common source of fatal injury among elderly people.

Elderly women fall more often than elderly men, even though there is no apparent sex difference in balance. Most falls occur in the homes of elderly people. Especially disturbing is the fact that more than one-fourth of home-related falls could be prevented by redesigning or modifying elements of their homes. Modifications include securing throw rugs from slipping, adding grab bars to bathtubs and showers, and adding railings to stairs. Floors both in the home and in other places present a particular hazard. If a floor is not level, elderly people should start walking slowly to make certain their bodies are balanced. Any slick surface should be approached cautiously. Caution should also be exerted when moving in areas where there are animals or small children whose sudden movements may produce tripping. If furniture in a familiar room has been moved, elderly people should be informed of the changes before they enter the room. A flashlight with fresh batteries should be kept by the bed. Lightbulbs should be at least 100 watt. Organize work areas at home to minimize excessive reaching and the need to climb a ladder to reach things.

Many seniors have serious visual impairments that increase greatly the risk of falls, such as diminished acuity, diminished depth perception, poorer dark adaptation, and greater susceptibility to glare (see Vision). Decreasing the risk of falls requires seniors to have their vision checked regularly. Steps should be taken to reduce the probability of falling while climbing stairs or descending from them. Stairways should be well lighted, with the light shining on the walls, steps, and ceiling. The edge of each step should be marked with a strip with a color that contrasts with that of the rest of the step.

Environmental factors and visual impairments are not solely responsible for the high incidence of falls experienced by elderly people. Other physical impairments associated with normal aging also play a major role. Some of these impairments occur in the inner ear where the receptors involved in the maintenance of an upright posture and balance are located (*see* Dizziness). The frail physical condition of people at a very advanced age and their declining ability to prevent swaying while standing (*see* Posture) are also factors. Declining muscle strength in the hips, knees, and ankle joints are related to loss of balance. Interventions that improve strength in the lower extremities may reduce falls due to ineffective or weak postural adjustments.

There is also a relationship between walking gait and the likelihood of a fall. Elderly people with a history of falls, especially nursing home residents, tend to have decreased walking speed, shorter stride lengths, and greater variability of the length of successive steps relative to elderly people without a history of falls. The staffs of nursing homes should be aware of gait abnormalities among residents and be prepared to exert precautionary measures to prevent falls.

Patients with Alzheimer's disease also have difficulty suppressing incongruent visual stimuli when they try to maintain their balance. However, these patients seem to have less difficulty than normally aging people in changing their postural position quickly to altered supporting conditions. Many of the falls by nursing home residents (50 percent of them have at least one fall each year) could be eliminated by the use of wheelchair seat belts.

Health experts recommend a number of steps for elderly people to help them avoid falls. For example, elderly people are advised to avoid fast changes of direction while walking and to walk with their feet turned outward to provide greater stability. Taking a single rapid step during a fall may help to regain balance (*see also* Fractures [Hip]). However, elderly people have difficulty doing this, probably because there is a slowing down with aging in the execution of responses (*see* Slowing-Down Principle).

They should also avoid wearing running shoes while walking. In their homes they should not wear only socks or smooth-soled slippers on their feet. While going up or down stairs, they should always move slowly, take one step at a time, and hold onto the handrail. Elderly people need to be especially attentive when moving in an unfamiliar outdoor area. A researcher at Pepperdine University has estimated that 60 percent of the falls experienced by elderly people result from inattention and engagement in hazardous activities.

One of the most common causes of falls for elderly people is tripping over some obstacle (estimated to be more than 50 percent), even though they slow down when they approach an obstacle and shorten their stride length. Researchers in Michigan discovered that the less successful avoidance of obstacles by elderly adults than by younger adults is related to elderly adults' difficulty in maintaining focused attention on the obstacle and tuning out irrelevant sources of stimulation (for example, a nearby child; *see* Selective Attention).

The risk of a fall was found to be reduced for older women (age fifty to seventy-five) who had nine months of exercises that strengthened their lower body muscles. Other researchers have found that power exercise training strengthened muscle power in their limbs, resulting in better balance. Still other forms of exercise have proved to be effective in reducing the risk of falls. They include gait-modifying exercise, balance exercise, and even walking forward and backward in a swimming pool.

Some fear of falling is probably desirable for elderly people as a means of alerting them to potentially hazardous conditions in their environments. More than 40 percent of the community-dwelling elderly adults surveyed by Yale researchers indicated some fear of falling. Another survey revealed that the activity that makes the largest percentage of elderly adults fear falling is going out when there are slippery conditions (65 percent). The second most feared activity is taking a bath in a tub.

Nevertheless, most elderly people express a high level of confidence in their ability to perform everyday activities without falling. Those with the greatest confidence tend to be those with the highest level of physical functioning. Fear of falling is likely to increase in intensity once a fall has actually been experienced. Not surprisingly, older adults who have chronic dizziness are especially likely to fear falling.

There is the danger that the fear of falling will become irrational and present its own disabling consequences. Intense and irrational fears are likely to restrict the physical activities of those who experience them. A decline in mobility is the likely result of diminished physical activity. Researchers at the Yale University School of Medicine have discovered various procedures that reduce irrational fears of falling. Especially important are interventions designed to improve elderly adults' self-efficacy (confidence) in controlling their own activities. Family members are also cautioned to avoid excessive remarks to competent elderly people that discourage their independence (for example, "Don't do that—you might fall").

Older adults who fear falling and are considered high risks for falling may benefit from interventions that strengthen muscles in the legs. Otherwise they are in danger of restricting their physical activities to the point of their virtual disappearance. They need to consult with experts in exercising to find the appropriate exercise to strengthen their legs.

Not surprisingly, falls are not uncommon among elderly residents with dementia living in nursing homes. Researchers in the Netherlands analyzed the incidence of such falls during a two-year period. The residents averaged about four falls per year, with the incidence being greatest shortly after admission to the home and after transfer to a different ward in the home. The incidence also varied with the severity of the dementia and the degree of physical impairment, and it was as high for men as for women.

Most falls were caused either by a disruption of equilibrium or by inadequate use of available facilities. Fortunately, most falls produced relatively minor injuries, although fractures were occasionally the result.

An important objective of aging research is to identify those older people who have a high risk of falling and possibly experiencing a serious injury. In addition to gait characteristics, there are other characteristics of older people that may help to identify those with a high risk of falling. For example, Canadian researchers followed a number of elderly volunteers, all of whom had received a series of postural balance tests, during a one-year period. "Fallers" were distinguished from "nonfallers" largely in the greater amplitude of their lateral sway. Once such high-risk individuals are identified, they could benefit from the kind of balance retraining developed by researchers at the University of Oregon. The program stresses greater control of balance by means of improving the use of sensory information of importance in maintaining balance.

In addition, researchers in Finland discovered that the level of sex hormones in older women is related to the incidence of falls (the lower the level, the greater the incidence). Perhaps older women should be tested to determine their level. Those with a low level could then be given a training program to improve their balance (such as power exercises to improve their muscle power).

False Memory

"I could have sworn that I heard on the radio that Bob White the actor had died." If it turns out that this is not true, then the person has a *false memory*. A false memory is a memory of an event that seems to have occurred when it really did not. Such memories are fairly common, and they do not usually mean that something abnormal is going on in one's memory system. They are usually produced by some form of association between the imagined event and an event that actually occurred. For example, the person having the false memory about Bob White may actually have heard that Bob Black the athlete had died. Note that when one thinks of "white" it automatically triggers the strong association of "white" with "black."

Research in the laboratory strongly suggests that elderly adults are likely to experience slightly more false memories than do younger adults. This is what happens when participants of different ages are given a list of words that may include, say, *beautiful* as one of the words. When later asked if *pretty* was in the list, elderly participants average slightly more "yes" responses than do younger participants (*see* Recognition Memory versus Recall Memory).

In addition, when participants are asked to remember a list of words that contains *glass, pane, sill, curtain,* and *screen,* older participants are more likely than younger participants to believe that *window* was one of the words in the list when it was not (note that the actual words are all closely related to *window*). Interestingly, participants with Alzheimer's disease seem to have as great an amount of false memories for words not presented as normally aging participants even though their memory for words actually presented is much poorer.

Family Values and Traditionalism

Many people believe that contemporary older adults are more conservative or traditional in their beliefs and values than are younger adults. This even applies to roles of family members. For example, older adults are more likely to believe that a woman's place is in the home than are younger adults.

However, researchers at the Georgia Institute of Technology discovered that there is no indication that traditional family values increase with age. In their study they found that older participants were no more traditional than were younger participants. Seniors seem to "modernize" their values by keeping up with changes in society. They also found that older men are no more traditional than are older women.

Fatigue and Mental Performance

It is popularly believed that elderly people are more susceptible to mental fatigue from performing demanding mental tasks than are younger people. There is evidence to indicate the validity of this belief, but only when the demanding task has been performed for some time. Both younger and older participants score lower on an intelligence test when the test has been preceded by a lengthy performance of another demanding task than they do when there has been no prior task, but the negative effect on intelligence-test performance is much greater for the older participants. However, when the prior task is a relatively brief one, few negative effects have been found on a subsequent task for older participants. To safeguard against the negative effects of mental fatigue, older participants in laboratory research or older patients in a clinic usually receive frequent rest breaks while performing a demanding mental task or test.

Fatigue (Clinical Syndrome)

Chronic fatigue syndrome has vague symptoms, sufficiently so that many physicians do not believe their patients with it really have a disease. It has been found to be related to abnormal changes in genes that cause blood changes that are symptomatic of a wide variety of diseases.

Fatigue (Physical)

If you get proper sleep and you are an older person, what causes you to feel fatigued? Should it simply be blamed on "aging"? That does not help much. One possible reason is dehydration. Another is low blood pressure. Sleep apnea may be the cause by depriving you of proper sleep (*see* Sleep Disorders). Low testosterone may be the cause, but not very often. Perhaps your body has too little thyroid hormone.

The list of possible causes seems endless. Anemia (insufficient hemoglobin or red blood cells) should be on the list. So should eye strain—when your eyes feel tired, so do you (*see* Computers). Fatigue is a side effect of many medicines, including some for blood pressure, depression, anxiety, and infection. Perhaps too much alcohol before going to bed could interfere with REM sleep (*see* Sleep). Boredom could also give you the blahs. To combat fatigue, go outside in daylight for a while. It may help the brain's sleep centers. Take a nap for twenty to thirty minutes, or take a walk that is slow and quiet with frequent pauses to smell the roses.

Finger Movements and Exercise

As people grow older they often find it difficult to perform daily tasks that require skilled finger movements, such as tying shoes and fastening buttons. Especially important is the ability to use the fingers to grasp, lift, and manipulate objects between the thumb and one of the four fingers on the same hand (called a finger pinch). Researchers at the Cleveland Clinic Foundation in Cleveland, Ohio, have found that the right exercise can improve functioning involving finger pinch. The exercise consists of holding two metal balls in the palm of the dominant hand and rotating them clockwise or counterclockwise. The older participants in their study performed this task for two daily ten-minute sessions for several weeks. Most of the participants showed significant improvement in their finger-pinching ability.

Fire

About 80 percent of deaths from fire occur when people are asleep. Elderly people are especially vulnerable to death or serious injury from a fire in their house or apartment. Their residence should have at least one smoke alarm. Most alarms are designed to awaken an individual by a loud sound. However, this presents a problem for hearing-impaired seniors. There are special smoke alarms available that either give a very loud sound or a strobe light. There are also alarms to place beneath your pillow or between the mattress and box spring. They vibrate when activated by smoke. Check with your local fire department.

If there is a fire, get out of your house immediately. Crawl on hands and knees if it is smoky. Be careful opening a closed door. Feel the temperature with the back of your hand. If warm, pick another route. If you have to stay in a room, open a window and signal by flashlight (you should always keep one by your bed) where you are (call 911 if there is a telephone).

Flaxseed

Flaxseed is highly recommended as a nutritional supplement. It lowers the bad cholesterol level, or LDL. In addition, it is believed to reduce the risk of a heart attack and stroke. The fact that it contains potassium means that it lowers blood pressure, and its fiber content helps to prevent constipation and diverticulitis.

Fluid Intake

One concern about the health of elderly adults is whether they have sufficient daily intake of fluids to maintain normal biological functions. A study at Georgia State University provided tentative evidence to suggest that perhaps they do. Several hundred adults ranging in age from twenty to eighty recorded in a diary every food they ate and every fluid they drank each day for a week. The diary records indicated little difference between younger and older participants in the amount of fluids consumed daily. However, it is unclear if the younger adults themselves were consuming sufficient fluids.

Also unclear is the amount of water actually available for older adults to operate normally. Some of the fluids they consumed probably consisted of caffeinated beverages that served as diuretics and caused the body to lose water through increased urination.

The critical health factor for elderly adults is actually the amount of water they consume daily. Water aids in maintaining the appropriate body temperature and serves to transport nutrients and oxygen to cells and waste products from cells. Older people, on average, need six to eight cups of water per day to maintain normal body functions. However, researchers in New Mexico found that consuming eight glasses of fluid per day is not needed for many seniors. Milk, juices, and coffee (*see* Coffee) consist mainly of water and may be counted as part of the daily intake. Certain foods, such as soup, ice cream, and canned fruits, also contribute water, as do some vegetables. Elderly people should keep a water bottle handy to drink from throughout the day, and it would not hurt to start each meal with soup.

Too little consumption of fluids may eventually result in hydration. Sufficient consumption tends to result in fewer falls, less constipation, improved orthopedic condition, and a reduction in bladder cancer for men.

Fluid Intake (Cold Weather)

When working outdoors in cold weather, you could become dehydrated just as in warm weather. To stay hydrated, drink about one liter of water for every one thousand calories expended. Avoid cold water while working outdoors. It could cause the body to chill faster. Instead of water, you could substitute seltzer, diluted juice, or decaffeinated tea. Drink even though you are not thirsty. If you feel sluggish or have a headache, pause and have a drink of what you brought with you.

Fluid Intake (Differences between Younger and Older Adults)

There is evidence indicating that healthy older adults take in sufficient fluids to maintain an adequate hydration status. They consume more coffee and less soda and alcohol than younger persons. Older adults consume most of their fluids along with solids at meals, while younger adults increase their fluid intake later in the day.

Food and Meal Services

It is estimated that millions of elderly Americans fail to eat enough to maintain their physical health. In an effort to solve this problem, the federal government passed the Older Americans Act of 1965. The act established two free food services for anyone age sixty or older, services that were eventually administered by community Area Agencies on Aging.

The first provided meals at senior centers to qualified individuals and their spouses once daily for five or seven days a week. Donations are likely to be asked from those who can afford to give them. Around 2.5 million meals were served in 1993.

The second service is Meals on Wheels. This service is for people who have a disability that keeps them homebound. More than 800,000 people received these meals in 1993. Unfortunately, in recent years these two services have not been able to keep up with the needs of many elderly people. The problem is that the money allotted for them has remained fairly constant over the years, while the number of elderly people has increased greatly.

Another problem is that a number of elderly people abandon the Meals on Wheels program within a relatively short time after beginning it. For example, a survey of participants in western New York State revealed that nearly 65 percent of them had stopped participating over a period of several years. The reasons given for stopping participation differed somewhat between white and African American participants. For example, the most frequent reason given by white participants (20 percent) was placement in a supervised facility, while the most frequent reason given by African American participants (28 percent) was dissatisfaction with the meals or their poor appetite. Elderly men and women also differed somewhat in their reasons. The most frequent reason for men was moving to a relative's home or finding someone to cook (23 percent), while the most frequent reason for women was placement in a supervised facility (23 percent).

Elderly people may also benefit from food stamps issued by the Department of Agriculture and redeemed at grocery stores. The food stamp program helps to provide nutrition for 25 million people monthly. It greatly helps to fulfill the needs of seniors, disabled adults of all ages, and many children. To be eligible you must be a U.S. citizen, a refugee, or a legal alien. Your income must be no higher than $798 per month for a single person or $1,066 for a couple. You must not own property or have savings valued at more than $3,000 if you are age sixty or older (for those younger it is $2,000). However, in 2005 Congress threatened to reduce greatly funding for the program.

In addition, food or meals or both are offered to needy elderly people by many churches and civic organizations. Elderly people who need food or meal services and are not receiving them should contact local agencies on aging, senior centers, churches, and so on to find out what services are available in their communities.

Foot Problems

It is estimated that 75 percent of Americans have a foot problem sometime in their lives. Elderly adults are major contributors to this alarming statistic, especially elderly women. An issue of *Perspectives in Health and Aging* (1993, vol. 8, no. 2), an AARP publication, was devoted to foot problems. Most of the information in this entry is derived from that publication.

Changes occur in the feet of many people as they age normally. The feet may tend to spread, they may lose some of their cushioning, and they may become discolored. The skin and nails may also become dry and brittle. Other problems may occur. One is the presence of athlete's foot, which is caused by a fungus. To avoid this condition, older adults should keep their feet dry and exposed frequently to the air. Corns and calluses are caused by pressure from bony areas of the feet that rub against shoes. Their prevention requires wearing properly fitted shoes. Removal of corns and calluses should be done by a podiatrist. Some bunions are inherited, but others may be caused by wearing ill-fitting shoes. For more severe and painful bunions, surgery may be required. Hammertoe, a condition in which the second toe slants toward and under the big toe, may accompany a bunion. Hammertoe may cause a problem with balance and may therefore be a contributing factor to falls. Mild cases are treated by wearing the correct shoes and stockings, but more severe cases may require surgery.

Calcium growths on the heels, known as heel spurs, can be very painful. They may be prevented by avoiding prolonged standing and by wearing well-fitted supportive shoes. Calcium growths are treated by wearing shoes with heel pads and heel cups and sometimes by drugs.

Plantar fasciitis is another painful heel condition. The plantar fascia is the tissue that stretches from the heel to the base of the toes. Wear and tear on the foot may result in prolonged pain in the heel, especially while walking. Rest is needed for relief of the pain, along with protecting the sole and heel of the foot by an insert in the shoe to relieve pressure. Soaking the foot in warm water for twenty minutes two or three times daily may also help.

Ingrown toenails consist of corners of nails that pierce the skin. A 1988 survey by the U.S. Department of Health and Human Services reported the incidence of ingrown toenails to be three times greater for people age seventy-five and older than for people in the eighteen-to-forty-four-year range. They are usually the result of improper nail trimming, but they may also be caused by an injury or a fungal infection. They may usually be avoided by always cutting the toenails straight across.

Unfortunately, foot problems may be aggravated in many elderly adults who use walking as their form of exercise. The difficulty lies in wearing improper walking shoes and socks. A podiatrist should be consulted before purchasing walking shoes. Among the things to look for are shoes with firm heel counters to cushion the impact while walking and soles that provide a high degree of shock absorption. Equally important is the wearing of the right socks. Podiatrists often recommend wearing two pairs of socks during strenuous walking. The thin inner pair should be made of silk or wool to prevent blisters, and the thicker outer pair should be made of a blend of acrylic fiber and either cotton or wool. A particular danger from improper walking shoes is a blister. One way to ease the pain from a blister is soak a cotton ball or a washcloth in cool milk and apply it to the blister for fifteen minutes, and repeat as often as needed. Applying the milk compress within twenty-four hours of getting the blister helps to reduce inflammation as well as the pain and may hasten healing of the blister.

Forgetting

"Mommy, my forgettery is better than my memory." The little girl in the comic strip who said this was displaying a wisdom well beyond her years. She reminded us that the imperfections of memory are present at all ages, and that many of these imperfections result from forgetting information that had once been acquired. *Forgetting*, like memory per se, is a fact of life, and especially for episodic memory (*see* Episodic Memory). Information in short-term memory is forgotten in a matter of seconds if it is not continuously rehearsed (*see* Short-Term Memory). However, the rate of short-term forgetting appears to be no greater for older adults than for younger adults.

But what about long-term episodic memory? Much of the information that has entered the long-term memory store does seem to be forgotten. However, an important distinction must be made between the unavailability of that information and the inaccessibility of that information. Unavailability means that the once-stored information has been "lost" and is no longer available for retrieval. Inaccessibility means that at least some of that information is still present in the store, but it cannot be retrieved at a given moment.

Consider a particular foreign-language word that you learned in high school but you cannot recall. For example, you may be trying to recall the Spanish word for "dog," and you cannot remember it. However, on seeing it, you may immediately recognize that it means "dog." This surely indicates that you have not fully forgotten the word. Moreover, even if you do not recognize the word, you may still have some memory of it. This is likely to be demonstrated if you took a refresher course in Spanish. The Spanish words you seem to have forgotten are likely to be learned faster than they were learned originally. This is called a savings in learning, and it clearly demonstrates that some memory remains even though it cannot be consciously recollected (see Implicit Memory). Most people have difficulty recalling the content of a college course after only a year has passed. However, they are likely to discover that they learn the same material much more quickly if they repeat the course. This again is a savings that indicates more memory persists than is within our conscious recollection.

We usually view forgetting in terms of our conscious recollection of information. If information can be neither recalled nor recognized, it is likely to be considered forgotten. Forgetting usually follows a normal progression, with most of it occurring shortly after acquisition, with further forgetting occurring at a slower rate until it levels off at some residue of retained information. This is the case, for example, with the foreign-language words you may have acquired in a high school language course. Most of the forgetting takes place within the first year after the course (see Very Long-Term Memory).

Why does such forgetting occur? The most important reason is the *interference* from other somewhat similar material acquired both before the language course and after the language course. Consider your memory of the names of television programs from ten years ago. You probably do not recall many of their names, and you probably would not recognize many more as well. In this case, interference comes from both the names of programs you viewed more than ten years ago and the names of programs viewed during the intervening ten years. The interference from prior information is called *proactive interference*, and interference from later information is called *retroactive interference*. The product of the two sources of interference is the loss from the long-term store of some information and the inaccessibility of the remaining forgotten information.

Forgetting is studied in laboratory situations by having participants learn successive lists of paired words (paired-associate learning; *see* Verbal Learning). Retention may then be determined for either the first list or the second list. The forgetting that occurs for the first list is largely the consequence of the interference produced by the second list. That is, it is the product of retroactive interference. The forgetting that occurs for the second list is the consequence of the interference produced by the first list. That is, it is the product of proactive interference.

As with real-life information, forgetting is rapid after acquisition. In this situation most of it occurs within a day after learning the lists and then slows until a residue of still remembered information remains. Of great importance is the general finding that the rate of forgetting is no faster for elderly participants than it is for younger participants, provided the material has been mastered equally at each age level. The implication is that new episodic information that has been well registered in the long-term store should not be forgotten, on average, at any substantially greater rate by older adults than by younger adults. This equality in forgetting rates is somewhat surprising in that elderly adults were once believed to be more susceptible to the effects of interference than younger adults (*see* Transfer of Learning/Training).

There are severe forms of forgetting known as amnesia that are produced by deterioration of the brain. One form of loss is in terms of the difficulty of acquiring new information and storing it in memory. The other form is in terms of the difficulty in retrieving memories that were stored before the onset of amnesia. The former is called *anterograde amnesia* (meaning forward in time); the latter is termed *retrograde amnesia* (backward in time; *see also* Alcohol [Physical and Mental Effects]).

Form Perception

When you look at a tree, you recognize it as a tree. Similarly, a dog is recognized as a dog, an automobile as an automobile, and so on. These are familiar examples of form perception. We are able to "make sense" of the "raw" visual information registered by our eyes, and perceive the forms initiating that information meaningfully. That is, we are able to name those forms.

Our visual system, including the visual areas of the brain, automatically extracts features of the object in question and matches it with information stored permanently in memory. Thus, the features of an automobile include four wheels and mechanical power. When a form has features matching these and other features we know that characterize an automobile, that form is recognized and identified as an automobile. Extracting features and matching them with what is stored in memory is known to psychologists as *pattern recognition*. Consider the form *A* that you immediately identify as the uppercase form of the first letter of the English alphabet. The form has two distinctive features, converging slanting lines and an intersecting horizontal line. Stored in your memory is information acquired during childhood that these features identify the letter *A*. Whenever a new pattern is encountered that matches these features, pattern recognition occurs rapidly and effortlessly. Even with some distortion of the features, as in the form or pattern ⌂, there is enough commonality with the basic features to identify the novel form as an *A*.

Are elderly adults less accurate in form perception (or pattern recognition) than young adults? Under normal circumstances, the answer is only slightly, if at all. When young and older adults are compared in the accuracy of naming pictures of objects, the age difference in average scores is small. Normally aging older adults, like young adults, rarely make misidentifications. However, when the circumstances make pattern recognition more difficult, there is a more moderate age difference. This may be seen when segments of the pictures are deleted. In a study by researchers at the University of Missouri at Columbia, young and elderly participants viewed drawings of such objects as a violin and a rabbit in which 90 percent of each form had been randomly deleted by means of a computer. The young participants were able to identify, on average, about 85 percent of the pictures, and the elderly participants identified about 75 percent.

Although the effects of aging on the accuracy of form perception are modest, the effects of aging on the speed of pattern recognition are much greater (in agreement with the "slowing down" principle; *see* Slowing-Down Principle). The age difference is demonstrated in the laboratory with simple materials in which participants view pairs of letters, and they decide whether they have the same name. Examples of such pairs are *Aa*, *BB*, *HK*, and *Tb*. Note that for the first two pairs the answer is yes. However, the answer will be given more quickly regardless of age for the second pair than for the first pair. This is because the letters in the second pair have completely overlapping features—and they must therefore have the same name.

This is not true for the first pair where there is no overlap of features. Therefore pattern recognition takes somewhat longer while memory is searched to discover that *A* and *a* do indeed have the same name. Elderly adults are slower than young adults for both *Aa*- and *BB*-type comparisons, but the magnitude of the age difference is greater for the *Aa* type. These are simple materials of little relevance to everyday form perception. However, they do suggest that elderly adults will, on average, be slower in identifying many forms in the everyday world. For example, is the object in the road ahead of the driver simply debris or an animal? The slower recognition by the older driver than by the younger driver could result in very different actions taken by the drivers (for instance, swerving the car or not swerving it).

Foster Grandparent Program

The Foster Grandparent Program in the United States is one of several programs established by the Domestic Service Act of 1973. The objective of the program is to encourage the participation of elderly people in activities that should improve the quality of their lives and enhance their mental health, as well as the lives of the recipients of these activities. Elderly participants are paid a small compensation for working with children in various settings, such as schools and homes for children with mental disabilities. Not only are the foster grandparents likely to benefit from their relationship with the children, but the children also are expected to receive attention that may otherwise be missing in their lives.

By the early 1980s more than eighteen thousand foster grandparents were employed in this program. Their average age was sixty-nine, and more than half were widowed. Among the reasons cited for joining the program were to make better use of their time, to help children, and to earn some badly needed money.

Fractures (Hip)

Ninety percent of hip fractures occur in people over age sixty-five (220,000 annually), mainly in women. The costs for hospitalization and long-term care are estimated to be between thirty-one billion and sixty-two billion dollars annually. There are two main kinds of hip fractures that together account for about 97 percent of all hip fractures. They are fractures of the femoral neck (the femur is the thigh bone) and fractures through the intertrochanteric region of the femur. The neck of the femur is the part that fits into the cavity of the hip bone, and the intertrochanteric region is between the two segments of the femur below the neck. There is recent evidence indicating that patients with intertrochanteric fractures are older, are sicker on hospital admission, have longer stays in the hospital, and are less likely to have recovered the activities of daily living (*see* Activities of Daily Living) two months after the fracture than patients with femoral neck fractures.

Osteoporosis (declining bone density with aging; *see* Osteoporosis), calcium deficiency, and vitamin D deficiency are important indirect causes of hip fractures, while the increased susceptibility of elderly people to falls (*see* Falls) is the most important direct cause. An excessive amount of thyroid hormone contributes to the risk of hip fracture in some women by accelerating bone loss.

Do regular supplements of calcium and vitamin D reduce the risk of hip fracture? This possibility was tested on thousands of women age fifty to seventy-nine who were participants in the Women's Health Initiative Study. Half of them took the supplements regularly; the other half did not. The results were only moderately encouraging. The participants with the supplements did have better bone density than those who did not, but the former did not differ from the latter in avoiding fractures of all kinds. However, those over age sixty who took the supplements did have a 21 percent reduction in the incidence of hip fractures, and women who adhered closely to taking the supplements daily had a reduced risk of 29 percent.

After surgery for a hip fracture, the patient's social support improves recovery only if present early in recovery. Low improvement in walking after surgery is likely to lead to depression. Within one year after a hip fracture about 20 percent to 25 percent of elderly victims die. Risk factors for death following a hip fracture include age over eighty-five, a deep wound infection, and postoperative pneumonia. About 10 percent to 20 percent of patients with a hip fracture will lose sufficient physical ability to require nursing home care.

The incidence of hip fractures in women varies greatly among countries. The countries with the highest incidence are those where daily animal-protein intake is highest (for example, Denmark and the United States), and the countries with the lowest incidence are those where the average daily intake of vegetable protein is the highest (such as Nigeria and Thailand). The evidence here suggests that an increased ratio of vegetable to animal food may offer some protection against hip fractures.

A diet with at least 109 micrograms of vitamin K daily has been found to reduce the risk of hip fracture by 30 percent. Foods high in vitamin K are cooked spinach, broccoli, and brussels sprouts.

There is the possibility of avoiding a hip fracture. When sensing you are about to fall forward, outstretch your hands to break the fall with your hands. Canadian researchers found that older women are able to outstretch fast enough to avoid landing on their pelvis. *See also* Falls; Nursing Home Discharge Outcomes.

Frailty as a Clinical Syndrome

How would you define "frailty"? It isn't easy to do. A team of researchers has established a definition of it as a clinical syndrome in which three or more of the following are present: an unintentional weight loss of ten pounds or more in the past year, self-reported exhaustion, weakness as measured by grip strength, slow walking speed, and low physical activity.

Frailty (Identifying Degrees)

Researchers at the Washington University School of Medicine have distinguished among three categories of frailty: not frail, mildly frail, and moderately frail. The distinction is based on scores obtained on a nine-item physical performance test (for instance, putting on and taking off a coat).

Frailty (Incidence and Causes)

The percentage of older Americans who are frail has been estimated to be about 25 percent. By contrast, French researchers have found it to be more than 30 percent in France.

Conditions producing frailty in late adulthood include years of heavy drinking, smoking, physical inactivity, and social isolation. During late adulthood itself, a primary condition is inadequate diet and nutrition. A survey of the food intake of nearly five hundred normally aging adults between the ages of sixty-five and ninety-eight revealed that 40 percent of them had energy intake from food that was well below the recommended amount. More than 20 percent reported that they normally did not eat lunch. In another survey of a large sample of women over age seventy, 16 percent were underweight, and nearly 30 percent failed to consume adequate amounts of the basic nutrients.

French Paradox

See Portion Size and Heart Health.

Frequency-of-Occurrence Memory

How many times in the past week did you see an advertisement on television for Budweiser beer? Which advertisement did you see more often in the past week, one for Budweiser beer or one for McDonald's? You are likely to be reasonably accurate in your answers to these questions (assuming you pay attention to television commercials). This is true even though you had no idea your memory for the frequency-of-occurrence of these events would be tested, and you therefore acquired the frequency information without intending to do so. That is, the frequency information was acquired incidentally and without your effort to rehearse the events in question.

Some memory theorists believe that the frequencies with which events occur are registered automatically in memory in the sense they do not require the intent to register that information. Presumably, we have been programmed genetically to record frequency-of-occurrence information for the events that occur in our everyday lives. If true, then we would expect frequency-of-occurrence memory to be as proficient for normally aging adults as for young adults.

To investigate these characteristics of frequency-of-occurrence memory, researchers use a laboratory task in which events occur different numbers of times. Participants are then asked to give judgments about those frequencies. The events usually are familiar words that appear in a lengthy series. Some of the words appear only one time, some two times (widely separated appearances), some three times, and so on.

At the end of the series participants may be asked questions such as "How many times did the word *apple* appear in the series?" Alternatively, they may be asked, "Which word appeared more often, *apple* or *pencil?*" Answers to questions of these kinds are usually rather accurate. Moreover, accuracy is usually as high when the participants do not know in advance that their memory will be tested (incidental memory) as when they do know in advance exactly what kind of memory will be tested (intentional memory).

This is true regardless of the age of the participants. Most important, older participants are nearly as accurate as younger participants. The magnitude of an age decline in frequency-of-occurrence memory proficiency does seem to be much less than the magnitude of the decline found in many other forms of memory (for example, spatial memory and temporal memory; *see* Spatial Memory; Temporal Memory). For whatever reasons, frequency-of-occurrence memory seems to be largely immune to any pronounced declines with normal aging.

Friendships

There are two kinds of friendships: interest related and deep. An interest-related friendship is one brought about by similar interests of the friends, such as a common hobby or playing bridge together. A deep friendship is one involving a more intimate relationship that goes beyond shared interests. There is a bond of closeness between the friends.

The number of friendships, particularly interest-related ones, may decline in late adulthood because of deaths, health problems, and other factors that constrain the opportunity for interactions with friends. There may be another important reason. Some gerontologists believe that many elderly people restrict their social interactions to longtime friends and avoid making new friends to conserve their physical energy and to minimize negative emotional states that might arise from social interactions with other than old and familiar friends. More elderly adults than young adults are satisfied with the size of their social networks, and elderly adults may not wish to enlarge them. They often see themselves as having only a few years left to live, and they believe they are better off spending time with a few close friends.

There is evidence that new friendships are relatively infrequent for elderly people, especially those in their eighties and older. The number of friends does decrease for those in this age range, relative to those in the sixty-to-eighty-year range. However, the number of close relationships for the very old remains about the same as for the younger old. Thus, the proportion of close, deep attachments increases during very late adulthood. In general, the quality of social contacts shows a stronger positive relationship with well-being than does the number of social contacts.

It should be recognized that the evidence on age differences in friendships has been gathered in cross-sectional studies and not in longitudinal studies. Conceivably, these differences could be the result of differences in friendships between different generations or cohorts, rather than the result of a change from early to late adulthood in the need for different patterns of friendships (see Cohort [Generational] Effect).

In general, older people appear to find greater satisfaction in their relationships with friends than with family members. The apparent reason is the greater sharing of leisure activities with friends than with family members. However, there are important sex differences in the friendships of older people. Older women, in general, have more friends than older men, and they are likely to place greater value on their friendships than do older men. Older women also seem to have a greater sharing of their activities and a greater emotional involvement with their friends than do older men. For older married couples, the wife is likely to have a friend as her closest confidant, whereas the husband's closest confidant is likely to be his wife. However, for both men and women, social connections with friends are very important as a factor in determining successful aging.

A theory widely applied to friendships is called equity theory. According to this theory, the satisfaction gained from a friendship depends on the mutual benefit gained from it. This theory has received considerable support when applied to the friendships of younger adults. However, it has received less support when applied to the friendships of older adults. A survey of older adults in Colorado suggests that for older adults the perception of equity or fairness in a relationship is relatively unimportant when applied to their best friends. However, perceived equity does seem to be an important factor in determining the degree of satisfaction from relationships with other "non-best" friends. Healthy older adults do seem to want a balance between giving and receiving with these friends. See also Loneliness; Social Networks; Successful Aging.

Frontal Lobe Functioning (Improving It in Dementia)

Researchers in Japan gave six months of training in reading out loud and doing simple arithmetic calculations to patients with Alzheimer's disease. Previous research had indicated that these tasks activate the prefrontal cortex of the brain (see Brain and Aging), an area critical for cognitive functioning. The patients in the Japanese study showed significant improvement in cognitive functioning after the training period.

Functional Age

"I may be seventy years old, but I have the handgrip strength of a man forty years old." If this statement is true, then the man making the statement has a physical functional age that is many years younger than his chronological age, at least for the specific physical function of hand strength. If someone's level of functioning corresponds to the level of functioning of an average forty year old, then the person's functional age is forty years. This would be the case whether the person is actually thirty, fifty, or seventy years old.

Of course, that same person's functional age is likely to be different for other physical skills and functions, and may even be greater than seventy for some. For example, his lung capacity may correspond to that of the average seventy-five-year-old man. In fact, for any given individual, there may be considerable variability in his or her various functional ages. It is this variability that makes physical functional age difficult to serve as an effective replacement for chronological age in defining the onset of old age (*see* Old [Defining Late Adulthood]).

The concept of functional age may also be applied to mental skills and abilities. Thus, a seventy-year-old person who has the memory proficiency of the average forty-year-old person would have a functional age of forty in regard to memory. However, that same individual is likely to have different functional ages for other mental skills and abilities, thus making functional age on any one ability an unlikely replacement for chronological age in defining late adulthood.

There is the argument expressed by various occupational groups (such as airline pilots, physicians, and professors) that it is functional age on job-related skills that should determine retirement and not some arbitrary fixed chronological age. Airline pilots have been required to retire as pilots when they reach age sixty. This practice seemingly conflicts with evidence indicating that the incidence of flying accidents for pilots of private airplanes is actually lower for pilots in their sixties and seventies than it is for younger pilots. Older pilots may continue to work as flight engineers. Some hospitals require physicians to retire at age seventy, and professors are usually urged to retire at age seventy or younger.

Pilots who are chronologically older than sixty have long argued that functionally (in terms of the skills needed to fly a large airplane) they may be much younger, and that it is their functional age and not their chronological age that should determine retirement. A similar argument has been made by many physicians, resulting in various legal cases, and even by a referee of the National Football League who was given duties off the field because of his age.

Surely, many college professors at age seventy have a functional age for professorial skills that is well below their chronological age. Unfortunately, the difficulties in reliably and thoroughly determining functional age for any given occupation have made its substitution for chronological age in determining retirement age unacceptable. This is likely to change in the future, however, as better understanding of aging abilities and their measurements is accomplished.

Funerals

Our coverage will focus only on what are generally considered to be traditional Christian funerals that do make up the vast majority of funerals in the United States. Prior to the funeral itself, some caskets are open fully for viewing, others halfway, and still others not at all. Caskets have guarantees of twenty-five years, fifty years, one hundred years, or forever. Most cemeteries require the use of a vault to prevent creating a depression in the ground and adding to groundskeeping costs.

Arranging for a funeral for a spouse or other close relative can be very traumatic for elderly adults. It is possible to make funeral arrangements for yourself in advance, including prepayment of the various costs. The assistance of an offspring or close friend is usually greatly appreciated, if advance arrangements have not been made. Funerals can be very expensive, and sometimes excessively so. For more information about funerals, contact the Funeral Service Consumer Assistance Program, National Research and Information Center, 2250 East Devon Avenue, Suite 250, Des Plaines, IL 60018 (or call 800-662-7666). *See also* Cremation.

G

Gallbladder Diseases

Gallbladder diseases, even when they are not life threatening, present a serious problem to many older people. It is estimated that about 35 percent of people over age seventy, compared to fewer than 20 percent of people between fifty-five and sixty-five years of age, have gallstones. Gallstones produce pain just below the rib cage or in the right shoulder. They can result in serious damage to the pancreas or liver. Treatment for gallstones is likely to be either surgery or medical treatment consisting of weight reduction, avoidance of fatty foods, and use of antacids. For surgery, a scope is inserted to pull out the stones. A liquid can be inserted through the skin into the gallbladder to liquify the stones. Sound waves may serve to break up the stones. Of concern is the evidence indicating that women who are on estrogen and progestin therapy have a greater risk of gallstones than women who are not on the therapy.

Gallbladder pain may result from a condition known as biliary dyskinesia. The condition is the result of the gallbladder not emptying its content of bile. The continuously full bladder causes pain on the right upper side of the abdomen. Stay away from fried foods and fatty foods. The usual treatment is removal of the gallbladder.

Gallbladder cancer is a relatively uncommon, but highly fatal, form of cancer. It affects about six thousand people in the United States annually. It is most frequently diagnosed when people are in their sixties. Women have the disease substantially more often than men. It seems to be associated with gallstone disease, estrogen, cigarette smoking, excessive alcohol consumption, and obesity. Symptoms include jaundice and weight loss. Successful treatment is difficult to achieve.

Gamblers (Differences between Younger and Older Gamblers)

A telephone survey in 1999 by the National Research Council revealed that only 0.4 percent of the seniors age sixty-five and older contacted admitted to obsessive gambling. The percentage today is probably much larger given the great expansion of casinos across the United States (even Boonville, Missouri, has one). Of the ninety-one seniors surveyed in gaming facilities by researchers in Nebraska several years ago, 11 percent were identified as being obsessive gamblers. This probably underestimates the percentage. Many older adults addicted to gambling may refuse to admit to their addiction.

How do older obsessive gamblers differ from younger obsessive gamblers? In a recent study of young, middle-aged, and older obsessive gamblers, only in the oldest group were there more women than men (23 percent, 40 percent, and 55 percent in the young, middle-aged, and older groups, respectively). The older women reported that they started gambling regularly at the average age of fifty-five, the older men at the average age of thirty-three. Comparable average starting ages for the middle-aged gamblers were thirty-nine and twenty-eight, respectively.

The average amount gambled in the past month was eighteen hundred dollars for older women and fifteen hundred dollars for older men. By contrast, the comparable averages were one thousand dollars and one thousand dollars for middle-aged women and men gamblers and eight hundred dollars and one thousand dollars for young women and men gamblers, respectively.

The age groups differed in their primary choice of type of gambling. For older gamblers it was slot machines (57 percent compared to 41 percent for middle-aged and 19 percent for younger gambler—card games were the primary choice for both of these age groups).

Garlic

Does garlic really have major positive effects on physical health? A review of many studies revealed that its positive benefits are rather slight. Some positive effect on total cholesterol level was reported, but no significant effect on blood pressure level. But it may chase away vampires.

Gender and Sex Differences in Aging

The terms *gender* and *sex* are often confused in the everyday world. A good example is in the issue of gender equity in college sports. What is really meant is *sex equity* in the form of equal funding and support for women's and men's sports. *Gender* actually refers to what are commonly considered to be traditional masculine and feminine personality characteristics and behaviors.

For years, men played the role of family providers, and women played the role of child caregivers. Men were also expected to be more assertive and aggressive than women, and women were expected to be more tender and sensitive than men. Thus, assertiveness and tenderness are masculine and feminine characteristics, respectively, that have traditionally been associated with the masculine and feminine genders. However, there have also been gender reversals at all ages. Many men possess feminine characteristics (tenderness), and many women possess masculine characteristics (assertiveness).

One of gerontology's most interesting debates in recent years has been whether men and women become increasingly alike in their balance of masculine and feminine characteristics as they age. Do elderly men become more sensitive than they were earlier in life and elderly women more assertive? If so, they have become androgynous persons who are no longer bound to rigid gender characteristics and rigid sex roles. There is evidence indicating that androgyny is more characteristic of elderly men than it is of elderly women (*see* Androgyny). The trend toward androgyny is likely to increase for future generations as sex-role stereotypes become increasingly relaxed with changes in our society, and it is likely to be found in many men and women long before they reach late adulthood.

Sex differences refer to differences between men and women in physical and mental abilities and in behaviors. An obvious sex difference is in longevity; women generally live some years longer than men (*see* Life Expectancy). There are other obvious biological differences between men and women as well (for instance, in strength). There are also others that are not as obvious (such as urinary incontinence; *see* Urinary Incontinence). Declines in sensory functioning in normal aging are fairly comparable for men and women. Hearing does show a moderate sex difference. Declines in hearing proficiency with aging are greater for women than for men with low-pitched sounds, and the reverse is true for higher-pitched sounds (*see* Hearing).

Elderly men and women perform at comparable levels on intelligence tests and on most tests of specific mental abilities. However, there are a few exceptions. Early in adulthood women score higher than men on tests of verbal ability, and men score higher on tests of spatial ability. These sex differences persist through late adulthood (*see* Sex Differences and Scientific Ability; Spatial Ability; Verbal Ability). Sex differences in long-term memory have usually been found to be slight. However, for both young-old and old-old participants in the Seattle Longitudinal Study (*see* Longitudinal Studies of Aging's Effects on Health and Cognition), women scored higher on a recall task than did men (*see* Recognition Memory versus Recall Memory). Elderly men may be slightly more proficient than elderly women in remembering long-past events (*see* Very Long-Term Memory).

There are many behavioral differences between elderly men and women. For example, elderly men are more likely to remarry than are elderly women. A number of these behavioral differences, along with other physical differences between elderly men and women, may be found in other entries in this book (*see* Index of Entries and Cross-References).

Generativity

Generativity is a term introduced to psychology some years ago by Dr. Erik Erikson. It refers to a person's concern about the next generation and how to help guide members of that generation through teaching, leadership, and example. Dr. Erikson assumed that generativity peaked in middle age and then declined.

Researchers at Northwestern University challenged the suspected decline in late adulthood. They measured generativity for adults of various ages by means of a number of psychological tests (for example, self-ratings on a questionnaire and writing sentences describing personal goals). Contrary to Dr. Erikson's assumption, they found generativity to be as high in their older participants as in their middle-aged participants—and higher for both groups than for young adult participants. They also found generativity to be related positively to life satisfaction for the older participants, that is, generativity was highest for those elderly people who were most satisfied with their current lives.

The questionnaire used to measure age differences in generativity is called the Loyola Generativity Scale (LGS). It has twenty statements that participants respond to in terms of how they apply to them (from never to very often). Among the statements are "I feel as though my contributions will exist after I die" and "I try to pass along the knowledge I have gained through my experience." Elderly women tend to score higher in generativity on the LGS than do elderly men. High scorers differ from low scorers in several important ways. For example, high scorers tell more stories about themselves that stress caring for young persons, a trait presumed to be part of greater generativity, than do low scorers.

Geriatric Depression Scale

The Geriatric Depression Scale is a test designed specifically to assess older adults for depressive symptoms. It attempts to correct problems found with other tests of depression when used with seniors. The Geriatric Depression Scale has much less somatic complaints than the other tests. The test contains thirty items with yes-no answers.

Geriatrics

Geriatrics is that branch of medicine concerned with the investigation of the medical problems encountered in late adulthood and with the application of knowledge about the biological and behavioral aspects of aging to the diagnosis and treatment of those problems.

Gerontology

Gerontology is a broad field of study concerned with every aspect of functioning in late adulthood. Thus, gerontology is concerned with the many facets of aging, but especially the biological, psychological, and sociological. Research in biological gerontology is directed at the discovery of the biological mechanisms responsible for aging and at the determination of the nature of age-related changes in various biological and physiological functions. Research in psychological aging is directed at the study of what happens to various psychological processes and functions (for instance, sensory, attentional, memory, personality, and coping with stress) with aging and the determination of the reasons for these changes. One of the main areas of research in social gerontology deals with the demographic characteristics of elderly people. Other major areas are concerned with the family life of older people, the services available for older people, and the factors influencing life satisfaction for older people.

Ginkgo

Ginkgo is an extract from the ginkgo tree that is sold as a memory enhancer for both patients with Alzheimer's disease and nondemented elderly adults who have concerns about their memory functioning. Researchers reported in 1997 a modest improvement in performance on mental tests and in social activities in patients with Alzheimer's disease. In a study by researchers at Williams College, 115 healthy older adults were assigned randomly to a group receiving six weeks of ginkgo therapy. Another 115 healthy older adults were assigned randomly to a placebo group. Participants in both groups received a number of verbal and nonverbal memory tests. They were then retested later. At retest both groups improved on all tests. However, this was simply a practice effect. There was no additional benefit for the group receiving ginkgo.

Ginkgo, like such herbs as garlic and ginseng, may inhibit blood clotting and should not be taken by people using blood thinners (for example, aspirin). Potential users should know that some brands may not contain the level of the active ingredient considered to be needed to improve blood flow in the brain. They should check with their pharmacists. *See also* Alzheimer's Disease.

Goals

Do you make New Year's resolutions? If so, you are setting goals or objectives you want to accomplish during the new year. Goals, of course, are not limited to such resolutions (which usually are minor ones that are soon abandoned anyway). Life goals are those that give direction to our activities and our commitments. Succeeding at one's profession or job is a common goal for younger adults, as is raising their children to a happy and healthy adulthood. But what about older people? Do they continue to set goals for themselves? If so, what kinds of goals do they have? Most important, do their goals affect their happiness and their adjustment to the demands of daily living?

Researchers at New York University have conducted studies that provide at least partial answers to these questions. They classified goals into such categories as "active improvement of one's life" (for instance, doing creative volunteer work), "maintenance of one's social values and relationships" (maintaining old friendships), "feeling safe and secure" (living in a safe neighborhood), "having an energetic lifestyle" (being able to do your own errands), and "disengagement" (having fewer family obligations). Not surprisingly, they found that older people vary greatly in their goals.

However, they also found that certain characteristics and living conditions of elderly people are related to their goals. For example, they found that being widowed is characterized by having safety and security as a goal. They also found that retirees increasingly have the goal of an energetic lifestyle as the duration of their retirement increases and that healthy elderly people are more likely than less healthy ones to have an energetic lifestyle as a goal. Moreover, they found that satisfaction with one's present life is greater for those older people who have maintenance of social values and relationships or an energetic lifestyle as goals than for those elderly people who have disengagement as a goal (*see* Activity Theory; Disengagement Theory).

Closely related to goals is the intention to meet those goals. Elderly adults have been found, in general, to have more frequent lapses and longer lapses than younger adults in maintaining goal-directed behaviors. Such lapses have been linked to the loss of neurons in the prefrontal cortex of the brain of some elderly adults (*see* Brain and Aging).

Grandparenting

About three-fourths of the elderly people in the United States are grandparents. As you might expect, they show differences in their styles of interacting with their grandchildren. More than twenty-five years ago, researchers at the University of Chicago identified five basic styles of grandparenting. The first is a *formal style* in which there is a sharp division between grandparent and grandchild. That is, the grandparent stays largely in the background with an occasional offering of a gift. The second is a *fun-seeker style* that is characterized by a leisurely, informal orientation, and mutual pleasure experienced by both participants in their interactions. The third is a *surrogate-parent style* in which the grandparent substitutes for the child's parents. Not surprisingly, few grandparents select this style voluntarily. The fourth style is one in which the grandparent serves as a *reservoir of family wisdom* and perhaps authority. The remaining style is that of a *distant figure* in which the grandparent emerges from the shadows briefly at birthdays and holidays.

A grandparenting style, however, may not be a fixture. A grandparent may exhibit one style with one grandchild and a different style with another grandchild. Alternatively, a grandparent may exhibit the same style for all grandchildren at one age, but may change the style as the grandparent (or the grandchild) grows older.

Other researchers have identified the meanings found by grandparents in their roles as grandparents. For example, some perceive themselves as gaining immortality through the perpetuation of their bloodline, whereas others perceive themselves as treasured and respected elders. Typically, the role of a grandmother is broader and more intimate than that of a grandfather. In general, grandparenting is not very important in determining the degree of life satisfaction experienced by older adults. That is, life satisfaction is fairly independent of the frequency of encounters with grandchildren.

However, there does seem to be a moderate tendency for grandmothers to derive more satisfaction from grandparenting than do grandfathers. Moreover, the degree of satisfaction expressed by grandmothers appears to be related to their responsibilities for caring and helping their grandchildren. Are new grandparents as satisfied in their grandparenting roles as they expected to be? The available evidence suggests that grandmothers have slightly greater satisfaction than grandfathers relative to their expectations. Maternal grandmothers are especially more satisfied than either paternal grandparent.

A number of factors are related to the frequency of contacts between grandparents and their grandchildren. As expected, the most important is their proximity—the closer they live to each other, the more frequent the contacts. Other factors include the quality of the relationship between the grandparent and the grandchildren (the better the quality, the more frequent the contacts), the sex of the grandparent (grandmothers have more frequent contacts than grandfathers), and the relationships to the parents of the grandchildren (maternal grandparents have more frequent visits than paternal grandparents).

In a recent survey of grandparents over fifty years of age it was found that 80 percent of them had seen a grandchild or had chatted on the phone with a grandchild in the previous month. The most popular activities grandparents have with grandchildren are eating, watching television, shopping, and attending a religious service. Only 12.5 percent reported little contact with grandchildren. There is evidence indicating that more religious grandparents are more involved in the lives of their grandchildren than are less religious grandparents.

In general, the more frequent grandparents have noncustodial contact with their grandchildren, the more satisfied they appear to be as grandparents. Grandmothers report more frequent contacts with their grandchildren than do grandfathers. Nevertheless, there seems to be little difference between grandmothers and grandfathers in the satisfaction they receive from grandparenting.

An important issue concerns the visitation rights of grandparents. Some states have ruled against those rights. This ruling was confirmed in the year 2000 by the Supreme Court. The Court decided against two grandparents in Seattle who were in conflict with the mother of their two grandchildren regarding their right to visit the grandchildren.

In general, younger grandparents have been found to feel greater responsibility for offering child-rearing advice to their children than older grandparents, regardless of the number or ages of the grandchildren. Mothers, in general, have been found to take seriously the advice of grandmothers in regard to the nature of the punishments and rewards their children should receive.

There is a tendency for the contacts between grandmothers and their grandchildren to increase after the divorce of the children's parents. The frequency of the grandmothers' participation in the children's recreational activities and the frequency of babysitting are also likely to increase after a divorce of the grandchildren's parents. Unfortunately, less is known about grandfathers and their grandparenting activities after the divorce of their children.

Which of a child's four grandparents is most important in that child's life? That question was asked of a number of children by researchers at Adelphi University. Maternal grandmothers were selected more than twice as often as the other three grandparents. Maternal grandmothers seem to be more involved in their grandchildren's lives than the other grandparents, probably because mothers of children visit with their own mothers more often than they visit with either their fathers or in-laws.

Grandparents Raising Their Own Grandchildren

Nearly one million grandparents are raising their own grandchildren in a parentless home. The typical grandparent raising a grandchild alone is a grandmother, with the average age of 59.4 years. Their median annual income is about eighteen thousand dollars, which is half of a traditional parental family. More than 90 percent of single grandparents who are their grandchildren's sole caregiver are women. Nearly two million children are estimated to live in a household headed by a grandparent. For about a third of these children, neither parent is present. Researchers in South Carolina studied a large sample of children raised by grandmothers alone. They were healthier and had fewer behavioral problems in school than did children living with one biological parent (including a remarried parent).

Households for which grandparents are the sole caregivers of their own grandchildren (that is, the parents of the grandchildren do not reside in the household) are the fastest-growing type of household in the United States.

Does the strain of being a caregiver for grandchildren create health problems for the grandparents? In some studies health problems have been reported. However, in other studies the caregiving was found to have little effect on the grandparents' health.

There are some negative consequences for grandmothers who are caregivers. Depressive symptoms are not uncommon in the early stages of caregiving. Surprisingly, long-term caregiving does not seem to increase further the depressive symptoms. Both grandparents report less satisfaction with their lives early in the caregiving process. However, here too the lowering of life satisfaction does not seem to increase as caregiving continues for a long period.

Grandmothers express both positive effects and negative effects from their caregiving. Satisfaction with their caregiving role provides the positive effect, and misbehavior of the grandchildren provides the negative effect. Important in determining positive versus negative effects is the relationship the grandmother has or had with the parents of the grandchildren. The better the quality of that relationship, the more satisfied grandmothers are likely to be as caregivers.

Grape Juice

Drinking purple grape juice regularly seems to have several health benefits, presumably from a substance present in the juice. It may increase antioxidant levels, prohibit blood clotting, and lower bad cholesterol (*see also* Nutrition and Diet).

Growth Hormone (Physical Effects)

Does the growth hormone known as somatotropin reverse the effects of aging? In a study conducted at the Medical College of Wisconsin, twelve men between the ages of sixty-one and seventy-three took somatotropin for six months. At the end of the six months they claimed that they felt stronger, more alert, and functioned better mentally than they did at the start of the study. However, they expected to get better with the treatment, and much of the improvement, if not all of it, could be due to suggestibility.

In a more comprehensive study at the University of California at San Francisco, fifty-six men between the ages of seventy and eighty-five were also given doses of somatotropin for six months (they did not know if they were receiving the actual drug or a placebo). Their muscle mass increased slightly, and their body fat decreased moderately. However, they did not get stronger (in handgrip or lifting ability). Their mental functioning did not improve. Side effects included swollen ankles and aching joints. There is later evidence to indicate that it strengthens the heart muscle and could be used to treat congestive heart failure.

Guardianship and Conservatorship

Guardianship refers to the determination by a court whether a disabled individual has the physical capacity to take care of himself or herself and the mental capacity to make important decisions regarding health care and personal care. Conservatorship is also determined by a court, but it is concerned only with the management of the afflicted person's financial assets. The decision by the court is made after a hearing in which testimony is given by those involved, including a physician. The guardian or conservator appointed by the court is usually a family member.

H

Handedness

Do right-handed people live longer than left-handed people? In a 1980 study 15 percent of twenty-year-old people were reported to be left-handed, but only 1 percent of people in their eighties were left-handed. The conclusion from this study is that left-handed people live less years than do right-handed people. Later studies continued to find a difference in longevity between left-handed and right-handed people. However, the magnitude of the estimated difference was much less (from eight months to three years) than originally estimated. We do live in what is basically a world geared for right-handed people. Machines are usually built with right-handed people in mind. Although left-handed people are equal to right-handed people in motor skills that are tested in the laboratory, they are, nevertheless, twice as likely to have automobile crashes and four times more likely to die from crash-related injuries.

Hands

Take a look at your hands. They are remarkable anatomical structures. Their importance is apparent from the large area of the central nervous system devoted to their control. This is especially true for our prehensile (grasping) thumbs.

Despite their importance, there is no "hands-off" principle that protects our hands from declining with aging in their functional ability. The decline is largely from diseases commonly associated with aging. They include osteoporosis, osteoarthritis, and rheumatoid arthritis. Also contributing to the decline are hormonal changes and external factors such as some sports and work-related strains, and traumatic injuries.

Tests of hand functioning reveal that the declines occur with age for both men and women, and they are most apparent after age seventy-five. Especially important to everyday functioning is the declining ability to use the fingers to grasp, lift, and manipulate objects between the thumb and one of the four fingers (called finger pinch). There is an exercise that appears to improve the ability to do finger pinches (*see* Finger Movements and Exercise).

Tasks involving precision dexterity and two-hand coordination become increasingly difficult as we age. Even handgrip tasks that require strength (opening bottles and jars) become increasingly difficult with aging.

Handwriting

Judges have difficulty in distinguishing age from samples of handwriting. This is contrary to the stereotyped view that elderly people have shaky handwriting (but they do write more slowly than younger people). The handwriting of normally aging elderly adults resembles only slightly that of patients with Parkinson's disease. *See also* Speed of Behavior.

Health Literacy

Do you have difficulty comprehending articles in newspapers and magazines about health-related issues? What about difficulty in comprehending information accompanying the new medication prescribed by your physician? If you do, you are not alone—especially if you are an older adult.

Of course, information about health-related issues is not the only source of complex material that seniors are likely to encounter. It is estimated that nearly half of Americans age sixty-five and older are functionally illiterate in the sense of having difficulty understanding unfamiliar terminology and complex material.

Progressive declines in health literacy with increasing age in late adulthood have been found in several studies. The task used is known as the Short Test of Functional Health Literacy. The test simulates the kind of reading material that patients are likely to encounter in a health setting.

There is a decline in test scores of about 40 percent from people in their sixties to people age eighty and older. Moreover, the extent of the decline is about the same regardless of years of education and regardless of the physical and mental health status of the test takers. Older adults who read newspapers frequently do score higher than older adults who never read newspapers.

Fortunately, procedures are being developed by health professionals to make it easier for seniors to comprehend the instructions accompanying their medications (*see* Medication Compliance and Comprehension).

Health Maintenance Organizations (HMOs)

Health maintenance organizations (HMOs) are a prepaid medical service in which members pay monthly or yearly fees for all health care, including hospitalization. Most HMOs involve physicians who are engaged in group practice. Preventive medicine is stressed to reduce costly hospitalization.

Patients are able to use only physicians and specialists who are associated with the organization to which they belong. Open-ended HMOs offer members the option of seeing a physician who is not part of the HMO, but the patient must pay additional costs.

One of the past problems with HMOs has been their denial of a second diagnostic opinion from another physician that will be paid for by the HMO. However, some states have laws that assure patients the option of obtaining a second opinion. Other states are likely to follow in the future. Second opinions often make it easier for patients to deal with a complicated medical diagnosis and treatment procedure. *See also* Medicare.

Health Promotion Programs

Health programs are designed to provide information or experiences intended to improve the health of the participants. Such programs may include instruction and training on weight control, smoking cessation, and exercise. Older people have greater health risks than younger people, and they are therefore a group most likely to benefit from participation in health programs.

Nevertheless, the percentage of elderly people who do participate is small (those who participate are more likely to be women than men). This is apparent from a study of a large sample of older people in western Washington. A number of elderly people received mailings of descriptive material for a health promotion program in which they would be visited in their homes by a nurse educator who would discuss health risks with them. In addition, they would have the opportunity to participate in other programs, such as having a pharmacist review their medications. Only 29 percent of the elderly people contacted consented to be participants.

Those who consented were found to be more educated, to have a higher income, and to be more involved in community organizations than those who did not give their consent. Other researchers have discovered that there are effective strategies that may increase the number of elderly people in health programs, such as selecting program recruiters who have characteristics resembling those of the elderly adults to be recruited and good publicity of the support of the program by influential community leaders.

Health-Risk Behaviors

There are a number of behaviors that if they are not performed present a health risk to the nonperformer. They include such behaviors as wearing a seat belt in an automobile, avoiding fat in one's diet, exercising properly, and conducting self-examinations for the presence of cancerous growths.

Are these behaviors as likely to occur for elderly people as they are for younger people? Researchers in Rhode Island surveyed a large sample of people in the age ranges of eighteen to fifty-four, fifty-five to sixty-four, sixty-five to seventy-four, and age seventy-five and older. They did find age differences for some of the behaviors. People age seventy-five and older were found to be as likely to wear a seat belt as younger people (65 percent compared to 62 percent, 69 percent, and 62 percent for the other three age groups, respectively). They were at least as likely to avoid eating fat as younger people (77 percent, compared to 56 percent, 74 percent, and 62 percent for the other three age groups, respectively) and to conduct self-examinations (68 percent, compared to 60 percent, 69 percent, and 71 percent, respectively).

However, people age seventy-five and over were less likely than the younger people to report exercising regularly (46 percent, compared to 50 percent, 48 percent, and 53 percent, respectively). It is discouraging to discover that at all age levels more people are not engaging in behaviors clearly relevant to their own health. This is especially disturbing for those who are in their seventies and beyond where health problems increase considerably. Health professionals need to find additional ways of encouraging elderly people to engage in health-relevant behaviors.

Health Span

See Life Span.

Health Status and Mental Performance

National statistics reveal that the health status of our elderly population is poorer than it is for younger people. Despite these statistics of poor health in many elderly people, about 70 percent of people age sixty-five or older in a national survey described their health as being excellent or good. This percentage does not differ greatly from the 75 percent of people in the fifty-five-to-sixty-four-year age range who reported their health to be excellent or good, or even from the 82 percent of people in the forty-five-to-fifty-four-year age range.

Self-ratings of health are fairly valid measures of older adults' true health status. Mortality rates during a three-year period have been found to be much higher for elderly people with low self-ratings (implying poor health) than for older people with high self-ratings (implying good health). For example, in a Canadian study elderly participants who rated their health as being bad or poor were more than twice as likely to die within three to three and a half years as those who rated their health as excellent. French researchers found that self-rated health is a better predictor of mortality for men than for women. The high mortality for those having low self-ratings of health is even true for those elderly people with low ratings who appear to others to be healthy.

A sizable percentage of people age sixty-five or older do perceive their health to be less than good (that is, average or poor). In most laboratory studies of normal aging and mental performances, these individuals are eliminated from participation. A standard procedure is to have potential participants rate their health status on a 5-point scale, with 1 being excellent and 2 being good. Only those participants who assign self-ratings of 1 or 2 are likely to have their scores included in age comparisons. Investigators are typically interested in how normal aging affects mental performances and not on how these effects may be complicated by disease and poor health.

What happens when health status is an uncontrolled study factor? Researchers at the University of Missouri at Columbia found that it had little effect on the relationship between age and performance on a variety of learning, memory, and reasoning tasks. That is, the strong negative relationship between age and performance scores was about the same regardless of whether participants with low self-reported health were excluded. Conversely, researchers at both the University of Michigan and the University of Victoria found that the relationship between age and fluid intelligence (see Intelligence) was much less pronounced when participants who reported their health to be less than good were excluded from their analyses. In addition, elderly people with poor health self-ratings have been found to perform more poorly on the Mini-Mental State Exam (see Mini-Mental State Exam) than those with good or excellent ratings.

The standard practice in research on the relationship between age per se and mental performance should be to continue to exclude participants who rate their health as poor. Of course, there is the important area of research in which the health status of older people serves as the focus, that is, the interest is in how elderly people in poor health compare in their mental performances with elderly people in good health. From the conflicting evidence to date, it is apparent that more research is needed to determine exactly how self-rated health is related to mental performances.

Except for cardiovascular diseases, diseases identified by standard medical procedures seem to be only moderately related to performances on most mental tasks and tests. However, researchers in the Netherlands did find evidence that diabetes in elderly people may be associated with poor performance on a number of cognitive tasks. See also Cardiovascular Disease and Mental Performance.

Hearing

Presbycusis is the diminished ability to hear sounds of high pitches, particularly those of 3,000 hertz (that is, 3,000 cycles per second of the sound waves) and higher. It is one of the most common consequences of aging. Nearly all individuals age sixty-five and older are affected to some degree by presbycusis. It is estimated that nearly 30 percent of these individuals have noticeable impairment, especially white men, and more than 10 percent have severe cases.

Diminished hearing of high-frequency sounds begins for people in their thirties. By the fifties the hearing loss is already moderate, and it increases greatly during the remaining decades of life. On the other hand, the loss of hearing ability with normal aging is much less severe for sounds of lower pitch, especially those of 1,000 hertz and lower.

There are sex differences in the rate of loss of hearing ability with aging for higher-pitched sounds. In general, the hearing loss for women is greater than that for men of sounds of 1,000 hertz and lower, but it is somewhat less than that for men for frequencies of 2,000 hertz and above. The sex difference is probably related to differences in exposure to environmental noise rather than to sex differences in the biological components of hearing. Prolonged exposure to noise causes damage to the hair cells in the inner ear that respond to sound waves. Older whites are more likely to have hearing loss than older African Americans.

The importance of environmental noise in producing hearing loss is apparent from comparisons between Americans and people from other cultures who live in isolated areas that are relatively free of intense environmental noise. For example, the hearing loss for Sudanese men in their seventies has been found to be half that of American men in their seventies. Given the loud music preferred by many young people, the threat of even greater hearing loss for future generations of older people is a definite possibility. People of all ages should limit their exposure to certain noisy environments, such as no more than thirty minutes in a noisy arcade (where the noise level is about 110 decibels).

Hearing acuity for a particular sound frequency is measured by determining an individual's absolute threshold for a pure tone at that frequency. To determine the threshold at 3,000 hertz, the participant would receive tones of that frequency at varying levels of loudness, beginning at a very low intensity (in decibels). The intensity is increased until the level of intensity at which the participant hears the tone half of the time it is presented (that is, in half of the trials). The decibels at that level define the absolute threshold. For people in their seventies, the threshold value at 3,000 hertz averages about 30 decibels greater than that of people in their twenties.

Impairment in the ability to discriminate between sounds of different pitches also accompanies normal aging. For example, can you detect the difference between tones of 3,000 hertz and 3,030 hertz? Between 2,000 hertz and 2,010 hertz? Although there are major losses with aging in the ability to discriminate between pitches, the losses are slight for tones less than 1,000 hertz. They become much greater for higher pitches, and they are especially large for sound frequencies of 3,000 hertz and higher. To determine pitch-discrimination ability at any given frequency, the difference threshold is measured. If that frequency is 3,000 hertz, a number of trials is given in which the 3,000-hertz tone is sounded first (at about 40 decibels) and is followed by a second tone. The frequency of the second tone is gradually increased until you are able to detect the difference in pitch from the first tone half of the time. The difference in frequencies at that point defines the difference threshold. For people in their twenties, the average difference threshold for tones in the 3,000-hertz range is about 15 hertz. It increases in magnitude with aging; for people in their sixties and seventies, the difference threshold averages about 40 and 70 hertz, respectively. Older people are obviously less sensitive to variation in pitch than are young adults.

Hearing impairment in late adulthood has obvious adverse effects on everyday living. Speech perception is affected to some degree by both declining acuity in hearing sounds and declining ability to discriminate among pitches (*see* Speech Perception). Older people are also likely to have diminished quality of the music they hear. There is also a more subtle effect of hearing impairment. Researchers have discovered that scores earned by elderly people on an intelligence test and on memory tests are related to some degree to the extent of their hearing impairment (*see* Intelligence). Elderly people with long-term hearing impairments have been found to have difficulty performing many physical functions as well as having higher levels of depression than the hearing unimpaired.

Elderly people should be aware that hearing impairment may be caused by factors other than environmental noise. Ototoxic drugs (that is, drugs that are damaging to hearing receptors) may produce impairment, or they may worsen an already existing impairment. Included among these drugs are certain diuretics, certain antibiotics (especially streptomycin) and cisplatin (a drug used in some forms of chemotherapy). In addition, tinnitus (*see* Tinnitus) may be caused by high doses of aspirin.

Elderly people should realize that some hearing impairments may be treatable. This is the case when the impairment is caused by excessive wax in the ear canal or by some forms of infection. Older people should be encouraged to have regular hearing tests to determine the probable cause of any new impairment.

Unfortunately, nearly two-thirds of the millions of Americans with hearing loss do not use conventional hearing aids. There are now new hearing aids that fit deep in the ear canal and are virtually invisible if fitted properly. They offer high-fidelity sound with low distortion even when the listener is in a noisy environment. There are also special forms of equipment for people with hearing impairment, such as louder doorbells and telephones.

Heart Rate

A beat of the heart consists of one complete contraction and relaxation of the heart's muscle. When individuals are at rest and in a supine position, the heart rate of beating does not differ between younger and older adults. When they are in a sitting position, there is a slight decline (about 10 percent) in the rate of beating with aging. With exercise, the decrease in the rate of beating with aging is more pronounced (about 25 percent).

Heat Stroke

Heat stroke occurs when outside weather conditions add heat to the body faster than the body can handle it. Older adults are at a much greater risk of illness or death from heat stroke during periods of high temperatures and high humidity than are younger adults. The risk is especially high for elderly adults with respiratory or heart conditions. Symptoms of heat stroke include difficulty in breathing, hot and red dry skin, leg cramps, headache, nausea, and exhaustion. One reason for the greater risk is that older people perspire less than younger adults, and perspiring is a primary way for the body to cool itself. A second reason is that older adults are more likely than younger adults to be taking medications that increase the risk of heat stroke. These medicines include many cold medicines, antihistamines, diuretics, and antidepressants.

Friends or family members of a victim should call for medical help when they observe symptoms of a heat stroke. While waiting for that help, they should keep the victim lying down in a cool place, remove the victim's clothing, cover the victim with a wet sheet, and cool the victim with a fan or air-conditioner.

Elderly people should avoid being outdoors during periods of extreme heat (especially when the heat index has been at least 105 degrees for two days), and they should stay in air-conditioned quarters as much as possible. They should also drink plenty of cool water and splash their skin with cool water. Unfortunately, many older adults cannot afford air-conditioning. Those who do not have air-conditioning should contact their local health authorities and social agencies to request help either in obtaining air-conditioners or for finding temporary air-conditioned quarters. They should also contact their utility companies for budget billing.

Heat exhaustion is milder than heat stroke. It usually occurs after several days of high temperature. Although it may require hospitalization, death is unlikely. The signs of heat exhaustion include heavy sweating, pale and clammy skin, and a slightly elevated body temperature. The victim should consume water and electrolyte fluids and sip a salt solution of one teaspoon of salt in eight ounces of water.

Heredity versus Environment as Determiners of Functional Health

What is important in determining whether older adults are able to maintain good functional health—their heredity or their environment? Functional health refers primarily to the ability to perform normal physical activities of daily living, such as bathing and toileting, and instrumental activities of daily living, such as shopping and visiting friends (*see* Activities of Daily Living).

To answer this question researchers have employed fraternal (nonidentical heredities) and identical twins (identical heredities) ranging in age from seventy to eighty (*see* Twins). If heredity is responsible for functional impairments, then the probability of one twin having it when the other twin does should be much greater for identical twins than for fraternal twins. If this is not the case, then the probability is high that the twins have had uniquely different environmental experiences. The evidence obtained in the twin studies clearly implies that it is unique environmental experiences, and not one's heredity, that is responsible for functional impairments in late adulthood.

The incidence of functional impairments presumably may be decreased by altering the environments of older people, such as moving them to less stressful neighborhoods.

Hiding Your Age

"You certainly don't look your age. You look great." Many older adults would be greatly pleased to hear these words—they would be happy not to look their age. In fact, some try to look younger than they are by hiding as many signs of aging as possible. For example, they may hide the graying of their hair by dyeing it. Women are judged more on their appearance than are men. Not surprisingly, looking old may be considered more unattractive for elderly women than for elderly men. Consequently, more older women than older men may try to hide their signs of aging. Evidence provided by researchers at the University of New Mexico provides strong support for this likelihood. They surveyed a number of people older than fifty years of age. Only 6 percent of the men reported coloring their hair, in contrast to 34 percent of the women. Similarly, only 1 percent of the men reported using wrinkle creams, in contrast to 24 percent of the women. *See also* Facial Appearance.

Hip Replacement

Total hip replacement (total hip orthoplasty) relieves joint pain and improves mobility and the quality of life for some elderly people with severe osteoarthritis or rheumatoid arthritis in the hip. Postoperative mortality is low, but the risk of death increases nearly threefold for every ten-year increase in age after age sixty-five. Sex and race seem to be unrelated to the risk of postoperative mortality.

Holiday Greeting Cards

The sending of greeting cards during the December holiday season is a long-standing practice. Of interest is the possibility of age differences in the practice of sending these cards. Some information about these age differences was provided by researchers at Pennsylvania State University. They surveyed young adults (twenty-four to thirty-nine years), middle-aged adults (forty to fifty-nine years), and older adults (sixty years and older) living in four different cities of various sizes.

The survey concerned the sending (and receiving) of greeting cards during two recent holiday seasons. The percentage sending such cards was 78 percent for the young adults, 97 percent for the middle-aged adults, and 74 percent for the older adults, and the percentage receiving cards was 100 percent for each age group. The average number of cards sent was twenty-four, thirty-seven, and fifty for the three age groups, and the average number of cards received was twenty-five, thirty-eight, and fifty-two. The most frequent recipients of cards sent were friends: 55 percent, 46 percent, and 56 percent for the three age groups. The younger participants viewed sending cards primarily as a means of maintaining or establishing friendships. The older participants viewed sending cards primarily as a means of connecting to their personal past.

Home Care

Home care is an alternative to assisted living facilities (*see* Assisted-Living Facilities) for older people who are living alone and are no longer physically functioning independently. They are still able to live at home, but they need help to do so. Services include shopping and transportation to medical and therapy appointments. The program ensures considerable independence, but it can be expensive.

Homeless Older People (Reasons for Their Homelessness)

Why do some older people become homeless? A study conducted by researchers in several different countries (including Australia and the United States) found basically the same reasons in each country. The reason given by the most older homeless participants (nearly 30 percent) was that they had difficulty paying the rent or mortgage. The next most frequent reason (20 percent) was the loss of their home by being sold or converted to apartments or because it needed major repairs. The next most important reasons were the breakdown of their marital or cohabital relationship (17 percent), death of a relative or close friend (12 percent), and a dispute with a landlord, other tenant, or neighbor (11 percent). Only very few gave as their reason alcohol problems, gambling problems, or drug problems.

Homeless Older People (Who Are They?)

Homeless people are usually defined as those people sleeping in shelters or public places. It is estimated that only 3 percent of the homeless are people who are age sixty-five or older. Those elderly adults who are homeless are mostly men, and they are more likely to be African American than white. Older homeless people are more likely to have a chronic illness or a physical disability than are younger homeless people.

Home Maintenance

There are more than fourteen million homeowners who are age sixty-five and older. Several surveys have shown a relationship between age and the maintenance activity of homeowners: the amount of money spent annually on the upkeep of a home is less for homeowners age sixty-five and older than it is for younger homeowners, and the amount spent decreases progressively, on average, with increasing age beyond age sixty-five.

This is apparent in a survey of homeowners in the Houston area. The average amount spent annually for home maintenance was about $466 for homeowners younger than age sixty and only about $145 for homeowners age seventy-five and older. Moreover, the percentage of homeowners age seventy-five and older who engaged in home upkeep was about 63 percent, compared with the 80 percent of homeowners younger than age sixty. The results from this survey also indicate that the major reason for the age difference is the decline in income during late adulthood.

Other factors, such as the health status of the homeowner, were found to have little effect on home maintenance. However, it was also found that elderly homeowners were just as likely as younger homeowners to maintain essential properties of their homes (such as roof repairs). The age difference is attributable largely to the fact that elderly homeowners spend less money than younger homeowners on what may be considered cosmetic home maintenance (like painting). On the other hand, more elderly homeowners pay for housecleaning help than do younger homeowners.

Home Medical Devices

Technology has made it possible for many elderly people to have health devices at home that enable them to monitor their own health. They include, for example, blood-pressure measurement devices and handheld battery meters that measure glucose levels for patients with diabetes.

Unfortunately, these devices could present some problems for older users. The devices are very complex, and they give little feedback as to their correct use. In addition, there is a good possibility of making an error in their use. Researchers at the Georgia Institute of Technology found that the instructions for many devices are inadequate for teaching their use. They have prepared instructional materials that make it easier to use some of these devices.

Home Ownership

According to the 2000 U.S. Census, 81 percent of householders age sixty-five to seventy-four owned the house in which they lived. This is the highest percentage of any age group.

Homosexuality

It is believed that the proportion of older people who are homosexual differs little from the proportion of younger people. This means that there are about three million elderly homosexual men and women in the United States. A myth of aging is that elderly homosexual men and women are, on average, more lonely and more despairing than elderly heterosexual men and women. This may have been true before the onset of the gay rights movement in 1969, but it seems unlikely today. Surveys during the past ten or so years have indicated that gay older men show diverse lifestyles and considerable well-being. The majority do not appear to be depressed, lonely, or sexually frustrated. Many of those interviewed revealed that they are still sexually active and that their sexual relationships are very satisfactory. Virtually all of the elderly gay men interviewed indicated that they preferred their sexual contacts to be men of similar ages rather than young men. Similar surveys of older lesbians reveal that, on average, they are comfortable with their sexual preference and that they appear to be in excellent mental health. There is some indication that lesbians may discontinue sexual activities at an earlier age than do gay men.

It has been argued by some gerontologists that homosexuality may actually be adaptive to the usual stresses of aging caused by society's frequent devaluation of its elderly population. A homosexual preference may help the individual to become more independent early in life and to avoid being entrapped in traditional sex roles. Homosexuals have become familiar with the stigmatization often associated with homosexuality, and may therefore be more adaptable than heterosexual elderly people to the stigma associated with aging. However, the little evidence available fails to lend much support to this belief. A study conducted in the mid-1980s revealed that more than 80 percent of the older lesbians interviewed felt positively about their sexual preference, but only about 50 percent felt positively about aging.

A problem facing homosexual older people is the fact that senior centers, retirement communities, and nursing homes are all traditionally heterosexually oriented. Homosexual participants and residents are therefore likely to feel constrained and isolated in these facilities. Of interest are the results of a survey of older lesbians in which only 5 percent of those interviewed said they attended a senior center, and most of them indicated a strong preference for lesbian or lesbian and gay facilities and services. This problem is likely to be resolved in the future as the rights and needs of homosexuals, including those of elderly homosexuals, are increasingly being recognized.

Hospice Care

The term *hospice* originally meant an inn or a way station for travelers. Since 1967, it has assumed another meaning, namely, a program of care for terminally ill patients, most of whom are older people dying of such diseases as cancer. The first hospice was founded that year in England by Dr. Cicely Saunders. The purpose was to provide services for the terminally ill that would allow them to be as free of pain as possible, provide emotional and social support, and fulfill as many of their desires as possible, as the end of life approached. In addition, patients were encouraged to maintain as many of their functions as they could. The concept spread to the United States in the early 1970s, and there are now thousands of hospice programs in the country. Such programs are either inpatient or outpatient. Inpatient programs may be located either within an established hospital or in a special facility designed only for hospice care. Outpatient programs are for terminally ill patients who remain in their homes while receiving care from hospice staff members. Outpatient programs are becoming increasingly popular, given their lower cost.

Patients in a hospice program are usually treated by a team consisting of a physician, a nurse, a social worker, and a counselor. A typical team also includes lay providers, many of whom are elderly persons. The patient's dignity and self-respect are given the highest attention by such practices as maintaining physical appearance and grooming at as high a level as possible. Most patients prefer a hospice center or program to that of a regular hospital. Hospice patients tend to be more mobile and less depressed and anxious than terminally ill patients cared for in a regular hospital. Those who are enrolled in both traditional Medicare and Medicare HMOs are entitled to hospice benefits in their own choice of Medicare-certified hospice programs. The benefits partially or fully include physician care, nursing care, therapy, home-health care, and drugs and medical supplies.

Hospital Infections

Elderly people have a much greater risk of postsurgical infections than do younger people. In general, hospital-acquired infections occur three times more in elderly adults than in the general population. This presents a real problem for elderly people in that they have more frequent and longer hospitalizations than do younger people. There obviously is great reason for hospitals to be especially cautious in preventing infections for their elderly patients.

Hostility

Hostility is characterized by a negative approach to other people. It may be expressed by abusive thoughts or statements or abusive actions or both. Psychologists have known for some time that expressions of hostility decline from adolescence to midlife, with the lowest incidence being among people thirty to sixty years of age. Less certain has been the frequency of hostility after age sixty. A cross-sectional study conducted several years ago found a moderate increase in the expression of hostility for people after age sixty. A more recent study by researchers at Duke University reported that the older adults in their sample were generally more suspicious of other people and more cynical in their beliefs about other people than were middle-aged adults. More hostile behavior was also expressed during an interview by the elderly adults than by the middle-aged adults. The greater verbal expression of hostility was true for both older men and women. However, violent acts as expressions of hostility tend to decrease in late adulthood.

The apparent increase in hostility in elderly adults has important implications for their health. There is considerable evidence indicating that high levels of hostility have adverse effects on physical health (for instance, increased risk of heart disease) and on longevity.

Household Expenditures

Running a household requires spending money—for food, clothing, entertainment, rent or mortgage payments, and so on. Do the percentages of monthly expenditures for various household needs differ for elderly adults compared to younger adults? What little is known about possible age differences in the allotment of household expenditures comes from a study by researchers at Northwestern University. They had available the results of a consumer survey conducted by the U.S. Department of Labor in the mid-1980s. Nearly four thousand members of households, age forty-five and older, were interviewed. The households were selected such that they represented a cross-section of all U.S. households.

The researchers found relatively few age differences in the percentages of expenditures on various items. This was true, for example, for food, recreation, and giving (to charities). However, people age sixty-five and older did allot more of their spending to health care than did younger people. By contrast, people in the forty-five-to-fifty-four-year age range devoted a larger percentage of their expenditures to clothing than did older adults. It seems likely that comparable results would be found for current households.

How Much Longer Do Seniors Want to Live?

"How many more years would you like to live?" "It depends" is your likely reply. You probably have in mind the fact that it depends on the status of your physical health, the status of your mental abilities, and how much pain you would have to endure.

Researchers at the Polisher Research Institute in Philadelphia investigated the number of years seniors wanted to live with functional limitations (performing the activities of daily living), mental limitations, and severity of pain.

Seniors were willing to discount years of life more with some conditions than with other conditions. This is apparent from the percentage of participants in their study (age seventy and older) who responded zero days to each condition. The highest percentages were for mental impairment (39 percent), confused at home (48 percent), and confused in a nursing home (62 percent). By contrast, the percentages of zero responses were 22 percent for functional limitations that kept you in bed, 22 percent for mild pain, and 12 percent for patient-controllable severe pain (*see* Pain Management). In general, the degree to which participants valued living was positively associated with the number of years they desired to continue living.

Human Growth Hormone (Antiaging Effects)

The human growth hormone is secreted by the anterior pituitary gland that is located at the base of the brain. It is essential for growth and other bodily functions. Its peak secretion is at adolescence, and the amount of secretion decreases with increasing age after that. It was first discovered in the 1930s, and it was first isolated in 1956. In 1990 evidence was published indicating its value as an antiaging substance. For example, it presumably improves skin texture and muscle mass. Users need to be cautious with it. It does have dangerous side effects, and many physicians strongly oppose its use as an antiaging substance (*see also* Growth Hormone [Physical Effects]).

Humor

The topic of this entry is not elderly people being the target of many jokes (which they are, frequently as victims of ageism; *see* Ageism), but rather possible age differences in the appreciation of humor and the use of humor. Humor researchers have identified two basic kinds of structure in jokes and cartoons. The first involves a situation in which there is an incongruity but a resolution is offered; the second involves a nonsense situation in which there is an incongruity and either no resolution is offered or a resolution is offered only to be followed by another incongruity.

Researchers have discovered that an important determinant of one's appreciation of humor corresponds with one's place on the conservative-liberal dimension. More conservative people tend to find incongruent-resolution humor to be funnier and less aversive than do more liberal people. The opposite is true for nonsense humor, that is, the more liberal individual is the one who is likely to find it funny and less aversive. The linkage of conservatism to humor suggests that we are likely to find age differences in people's reactions to jokes and cartoons, simply because the proportion of elderly people who are conservative is greater than the proportion of younger people (*see* Attitudes [Political and Social]).

This suggestion was tested in a massive cross-sectional study (different groups of people at each age level) by researchers in Germany. The participants in the study included more than four thousand individuals ranging in age from fourteen to sixty-six. Each participant rated a number of jokes and cartoons in terms of their funniness and their aversiveness. As expected, the average funniness rating increased progressively with increasing age for incongruity-resolution jokes and cartoons, while it decreased for nonsense jokes and cartoons. The participants also took several tests to measure their degree of conservatism. As expected, conservatism was found to increase progressively after the teens. Most important, a high correlation was found between degree of conservatism and the type of reaction to humor at all age levels. Age per se does not account for age differences in appreciation of humor. It is the higher incidence of conservatism in the elderly population that is responsible for the age difference.

The fact that older women usually have more sources of stress to cope with than do younger women probably accounts for an age difference in the use of humor. Researchers at the University of Nebraska at Omaha found that older women use more humor focused on coping with stress than do younger women. *See also* Laughter (Is It the Best Medicine for Seniors?).

Hypertension

Hypertension means you have blood pressure that is too high (*see* Blood Pressure [High and Low]). *Essential hypertension* means that there is no identifiable cause. The cause is most likely from genes, something wrong in your environment, or too much salt in your diet. *Secondary hypertension* means that the high blood pressure is caused by some other disorder, such as a kidney disorder, the use of certain medications, an adrenal gland tumor, and so on.

There usually are no symptoms of hypertension, although on occasion you may have a mild headache. If the headache is severe, or if you experience tiredness, vision changes, nosebleed, irregular heartbeat, or other unexpected disorders, you should see your physician as soon as possible.

There are a number of medications for treating hypertension. Changes in your lifestyle may also serve to lower your blood pressure. They include weight loss, a healthier diet, and especially a regular exercise program. Hypertension is a lifelong problem that requires frequent monitoring of your blood pressure to determine if your lifestyle changes are adequate. If not, adjustments need to be made.

Prolonged hypertension may lead to a number of physical disorders, including a heart attack, stroke, arteriosclerosis, kidney damage, brain damage, loss of vision, and other possible disorders. Your mental functioning may also be affected adversely (*see* Hypertension and Mental Functioning). You clearly should have your blood pressure measured regularly, even if you are not presently suffering from hypertension.

Hypertension and Mental Functioning

In 1971 Drs. F. Wilkie and C. Eisdorfer were probably the first to report the negative effects of moderately severe hypertension on intelligence-test scores. Their participants were in their sixties when diagnosed with hypertension and given an intelligence test. Ten years later they tested significantly lower on the test, relative to other participants of the same age with normal blood pressure. However, recent evidence has indicated that the adverse effect of hypertension on intelligence is not apparent until those with the disorder are in their sixties, and even then, the effect may not be apparent unless other cardiovascular problems are also present (*see* Cardiovascular Disease and Mental Performance).

Although some researchers have found adverse effects of hypertension on the memory performances of older adults, other researchers have reported only negligible effects. Perhaps the most serious effect of hypertension in late adulthood is on the performance of tasks involving executive or higher-order mental (cognitive) processes mediated by the frontal lobes of the brain (*see* Brain and Aging). One of these tasks requires the ability to switch rapidly from one task to a different task, such as on the Trail Making Test (*see* Switching Tasks; Trail Making Test). Older adults who perform well below average on tests of frontal-lobe functioning also tend to score well below average on such tasks as the Trail Making Test.

1

Illusions

Illusions occur when the senses are fooled in some way. They are usually associated with vision. In effect, you "see" something that is not consistent with physical reality (as when you are tricked by a magician). Age differences are studied in the laboratory through the use of simple materials such as those used to produce the Müller-Lyer illusion. The nature of this illusion may be seen by looking at the following: Which of the two horizontal lines appears longer? >————< ←——→ They are of equal length, but the one on the left probably appears to be longer.

Researchers have found that the illusory experience with these lines increases in magnitude steadily from early to late adulthood. This is true of some other visual illusions as well. They are known as *Type I illusions*. That is, for each, the magnitude of the illusory experience is greater for older adults than for younger adults. The increase in the magnitude of the illusion in later adulthood is the consequence of age changes in the eye, especially in the lens. The reduced amount of light reaching the retina by the "yellowing" of the lens seems to be the major reason. In fact, when young adults view the Müller-Lyer materials through goggles that reduce the amount of light reaching the retina, they experience the increased magnitude of the illusion characteristic of older adults (*see* Age Simulation).

There are other visual illusions, known as *Type II illusions,* in which the magnitude of the illusory experience decreases instead of increases from early adulthood through late adulthood. An example of a Type II illusion is the Uanadze illusion in which after viewing two circles of unequal diameters, you have the tendency to view two subsequently exposed circles of equal diameters as being unequal in size. It is suspected that age changes occurring at levels of the visual system beyond the eye (that is, in the brain) are responsible for these decreases in illusory experiences.

Illusions are of interest if only because they represent a quirk in normal visual sensory functioning. However, they are also of interest because of their potential diagnostic value. This is especially true for Type II illusions.

Conceivably, elderly people who show virtually no illusory effect for these illusions may be experiencing some abnormal form of brain degeneration.

Imagery

Imagine a map of the United States. Now name a state that has an outline similar to that of Oregon. You surely would not name Missouri or West Virginia. How would you select a state that does resemble Oregon? Many people will tell you that they are comparing *images* or *mental pictures* they have of various states with the image they have of Oregon. Which is bigger—a robin or a canary? To answer this question, some people will tell you they are comparing the image they form for each bird.

Consider a task that psychologists call mental rotation. You see a version of the letter **R** that is either the true letter or a mirror image of the letter. Your job is to determine which it is. The problem is that the letter you see is rotated, sometimes looking like this, **Я**, and on other occasions like this, **Я**. Participants performing this task, whether young or older adults, usually make few errors in judging whether the letter is true or a mirror image, although elderly adults are slower in reaching their judgments.

How do you know which form of the letter it is? We know that the more the letter is rotated, the longer it takes to make the judgment, again regardless of a participant's age. It is as if you have rotated in your mind an image of the object you see until it is "straight," and the time to rotate depends on how much you have to rotate it. We also know that lists of words that are easily imagined, such as *apple* and *cigar,* are easier to memorize than are lists of words that are less imageable, such as *mercy* and *justice,* regardless of the age of participants. Presumably, images enhance our memorability (*see* Memory Training) of episodic events.

We do seem to possess the mental ability of forming images of objects and events in our world. However, some people report that their ability to form mental images is much greater than that of other people. To what extent is this ability affected by aging? When asked about the vividness of their mental images, younger and older people report little difference. The existence of an imagery ability in late adulthood would seemingly be apparent from the evidence that elderly adults perform well on various tasks in which imagery seems to facilitate performance. They can do mental rotations, they benefit from the presence of easily imaged words in a word list, and so on.

However, there is also evidence of diminished proficiency of imagery in late adulthood. Elderly participants, for example, engage less in the spontaneous use of images than do younger participants when such use makes memorability easier. This occurs when participants are asked to learn word pairs such as *apple-pencil.* Young adults are likely to learn this pair by forming an image of a pencil stuck in an apple, even when they are not instructed to do so. By contrast, elderly participants are unlikely to make use of such images unless they are instructed and encouraged to do so. Even then, they are less proficient in generating the image than are younger participants.

The weaker imagery ability of elderly adults, in general, contrasts sharply with the high verbal ability of elderly adults (*see* Verbal Ability). Some researchers believe there is a reason for this difference. Verbal ability is largely a function of the brain's left hemisphere where language centers are located for most people, whereas imaginal ability is largely a function of the right hemisphere. The argument is that the right hemisphere of the brain "ages" at a faster rate than the left hemisphere. However, the evidence to support this argument is conflicting. Some studies suggest a differential rate of aging, but other studies do not (*see* Brain and Aging).

Immune Responses and Stress

Immune responses to the invasion of the body by viruses, bacteria, and other disease-causing agents called antigens consist of the production of antibodies by white blood cells called lymphocytes that are present in the spleen and the lymph nodes. Antibodies destroy the antigens and make them harmless.

The effectiveness of immune responses decreases with age, a decrease suspected to be one of the reasons for the adverse biological changes that occur with aging and the increased susceptibility of older people to such diseases as various forms of cancer and influenza (*see* Why Aging? [Biological Theories of Aging]).

Vaccinations usually consist of injecting a weakened or dead antigen into the body to stimulate the production of antibodies (*see* Influenza). The decline in the effectiveness of immune responses in late adulthood is exacerbated by the presence of psychological stress. There is evidence indicating that training in relaxation to reduce the stress also serves to improve the effectiveness of immune responses. Very positive social support, including strong family ties, serves to improve the immune responses of elderly people.

Surgical stress has been found to lower the effectiveness of immune response for older people. Training in relaxation before surgery and shortly after is likely to have positive effects on immune responses.

Implicit Memory

Several minutes after studying a lengthy list of common words, you are asked to recall as many of the words as you can. Not surprisingly, you discover that you can recall fewer than half of the words on the list. Perhaps somewhat more surprisingly, you also discover that you are even unable to recognize some of the words you could not recall. Does this mean that memories of the nonrecalled and nonrecognized words do not exist? Did memory traces of these words fail to be registered in your memory store? Or, alternatively, were they registered, but somehow were "erased" before you had the chance to test your memory? Not necessarily. Both recall and recognition are part of what memory researchers call *explicit memory*. Explicit memory is memory that requires conscious recollection of the events to be remembered in the sense of deliberately searching your memory store to find specific memory traces. Memory researchers have discovered that memories that are beyond conscious recollection may, nevertheless, be present and may become evident when the constraints of conscious recollection are removed. Memory without conscious recollection is known as *implicit memory*.

Suppose that *shade* was one of the words in the list you could neither recall nor recognize. To demonstrate the memory for that word's presence in the list, you are given another task to perform after your explicit memory for the list words has been tested. The task is really an indirect test of memory, but this information is not revealed to you. You are simply told that the investigator is interested in word productions to word stems (for example, the first two letters of a word). You are given a number of word stems, such as *cl, tr,* and *sh,* and you are asked to produce a five-letter word beginning with each stem. The question is, what word are you most likely to produce with the *sh*? There are many words beginning with *sh* that you could give—for example, *shape, shark, shoot, share,* and *shore.* However, the probability is quite high that you will come up with *shade,* the previously studied word that has not been consciously recollected.

Other procedures could be used to demonstrate your implicit memory in the absence of explicit memory. For example, instead of giving you word stems to complete, words could be flashed on a screen, and you could be asked to identify them. At first, the flash for a given word is too brief for you to identify it. The duration of the word's exposure is gradually increased until you are finally able to identify it. The duration is likely to be much briefer for previously studied words that are beyond recollection (such as *shade*) than for other similar words that had not been included in the study list. Again, implicit memory exists even when explicit memory does not. In this instance, it is your word identification rather than your word production that is facilitated by the implicit memory.

Normally aging older participants frequently perform, on average, moderately below the level of young adult participants on tests of explicit memory (*see* Episodic Memory). By contrast, age differences on implicit memory tests have been found to be slight and often nonexistent. That is, in the absence of the need for conscious recollection, older adults seem to manifest as much memory as do younger adults. Patients with organic amnesia, such as those with Korsakoff's disease (a brain disorder most commonly found in long-term alcoholics), also show as much implicit memory as do age-matched individuals without amnesia, even though the patients with amnesia show pronounced deficits in their explicit memory.

The fate of implicit memory with Alzheimer's disease in its early stages is presently unresolved. In some studies patients with Alzheimer's disease have been found to be quite deficient in implicit memory as well as explicit memory. However, other studies of patients with Alzheimer's disease have shown little deficit in implicit memory in the presence of considerable deficit in explicit memory, relative to normally aging elderly adults.

The existence of implicit memory helps to explain some puzzling memory phenomena. Have you ever had the experience of feeling you have met this person before, but you cannot recollect when it was or what the name of the person is (including not recognizing the name when you are told it)? Assuming you really did meet the person before, you are probably showing implicit memory. In fact, implicit memory may account for some of our experiences we refer to as déjà vu (the feeling you have been somewhere before or have experienced a particular event before, but you cannot recall the place or the prior experience).

As another possible phenomenon, consider the following scenario. You are doing your laundry, and you notice that your supply of detergent is low. So you make a mental note to buy detergent the next time you go to the supermarket. Several days later when you go shopping you make your list of items you need to purchase. Missing from the list is detergent. You failed to recollect consciously the event in the laundry room. However, at the market, as you pass through the soap department, the detergents seem to attract you to them, and you find yourself putting a box of your favorite brand in your shopping cart. Your implicit memory came through for you. It seems that implicit memory is as likely to benefit many elderly people as it is younger people.   .

Inactivity of Middle-Aged and Older Women

It is well known that physical activity has many positive health effects. This is especially true for older adults. Even moderate daily exercise or its equivalent has important positive effects on the physical health of older adults and on their mental health as well. Nevertheless, a majority of older Americans are not active enough to enjoy those benefits.

Middle-aged and older women are especially prone to inactivity. Older women commonly give many reasons they do not exercise regularly (for instance, they could seriously hurt themselves, or they have too many time-consuming responsibilities). Even when they join an exercise program, many drop out shortly after starting.

What are the real reasons for many older women to remain relatively physically inactive? A comprehensive study of these reasons was conducted by researchers at the Stanford University School of Medicine. The participants were more than twenty-nine hundred women age forty and older. In a telephone interview they identified the level of leisure-time or household-related activity engaged in during the previous two weeks. Based on the information they gave, they were assigned to one of three activity-level groups: active, underactive, and sedentary. Only 9 percent of the total participants met the criteria of being physically active. Nearly 60 percent were placed in the sedentary group. The older the age, the less the activity, and the less education, the less the activity.

There were many factors that contributed to being sedentary. They included tiredness, poor health, and self-consciousness about their physical appearance (they did not want to be seen outside walking). We hope future generations of older women will find fewer excuses for not being physically active.

Incidental Memory

You just finished watching a movie on television when your spouse (who did not watch it) asks you, "What was it about?" You are able to go into considerable detail about the movie's plot, even though you had no intention of committing it to memory. This is an example of incidental memory. The very act of comprehending the plot as it progressed was sufficient to transmit information to your long-term memory store. You probably would not have recalled much more, if any, if you had intended to remember the plot. It also would not matter how old you are. In general, incidental memory tends to be about as good as intentional memory for the same material for older adults as well as for younger adults.

This is quite fortunate in that much of our everyday memory does take place incidentally. Do you remember what you ate for lunch today? You probably do, but you surely made no conscious effort to get that information into memory. You did not find yourself rehearsing "I ate a peanut butter and jelly sandwich for lunch" over and over to ensure memorability. That would have been intentional memory. You did not need to do that. Automatism of some components of memory accomplished this for you without intent or rehearsal of the information.

Income of Elderly People

When adjusted for inflation, the average income for people age sixty-five and older in 1996 was $29,210. This was an increase of 57 percent from what the average income was in 1969. However, the increase would have been only 34 percent if the income of spouses was excluded. In 1996 the average income for people in the forty-to-sixty-four-year age range was $58,656. The poverty rate for people age sixty-five and older declined from 35 percent in 1959 to 10 percent in 2003. It is estimated that 40 percent of today's elderly people between sixty and ninety years of age will experience a year below the poverty level at some time in their remaining lives (*see also* Entitlements).

Influenza

Influenza (or flu) is a viral infection of the respiratory tract. There are two main kinds of viruses causing influenza, *Type A* and *Type B*, each type has many different strains. Type A viruses generally cause more severe illness than Type B. Symptoms of influenza include muscle aches, fever, headache, and, in some cases, nausea, vomiting, and diarrhea. These are symptoms that are usually not found with an ordinary cold. In addition, fatigue is mild with a cold, but severe with influenza. A stuffy nose, sneezing, and sore throat are common with a cold, but occur only sometimes with influenza.

Influenza is highly contagious, and it is spread by direct contact with an infected person or by airborne droplets when an infected person coughs or sneezes. To avoid influenza or to prevent it from spreading if you have it, wash your hands often, get a lot of rest, drink a lot of fluids, and call your physician if you are not feeling well. It may also be caught by handling material containing infected body secretions. Symptoms usually appear from one to five days after exposure to the disease. Treatment consists of bed rest, drinking a lot of fluids, and medicines to reduce the fever and discomfort from muscle aches. An antiviral prescription drug, Amantadine, may reduce fever and other symptoms of Type A influenza if taken when the symptoms first appear. In 1999 the U.S. Food and Drug Administration approved an inhaled anti-influenza drug called Relenza. It can reduce the duration of symptoms by one or two days. It may be used with either Type A or Type B viruses. To be effective it should be taken soon after symptoms appear and then taken twice daily for five days. Relenza may also be effective in keeping healthy family members from catching the flu when a relative has the illness. In 1999 the FDA also approved a capsule drug called Tamiflu. If taken within a couple of days of the illness, it may reduce the duration of symptoms by about one and a half days, and it may reduce the risk of bronchitis. Tamiflu may also prevent influenza if taken for six weeks prior to any flu symptoms (however, it is not as effective as a flu vaccination). Both Relenza and Tamiflu are effective in treating avian (bird) flu as well as influenza.

Influenza can lead to pneumonia, especially in older people, and become life threatening (*see also* Pneumonia). A vaccine is available every fall before the flu season (a new vaccine is needed every year). Elderly people should be encouraged to have the vaccination if it causes no serious complications. People who are allergic to eggs should not get the vaccine, nor should persons with a fever or an active infection of any kind. Amantadine may be substituted for those people unable to have the vaccine. Vaccination is not always effective in avoiding influenza for older people, but it should make the symptoms less severe in vaccinated people who contract the disease.

Despite the major health risk of not being vaccinated, at least 60 percent of elderly people who are at high risk for having influenza do not get the vaccination. Some elderly people are unduly afraid that the vaccine will make them sick. Others are either unaware of the vaccine or unaware of the risks of not being vaccinated. The cost would seem to be an irrelevant factor in that it is paid for by Medicare. Researchers have found that vaccination results in fewer hospitalizations, lower mortality, and considerable savings in health costs and may even reduce the risk of a second heart attack.

Influenza (Vaccines)

Vaccination for influenza is less effective for older adults than it is for younger adults. The reason for the decline in protection is the decline in the body's immune system for many older people (*see* Immune Responses and Stress). The vaccine is intended to trigger antibodies that enhance the body's immune system to ward off infection from the influenza virus. However, for those older adults with deficient immune systems, the triggering may not work.

Older people with healthy lifestyles that include regular exercise, healthy diets, and active social lives tend to have little age-related decline in the proficiency of their immune systems. They are the ones who have successful vaccinations. Those seniors with unsuccessful vaccinations need to improve their lifestyle to improve their response to influenza vaccines.

Evidence in support of this position comes from a study by researchers at Iowa State University. They compared adults age sixty-two and older who were classified as being either very active physically for the past year, moderately active physically, or sedentary. After their vaccinations the active seniors demonstrated significantly more benefit from the vaccine than the sedentary seniors, with the moderately active seniors falling between the two extremes.

In addition, researchers in the Netherlands tested the effects of nutritional supplements on the success of immunization with the influenza vaccine. The participants, age sixty-five and older, were in either the supplement group or a placebo group. For seven months prior to immunization, participants in the supplement group received a liquid supplement containing vitamins, minerals, and antioxidants, while those in the placebo group received a noncaloric neutral liquid. The seniors receiving the supplement had a significantly greater positive effect from the vaccine than did the seniors in the placebo group.

Insect Bites

Insect bites can result in infectious diseases. Stings by bees and wasps can incite allergic reactions caused by toxins placed in the skin. The best procedure for seniors to follow is to prevent bites and stings as much as possible. They should use insect repellant that is best applied to the clothing at the collar and cuffs. They should wear long sleeves, pants, socks, and closed shoes when in wooded areas. Avoid perfumes, scented cosmetics, hair spray, and cosmetics that attract insects. They should also avoid wearing brightly colored clothing that may attract bees and wasps. Do not walk in tall grass that may contain ticks. If bitten by a tick, remove the entire tick carefully with tweezers. If stung by a bee or wasp, remove the stinger with tweezers. If allergic, obtain a prescription for a self-administered adrenaline kit.

Intelligence

Intelligence is a frequently used term, but it is difficult to define. We refer to some people as being bright, others as being average, and still others as being dull. In what ways do these people differ from one another? More intelligent people seem to learn more easily, to have better memories, more proficient reasoning ability and problem-solving skill, and a greater store of knowledge about the world than do less intelligent people.

Intelligence is made up of a number of different abilities that collectively define *intelligence*, at least as it has been traditionally defined and investigated. However, it is the learning ability that has attracted the attention of psychologists who have studied intelligence. They constructed tests of intelligence with one objective in mind: to devise a test whose scores would predict scholastic success. Therefore, abilities believed to be related to academic achievement were tested. The test constructors were very successful in their endeavors.

The testing of intelligence as defined above began with the work of Alfred Binet in the early 1900s. He and Theodore Simon constructed a test that could identify low-achieving children in Parisian schools and predict the success of children in general in school. Eventually, Binet and Simon's test was modified and enlarged by Lewis Terman of Stanford University in 1916. The resulting Stanford-Binet test was subsequently revised several times, but its objective has always been to predict academic performances of children.

The first widely used adult intelligence test was the Army Alpha that was developed during World War I (*see* Army Alpha and Army Beta Intelligence Tests). The test was intended for use with adults rather than children, but its objective remained much like that of the Binet-Simon and Stanford-Binet tests: the prediction of academic success. However, in this case academic success referred to successful completion of army training programs. Other tests for adults, such as the Primary Mental Abilities Test and the Wechsler Adult Intelligence Scale (*see* Primary Mental Abilities [PMA] Test; Wechsler Intelligence Tests), have been similarly graded in terms of their success in predicting academic performances, whether it be in college or in an industrial or military training program.

Participants in such academic or industrial training programs are likely to be young adults. But what about older adults who have been away from academic or training situations for some years? The traditional intelligence tests were not developed for them. Intelligence in the daily lives of older adults is applied to the solving of everyday problems and the comprehending of information relevant to their lives, not to earning academic grades.

Over the years there have been attempts to construct intelligence tests that appear to be more relevant to the everyday lives of elderly people. In older tests questions were asked that probed their understanding of legal terms and documents or their ability to comprehend and follow the directions on a medicine bottle or an appliance. More recently, the concept of practical intelligence has resulted in tests of such abilities as tacit knowledge (knowledge derived from experience as contrasted with academic-type knowledge; *see* Practical Intelligence) and newer tests of solving everyday problems (*see* Problem Solving).

Psychologists view traditional, academic-success-related intelligence in terms of a top-to-bottom hierarchy in which abilities are ordered in terms of their specificity. At the top of the hierarchy is a very broad or general ability that is called *g* (for general). The amount of *g* one possesses is believed to be determined largely by familial inheritance. This general-ability factor is believed to influence, to some degree, more specific intellectual abilities.

General ability is "split" into two general, but distinctive, abilities that each encompass a number of specific abilities found at the bottom of the hierarchy. The two general abilities subsumed under *g* are called *crystallized intelligence* and *fluid intelligence.* Crystallized intelligence is influenced greatly by one's experiences, education, and social and cultural environment. The specific abilities derived from crystallized intelligence include vocabulary and general knowledge. Fluid intelligence is basically "raw" intelligence that is determined relatively independent of educational opportunity. The specific abilities derived from fluid intelligence include numerical ability and analogical reasoning ability.

Traditional intelligence tests include subtests that sample abilities related to both crystallized and fluid intelligence. From scores on these subtests, separate estimates may be given of the test taker's crystallized ability and fluid ability. In addition, all of the subtests may be combined to give an estimate of that person's *g* ability (often expressed as an intelligence quotient, or IQ, score).

In general, age-related declines in crystallized intelligence as measured by intelligence tests tend to be slight, if they exist at all, at least until very late in adulthood. However, declines in fluid intelligence test scores begin after early adulthood and progress in amount through late adulthood. When specific abilities are examined, considerable variability in age-related changes is found. Abilities identified with crystallized intelligence generally remain fairly stable throughout adulthood or may show either modest increases or modest decreases from early to late adulthood. Abilities identified with fluid intelligence generally show age-related declines; the extent of the decline is much greater for some abilities than for others. In addition, researchers at the University of North Texas found that elderly adults given training experiences to reduce stress and anxiety while taking fluid intelligence tests were able to reduce the amount of decline in their scores.

Intentional Forgetting

"I'll try to forget what a bad day I had to today." Can you intentionally forget events you want to forget? Evidence provided by researchers at Michigan State University suggests that elderly adults are less proficient at doing it than are younger adults. Their procedure called for a series of words in which each word was followed by a cue to either remember that word or forget it. Elderly participants had more intrusions of forget words than the younger participants, implying that they were less successful in intentionally forgetting events.

Internet

An estimated sixty to seventy million American households use the Internet for everything from chatting with friends to research and reading articles of interest. The fastest-growing segment of Internet users are women age fifty-five and older. Increasingly, more people over age sixty-five are joining the Internet community.

Researchers have provided modest support for a positive effect of Internet use on seniors' psychological well-being (see Well-Being [Psychological]). What is important is that older Internet users do not experience declining well-being. At one time it was thought that the use of the Internet would replace frequent direct social interactions, leading to feelings of isolation and loneliness. This does not appear to be the case. See also Internet (Differences between Users and Nonusers).

Internet (Differences between Users and Nonusers)

Older Internet users have been found to be significantly younger than nonusers (average ages of 69.8 and 76.7, respectively). Users have completed more years of formal education than nonusers (15 and 13 years, respectively). Also users have a significantly higher income than nonusers ($20,000 to $29,999 and $15,000 to $19,999, respectively). It does cost money to have a computer and to subscribe to an Internet service. Perhaps most important, users report being in good health, whereas nonusers tend to rate their health between fair and good.

Interpersonal Tensions

Adults of all ages are likely to have many daily interactions with other adults, such as spouses, their children, coworkers, friends, neighbors, and so on. Most of these interactions tend to be positive in nature, and cause little, if any, tension. However, some are likely to be negative in the sense of involving an argument or a heated discussion. The consequence is likely to be tension that affects the well-being of the individual.

Do older adults tend to have more or fewer tension-evoking events in their daily lives than do younger adults? When tension does occur, is it more or less stressful than it is for younger adults? Do older adults differ from younger adults in their reactions to interpersonal tensions?

Answers to these questions were provided in a study by Dr. Kira S. Birditt and associates of the University of Michigan. The participants in their study were young adults (twenty-five to thirty-nine years), middle-age adults (forty to fifty-nine years), and older adults (sixty to seventy-four years). The participants were interviewed for each of eight days. For each day they reported the interpersonal problems they had, the degree of tension they experienced from them, and their reactions to the tension. Older adults reported fewer interpersonal problems than younger adults, and they experienced less stress evoked by the interpersonal problems than did younger adults. Older adults were also more likely than the younger adults to do nothing in response to their tensions.

Both men and women seem to improve in their ability to deal with interpersonal problems as they grow older. They seem to become more mentally mature as they age, and they become increasingly concerned about maintaining close interpersonal relationships. Why damage these relationships by losing your temper—and then regret it later?

Ischemic Heart Disease

Ischemic heart disease is a general term that encompasses angina, coronary artery disease, and atherosclerosis. It refers to conditions in which there is a lack of blood supply to the heart from the heart arteries resulting from the clogging of those arteries.

J

Job Loss

The loss of one's job is likely to be a traumatic experience. This is true not only for younger adults but for older adults as well. The effects of job loss on the physical functioning and mental health of older workers were investigated by researchers at the Yale University Medical School.

The researchers followed two groups of older adults age fifty-five and older who involuntarily lost their jobs for a period of two years. About half of the participants managed to find a new job during the two years, but the others did not. All of the participants experienced some decline in both physical and mental health. However, the extent of the decline was significantly greater for the participants who were continuously unemployed over the two years. Physical functioning was measured by such tasks as kneeling and getting in and out of bed. Mental health was measured by answering questions about symptoms of depression (for instance, "How often in the past week did you feel sad?").

Job Training

Is it foolish for employers to consider giving job training to older individuals? The available evidence suggests that this is not the case. Adults ranging in age from twenty to seventy were given job training on such jobs as tailors, carpenters, welders, and electronic technicians. The quality of performance during training decreased with increasing age, and the time to complete the training program increased with age. However, the cost of extra time needed by older trainees was slight. Most important, the older workers were found to perform better than the younger workers once the job had been mastered.

Jurors

Are older jurors less likely to comprehend what evidence they receive at a complex trial and reach reasonable decisions than are younger adults? If so, are there interventions that may improve the comprehension and decision-making abilities of older jurors?

In an intriguing study by Dr. Joseph M. Fitzgerald of Wayne State University, some information to answer these questions, at least tentatively, was provided by having younger (nineteen to thirty-five) and older (fifty-five to seventy-five) participants view a two-hour videotape of a mock complex civil trial. Half of the participants in each age group were preinstructed at the start of the trial on complex legal issues and terms that appeared in the trial (for example, liability and compensatory damages). The other half received the same instructions, but after the evidence had been presented.

Both younger and older participants given preinstructions gave more detailed and cohesive accounts of the trial than those instructed after the trial. However, overall the benefit of preinstructing was greater for the older jurors. Posttrial instructions yielded relatively little benefit, and the limited benefit was no greater for the older jurors than for the younger jurors.

K

Kidney Cancer

Kidney cancer is not uncommon for elderly adults. It may go undetected until it spreads throughout the body. Blood in the urine may be an indication of the cancer.

Kidney cancer is a very deadly form of cancer once it spreads that kills half of its sufferers within a year. New experimental bone-marrow transplant treatment may help to cure some patients. Stem cells from the bone marrow are part of the transplant treatment.

Kidney Stones

See Physiological Functions.

Knee Replacement

Nearly four hundred thousand Americans have a knee replacement each year. Most of the recipients are elderly people suffering from severe osteoarthritis of the knees. The substance used for a replacement is made of high-grade plastics and metal alloys coated with a hard, resilient surface and cemented in place. The replacement is still effective in 97 percent of the cases after ten years and in 92 percent of the cases after twenty years. Many recipients can walk within twenty-four hours after surgery. After six to ten weeks of physical therapy most recipients can return to their normal activities.

Traditional replacement requires that an eight- to twelve-inch incision be made on the front joint and through the part of the quadriceps muscle and tendons. Damaged tissue is removed, and the replacement is inserted. There is a minimally invasive procedure requiring a smaller incision and moving the quadriceps muscle aside before removing damaged tissue and inserting the replacement knee.

L

Laughter (Is It the Best Medicine for Seniors?)

Do you laugh yourself silly watching old Laurel and Hardy movies? You probably do. There is an old saying—laughter is the best medicine for what ails you. If you are ill, will laughter aid your recovery?

Even in biblical times the medicinal powers of laughter were praised. Claims about its power have reappeared from time to time. They were heard most positively in a best-selling book by Norman Cousins (1979), the editor of the *Saturday Review of Literature*. Cousins had a very painful form of rheumatoid arthritis that he treated with daily exposures to laughter, such as hours of watching Laurel and Hardy movies. He eventually recovered from the disease, giving credit for his recovery to laughter. Of course, he also had daily massive doses of vitamin C. However, it was laughter and not the vitamin that was acclaimed. Since then laughter has attained even greater medical prominence. It is not uncommon to see clowns and comedy material in hospitals.

Does laughter really have medicinal power? There have been a number of studies examining the relationship between laughter and various forms of illness or poor health. One of the most intriguing areas of research involves laughter's potential analgesic effects, that is, relief of pain. In general, it has been found that exposure to comedy results in increases in pain threshold and pain tolerance. Perhaps physicians should show their patients a funny movie while they are receiving a painful treatment (such as a rectal examination).

Other areas of research have been less convincing in providing support for the health benefits of laughter. For example, whether laughter is an effective medication for treating high blood pressure is debatable. In fact, in one study laughter was found to produce short-term increases in blood pressure, without any long-term effects. Interestingly, the life duration of comedians and comedy writers does not differ from that of serious actors or writers.

Learned Helplessness

The concept of learned helplessness was introduced to psychology by animal researchers in the mid-1970s. Dogs were subjected to intense electric shock under conditions in which there was no way to escape the shock. Eventually, they encountered new situations in which electric shock could be avoided by performing a specified behavior. They were found to be very deficient in learning to avoid the shock even though they had the opportunity to do so. The researchers concluded that the dogs had actually learned to be "helpless." It was as if they had acquired a "what's the use?" attitude—no matter what they did, they had earlier found there was no escape from being punished.

Moreover, the dogs were observed to become distressed and passive in their behavior. The concept of learned helplessness was eventually extended to human behavior. Some people living under various negative and stressful conditions, such as poverty, may discover that there seems to be no relationship between their behavior and escape from the stressful conditions. That is, no matter how they try to cope with the negative events in their lives, they are unsuccessful in improving their lot in life, resulting eventually in a state of learned helplessness characterized by persistent passive behavior and even severe depression.

On the surface, older people might seem to be highly vulnerable targets for acquiring learned helplessness. More than younger people, they may be subjected to negative life events that are seemingly inescapable. However, various evidence suggests that older people are no more susceptible to learned helplessness than are younger people. For example, elderly people, in general, express satisfaction with their current lives that is no less than that expressed by younger people (*see* Life Satisfaction). Nor is their incidence of severe depression greatly different from that of younger adults (see Depression [Incidence, Symptoms, Causes]). In addition, many elderly people are very effective in coping with stressful events in their lives. *See also* Stress and Coping with Stress.

Learning (Overview)

If all new learning suddenly stopped for you, you would have no new acquisitions of knowledge. The name of a new president or a new senator would be unfamiliar to you in terms of their office every time you encountered his or her name. It would be impossible to acquire new words either in a foreign language or in your own native language. Strangers who were introduced to you would continue to be strangers on future encounters. There would be no hope of acquiring new recreational skills. If you did not already know how to play golf, operate a word processor, or play bridge, you would not in the future either. How to operate a new kitchen gadget would have to be relearned every time you used it. Finding your way around a new neighborhood would be a brand-new adventure every time you left your home. It would also be impossible to learn the meaning of new concepts, such as that of a black hole or AIDS.

Learning is essential for adaptation to our environments, and it is just as essential for older people as it is for younger people. Fortunately, elderly people remain active learners. They do learn new information, new recreational skills, new names with new faces, and so on. Of course, this does not mean that there are no declines in learning proficiency with normal aging. Given the importance of new learning to our everyday lives, it is essential that we discover the extent of these declines, the reasons they occur, and possible ways of reducing the declines in proficiency.

Our examples of new learning should make it apparent that there are many kinds of learning. Among the kinds of learning studied by psychologists are classical conditioning, operant conditioning, spatial learning, maze learning, motor skill learning, and verbal learning. A description of aging research on each kind of learning is found in separate entries.

The concepts of learning and memory are obviously related, and they are difficult to distinguish. Learning a task of any kind usually involves the intent to learn the task, practice the task, and progressive improvements in performance on the task with practice. This fits nicely with what happens when you *learned* to ride a bicycle. You had the intent to do so, you practiced it, and you gradually mastered the skill. This description of learning works less well for classical conditioning (*see* Classical Conditioning). Here there is no intent to learn, but there is practice and gradually learning occurs.

The fit is even poorer for the *memory* you have of the first bad spill you had with your bicycle. The memory of that spill required no intent, and practice was not needed (one occurrence only was involved). This is an example of episodic memory, that is, memory for personally experienced events in one's life (*see* Episodic Memory). There are many other forms of memory as well (*see* Memory [Overview]). *See also* Classical Conditioning; Concept Learning; Maze Learning; Motor Skill Learning; Operant Conditioning; Spatial Learning; Verbal Learning.

Legal Advice

The present generation of seniors has more reasons for wanting (and perhaps needing) legal advice than any earlier generation of seniors. Among the issues confronting many of them are: ensuring protection physically and financially during periods of incapacity (for example, having someone act as their agent through a durable power of attorney), recovering assets from someone who has cheated them, and ensuring understanding of long-term-care insurance policies. Many law firms now have an attorney who specializes in helping seniors resolve their legal issues. For information on locating an elder-law attorney in your state, visit the Web site of either the National Academy of Elder Law Attorneys (http://www.naela.com) or the National Elder-Law Foundation (http://www.nelf.org).

Leisure Activities

A leisure activity is usually defined as one in which individuals engage during their free time. Older people generally have more time available for pursuing leisure than do younger people. Of interest in gerontology is the nature of elderly adults' leisure activities and how they differ from those of younger adults. Not surprisingly, most elderly people decrease their strenuous leisure activities and increase their more sedentary activities (such as reading and watching television), relative to the activities engaged in earlier in their lives.

A survey of people living in a small midwestern city indicated that for people in the sixty-five-to-seventy-four-year age range the predominant activities were those involving social interactions and travel. Social activities were also reported by many of those surveyed who were age seventy-five and older, as were home-based and family-based activities. However, the percentage of those reporting travel as a leisure activity declined from 60 percent in the sixty-five-to-seventy-four-year range to 40 percent in the seventy-five-and-older age range. In general, the variety of leisure activities in which people engage declines progressively from young adulthood through middle age and into late adulthood.

Older adults, however, do not abandon physical activity as a form of leisure activity. According to the 2000 census, the most popular physical activity is walking. Less popular forms of physical leisure activities are swimming and exercising with equipment.

The choice of activities for many elderly people is surely restricted by their changing physical health status. This is true, for example, with elderly adults who have severe arthritis. They are likely to find that they are no longer able to participate in some of their physically demanding old leisure activities. Those who do not replace them with new, less physically challenging activities are most likely to have problems with their psychological well-being.

However, there is one physical activity that may not need to be replaced for older people with arthritis. It is gardening, one of the favorite leisure activities of many elderly people. Occupational therapists believe that if older people with arthritis make some changes in the way they plan and carry out their activities in their gardens, they may prevent pain and damage to their joints. For example, they should begin with a ten-minute warm-up period of stretching and exercising. While working in the garden they should sit down whenever they can. If they need to kneel, they should use knee pads. They should limit the amount of lifting they do, and they should bend their knees when they do have to lift. Tools such as hoes and rakes that have longer handles aid in reducing bending. They should use tools that reduce stress on their wrists and arms.

Most important, they should check with their physician to schedule an appointment with an occupational therapist at one of their local rehabilitation centers to prepare themselves for continuing their gardening.

Leisure Activities (Why Some Decline in Late Adulthood)

Canadian researchers found that participation in a number of leisure activities declines as seniors become older. Over an eight-year period the percentage ceasing an activity was 24 percent for dining out, 55 percent for attending a movie theater or sporting event, and 33 percent for travel. There were much smaller declines for watching television (7 percent) and reading (9 percent).

Why the declines? A number of factors were identified. They included self-rated health decline and limitations in performing the activities of daily living (*see* Activities of Daily Living).

Leukemia

Leukemia is a form of cancer in which white blood cells grow in a manner that harms the body. The most common form of leukemia in older people is chronic lymphocytic leukemia. It usually appears after age sixty. However, it may have been present for years without being detected. A blood test during a checkup may finally indicate its existence. Chemotherapy is the usual treatment.

Lexicon

As you read the words in this sentence, what enables you to do so? Each word in the sentence must have its own representation in your *semantic* or *permanent knowledge memory* (*see* Semantic Memory). The printed version of the word *what* is quickly read as the word *what* because the mental operations of reading ensure automatic contact with information in your memory that corresponds to that word. These representations are stored in a part of our semantic memory known as the lexicon (or mental dictionary).

Adults of all ages have difficulty *not* reading a word when it is in their visual fields. That is, contact with the word's representation in the lexicon occurs automatically and effortlessly regardless of an adult's age, and it is a process that is difficult to stop. The automatism of reading a word when it is physically present is clearly demonstrated by what psychologists call the

Stroop effect (named after the psychologist who discovered it). Suppose you are given a series of color patches (red, green, yellow, red, and so on), and you are asked to name each color as you see it. Regardless of your age, you will respond rapidly to each color (and, of course, correctly).

Now change the nature of the task. This time you are asked to name the color of the ink in which each word in a series is printed. The first ink color is red, and your response should be "red." However, the word written in red ink is the word *blue*. Similarly, the second ink color is green, but it is the color ink for the printed word *yellow*. Your responses of "red" and "green" will occur much more slowly than they do when you are simply naming red and green color patches (it is this slower responding that defines the Stroop effect).

The slower response occurs because you cannot avoid reading the color words, and by so doing you have to inhibit the name of the word in order to name the color of the ink. Older adults tend to show an even greater Stroop effect than do younger adults, because the added years of reading have increased the time needed to "turn off" reading the word. "Turning off" reading is one of the many behaviors that slow down with aging (*see* Slowing-Down Principle).

Our point is that color words have representations in our lexicons that are activated whenever they are encountered in printed form. Similar representations are present for every other word in our active vocabularies. Contact with representations in our lexicons also occurs automatically when we hear spoken words. Without such automatic contact we would be unable to engage in normal everyday conversations, listen to a lecture, or understand the content of a television program. Access to words in our lexicons is as automatic for normally aging people as it is for younger people, although access takes place a bit more slowly (at the level of milliseconds slower) in late adulthood.

Access to words is facilitated by the organized structure of our lexicons. Words are not stored randomly or haphazardly. Related words appear to be stored in close proximity to one another. The activation of a given word's representation in the lexicon spreads automatically to these nearby related words. When you read the word *doctor*, the activation of its representation spreads quickly to the representations of such related words as *nurse*. *Spreading activation* makes reading time faster for those words that have already been activated prior to their physical appearance. Consider the sentences "The doctor gave the instrument to the nurse" and "The carpenter gave the instrument to the nurse." Identifying the word *nurse* as "nurse" occurs more quickly in reading the first sentence than in the second sentence. This is because the activation of *nurse*'s representation in the lexicon began while reading *doctor* but not while reading *carpenter*. Numerous laboratory studies have revealed that spreading activation takes place to the same degree for elderly adults as for younger adults, although the time required for spreading to be completed is a bit longer for older adults (and much slower for patients with Alzheimer's disease).

The existence of spreading activation is not the only kind of evidence to indicate that the lexicon has an organized structure. The other major form of evidence is derived from the nature of word associations. Our associations of words to other words tend to show regularity and commonality among people of all ages. Most important, research on word associations indicates that the structure of the lexicon changes little, if any, with normal aging (*see* Word Associations). In fact, the most likely change in the structure of the lexicon with normal aging is in the number of representations of words it contains. Elderly adults typically have a larger vocabulary than younger adults (*see* Verbal Ability).

Licorice

Licorice, unlike chocolate with its positive physical health benefits, may actually affect physical health negatively. It may contribute to high blood pressure, whether it is in candy, tea, or capsules. It may also lower levels of potassium. Side effects from a high dose or prolonged consumption may consist of fluid retention or heart rhythm irregularities.

Life Expectancy

Life expectancy in any given year is usually defined as the average length of time an infant born in that year is expected to live, given that conditions present in that year stay unchanged. As conditions have changed over the years, so has life expectancy. In 1900, life expectancy in the United States was only 47 years. This does not mean that few people at that time lived beyond age 47. In fact, many individuals lived well into late adulthood.

The reason that life expectancy was so low was the high mortality rate for infants at that time. Their ages at death figured prominently in the calculation of the purely statistical concept of a life expectancy. As health conditions improved over the years, the incidence of infant deaths, as well as the deaths of adults below age 40, declined dramatically. The net effect has been a progressive increase in life expectancy. During the 1980s life expectancy had reached 74.5 years, and it reached 76.1 years in 1997. In 2005 life expectancy was reported to be 77.6 years.

However, the likelihood of living to an advanced age did not increase nearly as dramatically. People age 75 had a life expectancy of about 8 years (that is, on the average they were expected to live that much longer) in 1900 and about 11 years in the 1980s. This form of life expectancy may increase throughout this century as progress is made in the treatment of heart disease and cancer. The Social Security Administration anticipates overall life expectancy to increase to 79.3 in the year 2030 and to 81.5 in the year 2070. Longevity should also increase in the future with progress made in preventive medicine (*see* Longevity).

The figures above are for the entire United States and include both men and women. Life expectancy may also be determined separately for the sexes, for different races, for different geographical regions, and for different occupations. Life expectancy in 2000 was 74.1 years for men and 79.5 years for women. Life expectancy for African Americans (combined for the sexes) is about 5 years less than that of whites.

Life expectancy is also higher in some states (Hawaii and in the northern plains states) than in other states (South Carolina). Similarly, life expectancy is higher for some occupations (judges) than for other occupations (coal miners). In countries such as India and Ethiopia life expectancy is no greater than it was in the United States in 1900. The high incidence of infant mortality in these countries accounts largely for the low average life expectancy. By contrast, there are countries, such as Sweden and Japan, where life expectancy is greater than that of people in the United States. Life expectancy is the greatest for natives of Okinawa (81.2 years), presumably because of their healthy diet.

Life Insurance

You are seventy-five years old, and you believe that your life insurance may not even be enough to cover the rising cost of a funeral (*see* Funerals). Should you buy more life insurance, even though it is more costly than it would have been some years ago? Financial advisers generally recommend you should invest in more life insurance. The insurance could cover costs of a final illness as well as your funeral expenses. It could cover other remaining expenses, such as an automobile loan and a credit card balance. Of course, it could also leave funds for your heirs or favorite charity.

Life Satisfaction

How satisfied are you with your present life? Do you feel that your achievements come close to matching what you hoped they would be at your present age? Are you satisfied with your life now? On a 9-point scale in which 1 is very dissatisfied and 9 is very satisfied, where would you rank yourself? Your satisfaction with your life is a good index of your feeling of well-being.

Surprisingly, life satisfaction does not seem to be related to age. That is, older adults, in general, express no less or no greater satisfaction than do middle-aged or young adults. The average rating on the 9-point scale is about the same at each age level, and, in some studies, has even been found to be greater for older adults than for younger adults.

For example, in a 1995 survey of more than one thousand adults the percentages expressing satisfaction with their lives were 81, 87, 85, and 83 for adults in the eighteen-to-thirty, thirty-one-to-forty-eight, forty-nine-to-sixty-two, and sixty-three-and-older age ranges, respectively. However, the percentage happy with their lives may decline in very late adulthood. In a 1997 survey of people over age eighty, only 66 percent said they were very satisfied with their present lives. Other surveys, including one of Israeli citizens, ranging in age from their late teens to sixty-five and older, have confirmed the absence of any major effect of age on life satisfaction.

Our reference has been to present life satisfaction. Of further interest is what people believe their life satisfaction will be in the future. In the survey of Israeli citizens, the participants were asked to estimate their life satisfaction five years from the time of the rating. From the late teens through the early thirties, future life satisfaction was estimated to be considerably higher than present satisfaction. However, beginning in the late thirties, there was a progressive decline in rated future life satisfaction, such that by late adulthood future life satisfaction was rated, on the average, no higher than present life satisfaction. This trend suggests that people become increasingly less optimistic about the future as they progress through middle age into late adulthood.

The fact that elderly people differ little from younger people in their average degree of life satisfaction does not imply that all elderly people are satisfied with their present lives. There is considerable variability in life satisfaction scores—many older people are far less satisfied than other older people.

One of the most widely researched topics in gerontology is determining the reasons for this variability in life satisfaction among elderly people. What factors account for some elderly people feeling less satisfied than others? The most important factor, and one that should not be surprising, is health status. Older adults who perceive their health to be poor tend to be less satisfied with their lives than other elderly adults who perceive their health to be good or excellent. Socioeconomic status is another important factor, as is the amount of social interactions of elderly people. However, it is likely that the frequency and quality of social interactions are dependent on health status. That is, the more positive health is, the higher the frequency and quality of social interactions,

Numerous other factors have been related to the degree of life satisfaction expressed by elderly people. For example, Canadian researchers studied marital transitions (spouse present or absent) for a large sample of older people over a seven-year period. Women whose marital status remained unchanged reported a decline in life satisfaction. Men whose marital status remained unchanged reported no change in life satisfaction. For those with a loss of a spouse, there was a decline in life satisfaction for both women and men, with the decline being greater for men. In addition, men who gained a spouse over the seven years experienced an increase in life satisfaction. This was not the case for women who gained a spouse.

Similarly, elderly people who appear to be more religious tend to express moderately higher life satisfaction than less religious elderly people. Here too, however, it may be health status that is the more important causative factor. Church attendance is likely to be greater for elderly people who are in good health than for those who are in poor health.

There is evidence to indicate that elderly African Americans are less satisfied than elderly whites, undoubtedly because of the larger percentage of elderly African Americans living on poverty-level incomes. Extroverted elderly men tend to express greater life satisfaction than elderly men who are less extroverted, and evidence indicates that elderly men who score high in the personality trait of neuroticism score lower in life satisfaction than men who score lower in neuroticism (*see* Personality Traits). There appears to be little difference between elderly men and elderly women in life satisfaction scores. Wisdom is a cognitive ability that has been found to be related positively to life satisfaction for elderly people (*see* Wisdom).

The critical roles played by health status and socioeconomic status on life satisfaction in late adulthood suggest that future generations of older people will have fewer members who are dissatisfied with their lives. That is, medical progress in the years ahead will ensure good or excellent health for a larger percentage of elderly people than presently. Similarly, improved pension plans and improved preretirement economic planning should greatly reduce the percentage of elderly people with impoverished lives.

The life events one has experienced early in adulthood are also likely to affect one's life satisfaction in late adulthood. For example, a study of elderly women's life satisfaction found a relationship between the hardships they experienced during the Great Depression and their present life satisfaction. *See also* Disability (Psychological and Social Consequences); Racial and Ethnic Differences in Aging; Religion in Later Life.

Life Span

The life span of a given species is the length of time a member of that species could live if free of disease and accidents that prevent fulfillment of that duration. It may be estimated for a species by the oldest age a member of that species has been known to live. For human beings, that age is at least 122 years (a woman in France died in 1997 at age 122 years). There have been other reports of individuals who have lived longer than 120 years, but these claims have been difficult to verify. In general, other species have much shorter life spans than the human being. For some insects, the life span is only a few days. For the mouse it is about 3 years, and for the horse it is probably 30-plus years (although there have been claims, difficult to verify, of horses living to be over 60 years). On the other hand, the life span for the Galapagos tortoise may be as high as 150 years.

The human life span has apparently been the same for centuries. However, is it possible that the human life span can be increased in the future? Some scientists believe that this is a definite possibility. They have based their belief on research with rats. Rats that live on a restricted diet from birth have been found to have a longer life span than rats living on a normal diet. Restricting food intake seems to retard aging in rats. Whether similar food restrictions could increase the life span of human beings remains highly speculative.

Many scientists do believe that health interventions, such as regular exercise and nutritious diets, will serve to increase the number of people who are able to attain the full life span, but they are unlikely to increase the life span itself.

Perhaps what is more important is that greatly improved health practices could result in a longer health span, defined as the maximum number of years people live without suffering any of the chronic diseases associated with aging. The World Health Organization ranks countries in terms of their health span. Japan ranks first and Switzerland second.

Lifting Heavy Objects

Elderly people should avoid lifting heavy objects the wrong way. The result of doing so could be back pain and perhaps the loss of mobility for days. The right way to lift is to keep the object close to your body, bend your knees, and keep your back straight. For more information, write (with a self-addressed envelope enclosed) to Lift It Safe, American Academy of Orthopedic Surgeons, P.O. Box 1998, Des Plaines, IL 60017.

Liver Cancer

Primary liver cancer is uncommon in the United States. It is cancer that begins in the cells of the liver itself. Only about 3 percent of new cancers in the United States are primary liver cancers. On the other hand, *secondary liver cancers* are more common. They are secondary in the sense that they are metastatic cancers that spread from cancers of other organs, such as the colon, the stomach, or the lungs.

Primary liver cancer is rarely discovered early. This makes it difficult to control with existing treatments. However, the pain from the disease can often be controlled, which improves the quality of life for the patient. The most effective procedure is the effort to prevent primary liver cancer by protecting oneself from hepatitis infection and cirrhosis, the leading causes of primary liver cancer. Coffee drinkers may be interested to know that Japanese researchers in their study of thousands of adults found that habitual coffee drinkers were 29 percent less likely to develop liver cancer than occasional coffee drinkers.

Locomotion

Elderly adults, in general, walk more slowly than young adults. The age difference in velocity is already apparent by age sixty-five. Further decreases in
velocity occur after age sixty-five, such that people in their eighties walk
considerably more slowly than people in their sixties. Researchers in France
have determined that the reduction in walking rate is almost entirely the
consequence of the shorter strides taken by elderly people. This may be
seen in the fact that stride length averages 1.09 meters for participants in
their sixties and 0.71 meters for participants in their eighties, and speed of
walking averages 1.00 meters per second and 0.60 meters per second at the
two age levels. These researchers also discovered that adults of all ages are
capable of increasing their walking speed when required to do so. Regardless of age, the increase in speed is accomplished by both increasing stride
length and decreasing cycle time (that is, time from left-foot placement to
the next left-foot placement).

Sedentary elderly people have a more cautious walking style than active
elderly people, as shown by their shorter stride length and slower velocity.
Those elderly people who are confident of their capability of performing
the physical activities of daily living have a faster gait velocity than elderly
people with less confidence. Researchers at the University of Alabama at
Birmingham found that depression, falling, and lack of exercise play roles
in loss of mobility among African Americans, whereas incontinence and
poor vision may play roles among whites.

Whether exercise improves the gait of elderly people is inconclusive.
Researchers at Indiana University found that participants age sixty-five and
older who received twelve weeks of dynamic-resistance strength training did
not differ from other participants in a nonexercise control group at the end
of twelve weeks. Nor did the researchers find exercise to improve balance
for participants in the exercise group, again relative to those in the control
group. Older adults have lower ankle planter-flexor power than younger
adults. This suggests to some experts that a more appropriate form of exercise for maintaining stride length in late adulthood is one that strengthens
the planter-flexor muscle.

Some adults do seem to walk faster than they did when they were
younger. A faster gait is apparently their way of compensating for their relatively poor balance and the shift forward in their body's center of gravity.

Loneliness

Feelings of distress, separation, and isolation—these are the feelings that
define loneliness. A Harris survey revealed that the proportion of elderly
people experiencing loneliness is substantial. In fact, loneliness is ranked
high among the most serious problems older people believe to confront

them. Elderly people who perceive themselves as being lonely are likely to evaluate their physical well-being much lower than elderly people who do not perceive themselves to be lonely. Especially a problem is the high blood pressure experienced by many lonely elders.

The probable causes of loneliness for elderly people were investigated by researchers at the University of South Carolina. Information was obtained from nearly three thousand individuals aged sixty-five and older. A number of conditions were found to contribute to the loneliness experienced by many elderly people. However, the most important contributor was a low level of social fulfillment. Reduced social fulfillment means that they do not have enough to do to keep busy, and they do not feel needed. Among the other conditions contributing to loneliness of elderly people are changed marital status, reduced income, frequency of telephone contact, and poor health. However, the effects of these other contributors are largely indirect; that is, they affect loneliness largely by way of their negative influences on social fulfillment. Anxiety tends to increase feelings of loneliness. Introverted older people generally report more feelings of loneliness than do extroverted older people.

Loneliness is reduced for seniors by the affection they both give and receive from their adult children. Frequent contact is often needed by telephone for adult children who live far from their parents.

Especially likely to feel lonely are caregivers of patients with Alzheimer's disease who are unable to leave them alone. Friends of the caregivers would be doing them a great favor by arranging regular visits with them.

Longevity

Elderly people obviously differ greatly in the number of years they actually live. Viewers of the *Today* television program are reminded constantly that some lives continue well past the century mark. However, we all know older people who died long before attaining that mark. The average expected length of life for people of a given age is called their life expectancy, and the maximum number of years people are believed capable of living under the most favorable circumstances is called the life span (*see* Life Expectancy; Life Span). But what about individual persons? What determines their greatly different *longevities*? Scientists have long believed that heredity is a major determinant of individual differences in longevity.

Alexander Graham Bell conducted a genealogical study years ago of a single family that had thousands of descendants. He found that children of parents who lived to be eighty years or more lived about twenty years longer than children whose two parents died before they were sixty years old. A study in the 1950s reported that identical twins (who have identical heredities) die several years closer together than do fraternal twins (who are like ordinary siblings and do not have identical heredities). A similar difference in longevities between identical and fraternal twins was found recently for Danish citizens who were born between 1870 and 1880. Nevertheless, it should be noted that the relationship between parents and children in years lived is only slightly positive. That is, the correlation is positive, but not much greater than zero.

There are, of course, other factors that are major determinants of individual differences in longevity. Regular exercise and good health practices are likely to add years to one's life. Obesity and smoking are likely to subtract years from one's life, as is prolonged exposure to various pollutants in the environment. Excess weight moderately increases the risk of death from age thirty-five to age seventy-five, but at a declining rate with aging. By age sixty-five the risk is slight, and by age seventy-six virtually nonexistent.

There are also more subtle factors that influence longevity. For example, married people tend to live several years longer than unmarried people. Occupational/income level and educational level are related to longevity. In general, longevity is greater for people with higher levels of both than for people with lower levels. Perhaps the reason is that people with higher income or greater education have better health habits than those with less income or education. However, evidence from a major longitudinal study (*see* Longitudinal Studies of Aging's Effects on Health and Cognition) has indicated that people who score lower on most tests of cognitive abilities (for instance, verbal memory and word fluency) do not have an earlier mortality than people who score higher on those same tests. The exception is for those who score lower on tests requiring perceptual speed and have an earlier mortality. This is seemingly part of the general principle of processes slowing down with aging (*see* Slowing-Down Principle). Those who show greater slowing down are presumably in poorer health than those who show less decline in speed with aging.

Social activity may also be a factor related to longevity. Researchers at Harvard University followed a group of people age sixty-five and older at the start of their study for thirteen years. Those who were most socially active lived two and a half years longer than those who were least socially active. Social activities were identified as such activities as eating out, attending religious services, and participating in recreational games (such as bingo).

Other possible factors have been discovered by researchers in California who have been following the lives of more than fifteen hundred intellectually bright children who were first studied in 1921. Perhaps the most obvious factor determining longevity among these individuals is their sex. By 1991 50 percent of the men but only 35 percent of the women were known to be dead. Why do men average less longevity than women? It isn't just their greater drinking of alcoholic beverages and smoking nor their greater risk of violence. Men tend, on the average, to see physicians less often than women, and when they do, they talk less with their physicians about their problems (*see also* Barriers to Health in Older Men).

In addition, in the California study the participants who were more conscientious and socially dependable as children tended to live longer than those who were less conscientious and socially dependable, and those children whose parents had divorced when they were children tended to die at an earlier age than those whose parents had remained married. There is other evidence to suggest that certain personality characteristics are related to longevity. For example, people who live to age ninety and beyond tend to have a flexible attitude toward life in general. They are also unlikely to be extreme in their habits (for example, excessive eating of junk food or excessive drinking of alcoholic beverages), and they tend to adapt readily to sources of stress in their daily lives. *See also* Obesity (Effects on Longevity and Disability).

Longevity (What Determines a Long Life?)

Why do some people live to be one hundred years old or older? This is many more years than the normal life expectancy. Researchers at the Ohio State University Medical School studied the medical histories of four hundred centenarians. They discovered that many of them were successful in coping with life-threatening diseases long before they became centenarians. The most important contribution to a long life was found to be their heredity. Brothers of centenarians are seventeen times more likely and sisters eight times more likely to live to at least one hundred years than the general population (*see* Centenarians).

Researchers are presently searching for the gene or genes that seemingly determine a very long life span such as that of centenarians. Dr. Nir Barzilai, director of aging research at Albert Einstein College of Medicine in New York and a prominent geneticist, is confident that the search will be successful within the next ten years. The discovery could lead to the creation of medications that could enable seniors to extend their resistance to such life-threatening diseases as heart disease and cancer.

Researchers at the University of Chicago discovered that another factor appears to be the age of mothers at the time they give birth to their children. Children of younger mothers tend to live longer than children of older mothers. For example, more centenarians have been born to younger mothers than to older mothers.

Longitudinal Method

John's parents have been measuring his height on every birthday through age eighteen. Not surprisingly, they have discovered that John has grown taller with age. John's parents may not realize it, but they were using one of the major methods employed in aging research to determine the presence and nature of age differences on whatever characteristic or behavior is being measured. That method is called the *longitudinal method*. Assuming that John is a fairly representative child, we may conclude that children grow taller as they become older. This is a true age change for every normally developing child. We could have reached the same conclusion if we examined the heights of representative one-year-old children, two-year-old children, and so on through age eighteen. In this case, however, we have conducted a cross-sectional study in which the same individual is tested only once, and all individuals are tested at about the same time (*see* Cross-Sectional Method). Our cross-sectional study, however, runs the risk of falsely concluding that the age difference in height is related to a true age change in height. There is the possibility (very slim, of course) that the two-year-old was born with his or her current height, the three-year-old with his or her current height, and so on. If this were true, then the observed age difference represents a cohort or generational difference and not a true age change (*see* Cohort [Generational] Effect).

When the interest lies in determining if an age difference represents a true age change, then the longitudinal method has a decided edge over the cross-sectional method.

In aging research the longitudinal method uses a group of individuals rather than a single individual. The basic procedure calls simply for testing and retesting the participants in the group. Ideally, we would like to recruit participants who are young adults and test them on the characteristic or behavior in question (for example, intelligence). We would then retest them every few years until they reach late adulthood. The change in average scores with increasing age would identify a true age change. Because all the participants came from the same generation, the observed age difference could not be related to a cohort or generational effect.

Unfortunately, there have been very few longitudinal studies in which participants have been tested and retested for a period of many years. The studies with the best retesting records have been concerned either with intelligence or physical health. Most longitudinal studies have been directed at a relatively short span of years, but often that span is a critical period when true age changes may be expected to occur (for example, participants tested originally at age sixty-five and then retested at age seventy-five (*see*, for example, Victoria Longitudinal Study in the entry Longitudinal Studies of Aging's Effects on Physical Health and Cognition).

The longitudinal method is not without its problems. One problem is that many participants are likely to withdraw from the study because of death, illness, lack of interest, relocation, and so on. There is often a disportionality among the dropouts relative to the nondropouts in terms of ability as measured on the initial test. If the test was boring and uninteresting, the dropouts are more likely to be participants of high initial ability than participants of lower initial ability. By contrast, if the test was very challenging and demanding, the dropouts are more likely to be participants of low initial ability than participants of higher initial ability. In either case, a bias is introduced in terms of the nature of the remaining participants (that is, they would consist mainly of either initially low scorers or initially high scorers).

An additional problem arises from what is called progressive error. Retesting obviously leads to increasingly greater familiarity with the test in question. Consequently, scores on the test may increase simply from familiarity and disguise what the participants would have scored at a later age in the absence of such familiarity. This is why there are alternate forms of some tests. Form A is taken the first time and Form B the second time. The forms differ in specific content.

Finally, there is the possibility in some cases of the presence of a historical time effect. Social and cultural conditions change over the years. Consider, for example, young adults tested for the presence of depressive symptoms in the mid-1920s during a period of economic prosperity, and then retested in the mid-1930s during the time of the Great Depression. The presence of transitory depressive symptoms brought about by the sad economy of that time would not be surprising. An age difference in depression for twenty-five- and thirty-five-year-old people would be the likely outcome. However, it is unlikely to be a true age change. The greater number of depressive symptoms for the thirty-five-year-old participants was undoubtedly a temporary phenomenon, and the symptoms surely decreased when economic prosperity was restored. The possibility of a historical time effect is avoided in a cross-sectional study in that all of the participants at each age level are tested at the same historical time.

Longitudinal Studies of Aging's Effects on Health and Cognition

The Baltimore Longitudinal Study was begun in 1961 to examine aging's effects on both physical health and cognition (*see* National Institute on Aging). However, it was not the first major longitudinal study on physical health. That was the Framingham Study of Heart Diseases.

The town of Framingham, Massachusetts, was selected by the U.S. Public Health Service in 1948 to provide the participants in a study of the effects of aging on cardiovascular diseases. Initially, nearly five thousand male and female participants were selected randomly from the town's ten thousand inhabitants in the age range of thirty through fifty years. The survivors have been examined every two years to determine the beginning of cardiovascular diseases. In 1971 the spouses and children of the original participants were added to the study. Much of what is now known about aging's effects on cardiovascular diseases has been derived from this study.

Another well-known study of aging's effects on health is the Nurse's Health Study. It began in 1980 with more than seventy-five thousand nurses as participants, and it has been continuing now for many years. Among the findings from the study is that a diet rich in vegetables and fruits reduces the risk of a stroke from the blockage of a blood vessel (*see* Stroke). Another important study is the Women's Health Initiative Study, which has contributed important information about aging and breast cancer, nutrition and diet, and osteoporosis (*see* Women's Health Initiative).

Not as well known are the Veterans Health Study and the Normative Aging Study. The Veterans Health Study is gathering information about the health status of veterans and the care they receive. The Normative Aging Study is a program of longitudinal research that began in 1968. The study is concerned with aging's effects on both physical and mental health (psychological well-being) and with the factors that lead to declines with aging. One important finding has been the evidence revealing the negative health effects smoking in early adulthood has on health in late adulthood.

Understanding better the effects of aging on cognitive or mental functioning has been blessed by two very important studies, one on intelligence, the other on memory. The one on intelligence is the Seattle Longitudinal Study begun in 1956 by Dr. K. Warner Schaie. In that year a large sample of adults in the Seattle, Washington, area was tested on five of the subtests of the Primary Mental Abilities Test, a widely used test of adult intelligence (*see* Primary Mental Abilities [PMA] Test). Many of the original participants were subsequently retested every seven years as they aged. In addition, new participants from the same population were tested in 1963, 1970, 1977, and 1984, and also retested every seven years.

The longitudinal reassessments of intelligence indicate that intelligence does not change uniformly with aging. Fluid intelligence abilities (for instance, reasoning) tend to decrease in proficiency at an earlier age than crystallized abilities (verbal abilities; *see* Intelligence; Wechsler Intelligence Tests). Women appear to experience decline earlier than men in fluid intelligence abilities, but the reverse is true for crystallized abilities. Perhaps the most striking observation in the study is that fewer than half of the individuals retested at age eighty-one showed any significant decline in abilities from the previous testing at age seventy-four.

The longitudinal study of aging's effects on memory is the Victoria Longitudinal Study conducted by researchers at the University of Victoria in Canada. The components of memory investigated in the study are episodic long-term memory, implicit memory, and semantic memory (*see* Episodic Memory; Implicit Memory; Semantic Memory). The study began in 1986, and new samples of participants of different ages continue to be tested and retested several years later.

In agreement with most cross-sectional studies, no effect has been found for implicit memory, but an age-related decline has been found for word recall (a form of episodic memory). Contrary to most cross-sectional studies, no longitudinal decline has been found for discourse memory (*see* Discourse Memory). Surprisingly, a fairly large decline has been found for a fact-recall task (a form of semantic memory), in contrast to most cross-sectional studies that have reported little effect of aging on semantic memory.

Longitudinal research is not perfect. It does have problems (*see* Longitudinal Method). However, the problems are probably less troublesome than those found with the cross-sectional method (*see* Cross-Sectional Method; Recognition Memory Versus Recall Memory).

Long-Term Care

As longevity increases for Americans (*see* Longevity), so will the number of seniors needing long-term care increase. Dr. Peter Kemper of Pennsylvania State University and his associates have estimated that current adults turning age sixty-five will need an average of three years of long-term care before they die. Nearly one-fourth of them will rely on care provided by family members for at least two years, 35 percent will have nursing home care, and 5 percent will spend more than five years in a nursing facility.

The researchers estimate that those now turning sixty-five would need to invest forty-seven thousand dollars to cover the future costs of long-term care. About 53 percent of these future costs should be covered by government programs, 2 percent by private long-term insurance, and 45 percent by the recipient's own funds.

Lung Cancer

Lung cancer is the leading cause of death from cancer among men, and it is becoming a major cause of death among women as the number of women who smoke has increased greatly in recent years. It kills about 160,000 Americans a year, more than breast cancer, colon cancer, and prostate cancer combined. There are two kinds of lung cancer: non-small-cell lung cancer and small-cell lung cancer. Non-small-cell lung cancer is the typical type in late adulthood, with its incidence peaking around seventy to eighty years of age. It is hoped that the campaign being waged against smoking will greatly reduce the number of deaths of elderly people from lung cancer in the future.

Smoking tobacco is the leading cause of the disease. Other possible causes are secondhand smoke, radon, asbestos exposure, air pollution, and tuberculosis. There is the possibility that some genes make some people more susceptible to the disease than other people. Warning signs of the disease include a chronic cough, hoarseness, coughing up blood, weight loss, loss of appetite, and fever.

Unfortunately, at the present time the five-year survival rate for those diagnosed with lung cancer is only between 12 percent and 15 percent. One of the major problems in increasing the survival rate is having better early detection of the disease than that offered by the standard chest X-ray.

However, there is now hope of greatly improving the survival rate through early detection by improved computerized scanning procedures.

Usually symptoms of the disease do not appear until the disease is in an advanced stage. However, some lung cancers are detected early as a result of tests for other medical conditions, such as pneumonia or chronic bronchitis that involve microscopic examination of cells in the lungs.

Treatment of lung cancer consists of surgery to remove portions of a lung or all of a lung, followed by chemotherapy or radiation therapy. Improved technologies are reducing the risk of chemotherapy or radiation therapy to healthy tissues.

M

Magazine Reading

The magazine read most frequently by elderly adults, both men and women, is *Reader's Digest*. The magazine surely received by more elderly people than any other magazine is *AARP the Magazine,* a publication of AARP and received by its members. Unknown, however, is the percentage of elderly adults who read it regularly. Other popular magazines for both elderly men and women are *TV Guide* and *National Geographic.* There are some obvious sex differences in preferred magazines. For example, *Sports Illustrated* is read regularly by many elderly men, but few elderly women. The opposite is true for *Better Homes & Gardens.*

Managerial Ability

It is not unusual to find older people in managerial positions in business and other settings. However, relatively little is known about the effects of aging on managerial ability. Studies conducted in the 1970s suggested that older managers are slower in making decisions than younger managers, but they may be more thorough than younger managers in the amount of information they use in making those decisions.

A more recent study compared teams of midlevel managers of different age levels in making decisions in situations that simulated in the laboratory various situations encountered by managers in business and industry. The researchers found the performances of young participants (twenty-eight to thirty-five years of age) and middle-aged participants (forty-five to fifty-five years of age) to be similar. Older participants (age sixty-five to seventy-five years) were less proficient than the younger participants in some aspects of utilizing information effectively, and they tended to make fewer decisions than the younger participants. However, the older participants handled simulated emergencies as effectively as the younger participants. The researchers who conducted this study believe that the skills that appeared to be somewhat deficient in their oldest managers could be taught by use of laboratory simulations employed in their study (*see also* Work).

Marriage and Marital Satisfaction

There are more married elderly men than there are married elderly women. According to the 2000 census 67 percent of men and 29 percent of women age seventy-five and older were living with their spouses. For those age sixty-five to seventy-four, 74.7 percent of men and 53 percent of women lived with their spouses.

There are several reasons for this gender imbalance. In general, men marry women younger than themselves, and therefore married men are likely to reach late adulthood earlier than their wives. In addition, women live longer than men and therefore are more likely to experience loss of a spouse than are men (*see* Widowhood and Widowerhood). Moreover, older men are more likely than older women to marry for a second (or more) time, and often to a younger woman. The most likely members of the elderly population to be married are elderly white men, and the least likely are elderly African American women. Elderly African American men and women are more likely to be single than elderly white men and women.

Various surveys indicate that married older people have better physical and mental health than unmarried older people. The physical health benefits of marriage tend to be greater for elderly men than for elderly women. Married elderly people also tend to express greater life satisfaction and to have greater social support, greater economic resources, a lower incidence of entering nursing homes, and lives several years longer than those of unmarried elderly people.

Happiness about one's marriage tends to decline over the first twenty-five years of marriage. However, after that it tends either to remain stable or to increase slightly as the marriage continues. In general, the older the spouses are, the more likely they are to have a good marriage.

There are several reasons marriage often has such positive effects in late adulthood. One reason is that older married people are more likely to avoid behaviors that risk their health than are unmarried elderly people. Another reason is that a spouse is available as a caregiver in times of need. Continuing marriage into late adulthood also provides continuing opportunity to work together toward shared goals (for instance, trips that have long been postponed) and to share such positive events as the births of grandchildren.

After retirement, the marital satisfaction present before retirement should continue if the husband and wife share household tasks, show respect and caring for one another, give each other emotional and physical space, conduct occasional reviews of their marriage, and maintain their sense of humor. After retirement men tend to become dependent on their marriage to fill the void from work. This is less true for women after retirement. Most married elderly people consider their marriages to be happy and often very happy. In general, marital satisfaction appears to be greatest for young adults and elderly adults and least for middle-aged adults. Of course, divorces do occur among elderly people (*see* Divorce).

Mattis Dementia Rating Scale

The Mattis Dementia Rating Scale is a test that measures the general cognitive ability of people displaying neurological dysfunctioning. There are five separate scales measuring attention, initiation and perseveration, construction, conceptualization, and memory. It may be used for both whites and African Americans.

Maturity (Psychological)

Psychological maturity means setting mature goals for oneself and initiating tasks that realistically enable you to achieve those goals. Researchers at the University of Missouri at Columbia provided evidence indicating that older people may be more mature than younger people and therefore happier as a result.

Maze Learning

A maze consists of a pathway from a starting point to an end point or goal. Along the way are left-right choice points. At each choice point, one path (for example, left) continues in the direction of the goal; the other (right) is a blind alley or cul-de-sac. A learner moves through the maze a number of times. Gradually, the number of errors (entries into blind alleys) is reduced until the learner eventually moves through the maze without making an error. Most psychologists believe that learners are, in effect, acquiring a "map" or mental representation of the maze rather than simply a series of left and right turns. When all the choice points have been learned, the map is complete. Maze learning simulates the kind of learning needed to find one's way around a novel environment (like a new neighborhood) and is therefore of interest in aging research.

Most aging research on maze learning has used rats as participants and a three-dimensional maze in which the rats move their entire bodies. This research has revealed that age differences in the number of errors made while learning a maze are slight when there are only a few choice points to master (two to four), but they are quite pronounced when there are as many as fourteen choice points.

With human participants, a paper-and-pencil maze is used in which participants see only one choice point at a time, and they respond verbally with "left" or "right" at each one. Several studies have indicated that both middle-aged and elderly adults make many more errors than young adults in learning a complex (many choice points) paper-and-pencil maze.

Maze learning has gradually lost favor with gerontological researchers as other tasks have been found to represent more closely "map" learning in the everyday world. These other tasks usually require participants to travel in some way through a novel environment (such as a strange neighborhood; *see* Spatial Learning).

Medicaid

The Medicaid program was designed to be a joint federal and state program for assisting low-income people in payment of their medical costs. It began in 1965 as a companion program to Medicare. The intent of the program is to serve as third-party insurance. Among its many services are the payment of nursing home care, skilled nursing care, and physician's services. More than one-third of Medicaid's funds are spent on services for elderly people.

Medicaid is a state-administered program. Each state sets its own criteria for eligibility, subject to federal rules and guidelines. Certain services must be covered by the states in order to receive federal funds. Other services are optional and are selected by the individual states.

An old law made it a federal crime for people who wanted to qualify for Medicaid benefits by transferring deliberately their assets within three years (or five years for assets in a trust) of applying for benefits. A new law changes this so that only lawyers and others who receive pay for assisting Medicaid applicants will be subject to criminal charges. Applicants who have no paid advisers but who knowingly break Medicaid qualification rules will be charged with civil but not criminal violations. The new law expands Medicaid to include cancer screening, bone density testing, and diabetes services.

Medicaid pays the greatest amount of long-term care costs (in 1996 it was $40.8 billion; about 50 percent to 60 percent of the rest is paid by the residents and their families). To be eligible a patient must have a limited income and assets. The patient's spouse is allowed to keep some modest amount of income and assets, the amount being dependent on the state of residence. Two-thirds of elderly people who have been living alone spend all of their assets on nursing home care within an average of thirteen weeks of admission to the nursing home. Consequently, residents who are not eligible for Medicaid on entry into a nursing home soon become eligible after their admission.

Medical Records

Would you like to keep a copy of your medical records? Possession is determined by state law, which differs among states. However, in most states the records belong to your physician. You are entitled to a copy of your records.

The copy may be obtained by requesting it orally or in writing from your physician, preferably in writing. If the physician does not comply, you may file a complaint with the appropriate medical society. If you spend much time each year away from your home city or town, it would be a good idea to have a copy of your records with you in the event you need to see a physician while away.

Of course, you may be away from home by yourself when you become very ill and you are sent to an emergency room. You are without your medical records, and the emergency physicians are uncertain as to what medications you take and to what medications you are allergic. Modern technology now makes it possible for you to have digital medical records that the physicians can immediately retrieve on the Internet. Some communities (such as Boston and Indianapolis) enable you to have electronic medical records. Many other communities are likely to have that possibility in the near future.

Medicare

Title VIII of the Social Security Act established the Medicare program in 1965. From its beginning, the program was intended to prevent elderly people from suffering financial disaster produced by the costs of major illnesses. There are two original parts to the Medicare program: a compulsory program, Part A, and an optional program, Part B. For Part A no premiums are charged for workers and their spouses who have had at least ten years of employment covered by Social Security. For Part B there is a monthly premium that is deducted from Social Security monthly payments or is billed quarterly for those people who do not receive Social Security payments. About every dollar in premiums is matched by three dollars of government subsidies. Most people who participate in Part A also participate in Part B. Most people on Medicare are age sixty-five and older. Also eligible are people with kidney disease who need dialysis or a transplant and disabled persons who have received Social Security benefits for two years.

Part A provides coverage of hospital costs and related services, certain skilled nursing facilities, and home care under some conditions, provided the patient is able to pay for the first day of care. Medicare pays all covered hospital costs except the Medicare Part A deductible ($912 in 2005) during the first 60 days and coinsurance amounts for hospital stays that last beyond 60 days and no more than 150 days. An additional 60 days in a hospital or 20 days in nursing facilities may be paid, but there are substantial deductibles and coinsurance payments. Part A also pays for most of the care received in a Medicare-certified hospice center for the terminally ill, and the full costs of home visits for patients who need physical therapy, speech therapy, or part-time skilled nursing care. Part A does not cover full-time nursing care at home, Meals on Wheels, or home services that are needed for personal care or housekeeping.

Part B is designed to pay for physician's bills, outpatient care, an annual mammogram, and durable medical equipment, such as wheelchairs and oxygen apparatus. There is a yearly premium of $110. You pay 20 percent of the Medicare-approved amount for services after you meet the $110 deductible premium.

The Balanced Budget Act of 1997 reduced future Medicare spending by more than $115 billion over the next five years but then stabilized spending until the year 2007. This act also created a new program called Medicare + Choice. The new program gave new health care options, that is, joining health maintenance organizations (*see* Health Maintenance Organizations [HMOs]) to Medicare beneficiaries.

From December 8, 2003, through December 31, 2005, outpatient therapy services (physical therapy, speech therapy, language pathology therapy, and occupational therapy) were not limited by a dollar amount. Prior to that time there were limits for each.

A significant addition was made to Medicare by the Medicare Modernization Act of 2003. One part of the new law provided the approximately forty million Medicare-eligible people access to prescription drug service. Starting January 1, 2006, Medicare offered prescription drug plans to help pay for prescription drug use. The Medicare Prescription Drug Benefit program is also known as Medicare Part D. It presumably gives eligible people the opportunity to save on the prescription drug costs. Unlike Medicare Part A and Part B the drug prescription plans are offered by insurance companies throughout the United States. Those eligible began enrolling on November 15, 2005. Are medication costs likely to be less than the costs of buying medications from Canada? An analysis reported in AARP's *Bulletin* (vol. 45, no. 1) reported that they may be for many seniors.

Medicare Fraud

There are three kinds of Medicare fraud. The first consists of a treatment that was not medically necessary, resulting in improper Medicare payments. For the second, billing codes are upgraded to give the recipient a higher payment. The third consists of payment for services not covered or allowed by Medicare. Improper payments cost the U.S. government $13.5 billion in 1999.

Elderly people covered by Medicare can help fight fraud in several ways (remember, Medicare fraud is costing taxpayers a great deal of money). They should review their Medicare statements to determine if they received the service or product listed. They should decide if the service or product received is relevant to their illness. If they are not sure, they should call the Medicare Hotline (800-447-8477). They should not reveal their beneficiary number in conversations on the telephone, and they should report if their card is missing. AARP has available a booklet that provides more information on how to combat Medicare fraud. The booklet is titled *Your Three-Step Plan to Fight Medicare Fraud*. To receive a copy, write to AARP Fulfillment, EE01326, 601 E Street Northwest, Washington, DC 20049.

Medicare Hospital Patients

Medicare hospital patients have the right to receive all of the hospital care necessary for the correct diagnosis and treatment of their illness or injury. A federal law states that their discharge date must be determined only by medical needs. They have the right to be fully informed about decisions affecting their Medicare coverage and payment for their time in the hospital. They also have the right to request a review by a peer-review organization (PRO) after receiving written notice from the hospital that Medicare will no longer pay for their stay in the hospital. A PRO is a group of physicians who are paid by the federal government to review the hospital treatment received by Medicare patients. If patients believe they are being discharged too soon, they must have a written notice from the hospital before their case can be reviewed by a PRO. The patient's bill is not paid until the PRO's decision is made. If the hospital and the patient's physician disagree about discharge or treatment, the hospital may also request a PRO to review the case.

Medication Compliance and Comprehension

Illness usually requires taking medications. The frequency and length of time for which the medications are to be taken vary for different kinds of illnesses. Compliance with the doses of medication and the schedule of administration of those doses is essential for the medication to be effective. Are elderly people likely to be less compliant than younger adults? The results of several surveys have not been very helpful in answering this question because they have yielded conflicting results. Some surveys indicate less compliance within the elderly population, and other surveys indicate comparable compliance relative to younger adults. Noncompliance usually means underadherence in the sense of taking less medicine than is needed. It is estimated that about 90 percent of the noncompliance of elderly people consists of underadherence. Researchers have found that middle-aged adults may actually adhere less to their schedule of medications than do elderly adults.

There are a number of factors suggesting that elderly people are at a greater risk of harm from noncompliance than are younger people. One factor is that the incidence of diseases and illnesses requiring treatment by medication is higher among the elderly population than among the younger population. Moreover, more elderly people than younger people take several different medications daily. It is estimated that adults age sixty-five and older take an average of four and a half prescription medicines and two nonprescription medicines daily.

The more medications needed per day, the easier it is to mismanage the schedule. The sensory impairments experienced by many older people add to the possibility of their noncompliance, as does the fact that as many as 25 percent of elderly people live alone and have no one to check regularly with their compliance.

Compliance, regardless of one's age, tends to decrease the longer medications are needed. Elderly people are likely to have illnesses of longer durations than are younger people. Perhaps the most important reason is that elderly people are more hesitant, in general, than younger people in asking their physicians and pharmacists for information about their medications. The most likely elderly people to be compliant, according to a survey by a British researcher, are those whose self-rated health is the highest—the higher the rated health, the greater the compliance. Thus, those who need compliance the most are the least likely to be compliant and therefore the ones in greatest need of efforts to make them compliant.

The consequences of noncompliance are likely to be more serious for elderly people than for younger people, given the likely difference in the severity of the illness being treated in each age group. These consequences include further medical complications for the noncompliant elderly person and the possibility of an untimely and needless death. It is estimated that about 15 percent of admissions of elderly people to hospitals result from noncompliance with a medication regimen.

Seniors who believe their lives are controlled externally, including their health (for instance, by chance or powerful others; *see* Control over Life's Events), report less adherence to a medication schedule than seniors who believe they have control over their lives, including their health status.

Forgetfulness is a major reason for noncompliance by older people. Fortunately, steps have been taken in recent years to increase the rate of compliance by elderly people. These steps include special packaging and labeling of medications to make it easier to follow a regular schedule in their use and the application of various memory strategies to help elderly people remember when to take their medications. One memory strategy is the use of color-coded pill trays over an extended period of time. Another strategy is the use of a portable bar-code reader in which the exact time the medication is taken is measured. One such recording system is the Medication Event Monitoring System manufactured by the Apex Corporation. A microcomputer in the pill container's lid records the date and hour each time the container is opened. Data are fed to the computer, which generates a compliance report that is available to the patient's physician.

Another system is the Electronic Pill Box Timer-Clock that sells for less than twenty dollars. It has two separably programmable timers that sound an alarm at medication time. The patient then resets the timer for the time of the next dose. Researchers in California have also discovered that compliance may be increased by the use of a voice-mail system.

Some elderly people are likely to have a problem in compliance created by their difficulty in comprehending the instructions given with medications (*see* Health Literacy). Researchers have found several ways to improve their comprehension. One is to include pictures with written instructions (for instance, a picture of one pill or half a pill as needed). Another way is to format the instructions in a list rather than in a paragraph. For example, one list could contain possible side effects. A third strategy is to expand the limited space available on medicine bottles for instructions by including additional information on the cap of the bottle.

Medications

Americans spend billions of dollars annually on both prescription and non-prescription medications. Older individuals account for more than a third of the dollars spent on prescription medications. They pay more for drugs annually than they do for physician care. A large-scale survey revealed that prescription drugs are used by nearly 70 percent of men age sixty-five and older and about 75 percent of women age sixty-five and older. Moreover, the percentage of elderly people taking prescription drugs increases with age after age sixty-five.

Nevertheless, it is estimated that annually one-third of the prescriptions written by physicians are not filled. Unfortunately, most of the unfilled prescriptions are for elderly patients. Seniors between the ages of sixty-five and eighty are slightly more likely to delay taking filled prescriptions than seniors over the age of eighty. By contrast, the percentage of elderly people taking nonprescription drugs seems to show little increase with age beyond age sixty-five. The percentage of seniors overall reporting not eventually taking all of their filled prescriptions is small.

The use of medications among the older population is greater for those who smoke and drink alcoholic beverages than for those who do not. More frequent use of medications is also associated with symptoms of depression and with impairment of physical functioning.

The use of medications may present a number of problems for elderly people. According to a study conducted in 1987 by Harvard University researchers, one of the major problems for as many as a fourth of Americans age sixty-five and older is the prescription for drugs that should not be taken. For example, nearly two million elderly people had prescriptions for dipyridamole, a blood thinner useful only for people with artificial heart valves, and more than a million had prescriptions for propoxyphene, an addictive narcotic, in place of aspirin.

Elderly people should know about harmful drug interactions. Unfortunately, most of them do not. They should always check with their physician and pharmacist before taking a new drug, including nonprescription drugs. Seniors are the leading consumers of nonprescription drugs, with many of them suffering ill effects from interactions some of these drugs have with other medications they are taking. Their physicians should make sure they know what other medications elderly patients are taking whenever they prescribe a new medication. An excellent idea for elderly people is to have an annual review of their medications with their physicians. They should bring with them every medication they are taking, including over-the-counter drugs. They should also throw away expired medications, and never take a borrowed medication. Some of the other major problems related to medication are described in other entries (*see* Medication Compliance and Comprehension; Medication Sharing; Overmedication).

Another major problem is the high cost of prescription drugs. The average Medicare beneficiary age sixty-five and older who has no supplementary insurance that helps pay the cost of prescribed drugs spends an average of $1,205 annually for his or her prescriptions. The wholesale prices for the fifty prescriptions most commonly used by elderly people increased by 6.6 percent in 1998 (compared to the inflation rate of 1.6 percent for that year and a 5 percent increase for drugs overall). From January 1994 to January 1999 prices for those fifty drugs increased by 25.2 percent compared to the inflation increase of 12.8 percent for the same period. Only 14 percent of Medicare beneficiaries have private insurance plans such as Medigap. Even these plans usually require a large copayment for the purchase of prescribed drugs.

Medication Sharing

Elderly patients are advised to take only medications prescribed by their physicians and to destroy the remaining medicine after the schedule is completed. However, too frequently this destruction is not carried out, and leftover medicines are free to be shared with other older people. A survey conducted by researchers at the University of Iowa revealed that 40 percent of the elderly people interviewed had shared medicines with someone else. Especially likely to have engaged in this dangerous practice were younger elderly adults, elderly adults who had frequent contact with friends, and elderly adults who had difficulty making an appointment with a physician.

Memory Complaints

Human memory is imperfect at all ages. Nevertheless, older people tend to complain more about their memory problems than do younger people (*see* Diary Studies of Memory Failures). It is true that episodic memory proficiency tends to decline moderately with normal aging. However, some elderly people are unusually upset about their memory ability and complain frequently about it. Others take it in stride and complain infrequently, if at all.

Researchers in the Netherlands surveyed more than four thousand people age sixty-five to eighty-five and found that 22 percent of the non-depressed and nondemented individuals were memory complainers. What happens when "complainers" are compared in memory performances with "noncomplainers"? Researchers at Washington University in St. Louis recruited a number of elderly complainers through newspaper advertisements. They found that the complainers differed little in their laboratory memory performances from those of age-matched noncomplainers. The researchers also found that memory training improved the memory proficiency of the complainers, but it had little effect on their complaints about their memories.

Especially convincing is a four-year longitudinal study with participants between the ages of sixty and eighty-five years, all of whom expressed the belief that they were experiencing serious memory loss. They evaluated their memory proficiency several times with such questions as "How often do you have a memory problem with names?" They were also tested several times on a word-recall test. Self-reported memory proficiency scores declined over the four years, as did their scores of the word-recall test. However, the correlation between degree of self-reported decline and objective test-score decline was basically zero.

Australian researchers found that even a brief memory-training experience improved the memory performance of older memory complainers. Much of this improvement could simply be due to the power of suggestibility rather than to training per se. In contrast to the study by the Washington University researchers, the Dutch researchers found that the memory complainers in their study did perform somewhat more poorly on a memory test than did the noncomplainers. It seems likely that some elderly people believe their memory must be functioning poorly simply because they are old, and that memory must suffer greatly in old age. They therefore tend to exaggerate their minor to moderate memory problems.

Memory for Newsworthy Events

The moderate memory problem many elderly people have seems to apply to memory for newsworthy events. Three stories were selected by researchers in Georgia from actual news programs (ones that had received minimal or no national press coverage). They were presented to both young and elderly participants for study either in print, audio, or television format. The young adult participants recalled moderately more of the content than the elderly participants. The amount recalled was about the same for each format regardless of age.

Memory for Television Programs

Elderly adults watch several television programs daily. Do they remember less of their contents than do younger adults who watch the same programs? Memory that occurs for the content of television programs (including commercials) is almost certain to be incidental memory. People do not ordinarily watch television with the intent to remember what they are watching, nor are they likely to rehearse that content to themselves in an attempt to ensure its memorability. Nevertheless, the very act of attending to and comprehending the content ensures the automatic memory of much of what is seen and heard.

This is apparently as true for older adults as for younger adults. Surely, regardless of your age you still remember much of the content of the *ER* episode you watched last night. (However, much of the content is likely to be forgotten over time, to the point that when you watch the rerun you may not remember who had the brilliant idea that saved the little boy's life). In several studies, young adult and elderly adult participants have watched television programs (with commercials inserted) in the laboratory and were then tested for memory of their contents shortly after viewing the programs.

In general, age differences in accuracy of memory for the contents have been found to be slight. This should provide some comfort to those advertisers of products relevant to elderly consumers. Unknown is the extent to which elderly adults may forget the contents more rapidly than younger adults. Because elderly adults, on the average, watch more television than younger adults, they might be expected to experience more interference from other programs they have viewed and therefore forget more of the content of specific programs (*see* Forgetting).

Memory (Overview)

Imperfections of memory are found at all ages. Memory psychologists studying the effects of aging investigate the extent to which these imperfections increase during late adulthood, the reasons for their occurrence, and the discovery of means by which elderly adults may compensate, at least partially, for whatever declines do occur in memory proficiency.

The study of memory and aging is complicated by the fact that diseases that are more often found in late adulthood than in earlier adulthood may be related to the presence of memory problems. This is especially true of cardiovascular diseases (*see* Cardiovascular Disease and Mental Performance). Most aging research on memory is concerned with normal aging's effects on memory, independent of disease complications. For this reason, most research on adult age differences in memory is conducted with older participants who report their health to be good or excellent (*see* Health Status and Mental Performance).

It is most important to realize that memory proficiency in late adulthood shows great variability, more so than in earlier adulthood. On most memory tasks, the extent of individual differences is greater for elderly participants than for younger participants. As a result, it is not unusual to discover elderly participants who perform at a level above the average level of performance of even young adults.

The most difficult problem in determining the effects of normal aging is that created by the extreme complexity of the human memory system. The memory system consists of two main components: *semantic memory* (*see* Semantic Memory; Lexicon) and *episodic memory* (*see* Episodic Memory). There is a third component known as *sensory memory* (*see* Sensory Memory). The distinction between the two main components is an important one in that aging has little effect on semantic memory and moderate effects, in general, on episodic memory. However, even with episodic memory there are different forms of memory that vary greatly in the extent of their age sensitivity.

Semantic memory is the permanent knowledge of information that is stored without regard to the context (where and when) in which it was acquired. Your knowledge of the capital of Illinois, the square root of sixteen, and the name of the first president of the United States is stored in semantic memory. Such information is stored without personal reference in terms of when you acquired the knowledge and where the acquisition occurred.

An especially important part of your semantic memory is your lexicon or mental dictionary (*see* Lexicon). Stored here are the representations of the words in your vocabulary that you gain access to automatically and rapidly as you read them in a text or hear them in a conversation. In general, we expect to find little change in semantic memory with normal aging. In fact, we are likely to find increases in the amount of information held in our semantic store as we progress from early to late adulthood (*see* Verbal Ability). Gaining access to the information in the semantic store does slow slightly with aging. Consequently, older adults are likely to be a little slower in reading than younger adults, and they are more likely to have difficulty understanding sentences spoken at a rapid rate (*see* Reading and Reading Skills).

Episodic memory is memory for personally experienced events or "episodes" in your life. These episodes are stored in memory as memory traces that are in reference to "when" and "where." That is, the time and location of episodes are contextual components of the information stored. What did you eat for dinner last night? What did you receive as gifts on your tenth birthday? Your correct answers to such questions are possible only because of the record (memory traces) of these events in your long-term episodic store.

When elderly people complain of their "memory problems," they are usually referring to their episodic memory system. The extent to which episodic memory is affected by normal aging cannot be determined simply. Episodic memory has its own variations and forms. Essential to episodic memory is a piece of "mental equipment" memory researchers call *working memory* (*see* Working Memory). Working memory is where limited amounts of information may be recalled immediately or where that information may be rehearsed for transmission to the long-term store for more permanent storage. Information recalled directly from working memory is called *short-term memory* (*see* Short-Term Memory).

A familiar example of short-term memory is your retention of a telephone number from a directory that you remember just long enough to dial. Unless actively rehearsed, this kind of information will be lost within fifteen to twenty seconds. In general, the capacity of short-term memory declines only slightly with normal aging, and the rate of short-term forgetting is about the same for younger and older people. For example, the digit span of elderly people, on the average, is only about 5 percent less than that of young adults (*see* Memory Span).

Information that is rehearsed, encoded as a memory trace, and stored in a long-term store makes up *long-term episodic memory*. It is the current functioning of this form of memory that is of greatest concern to elderly people ("I remember well the events of fifty years ago, but I have trouble remembering events that happened yesterday"). How age sensitive is long-term episodic memory, and what is responsible for declines that occur with normal aging?

Again, simple answers are not possible. Some forms of long-term episodic memory are more age sensitive than other forms. For example, recall of information is likely to show greater degrees of age differences favoring younger adults than is the recognition of the same information (*see* Recognition Memory versus Recall Memory). This suggests that the retrieval of information from the long-term memory store is an effortful process that is especially difficult for older people. The effort required, and therefore the difficulty, is greatly reduced when only recognition is needed.

It is effortful memory that is most often studied in gerontology—for example, memory for lists of words and memory for face-name pairings. In addition, some information is recorded and stored in long-term memory without much effort. It seems to be registered automatically without intent to remember and is brought about either by the simple act of the comprehension of incoming episodic events (for example, your memory for conversations with other people or your memory for television programs watched and stories read; *see,* for example, Conversation Memory) or by the execution of actions (turning off the gas on the stove; *see* Action Memory).

Such automatic memory functioning is especially important in our everyday lives. The imperfections of memory are apparent at all ages. Most important, the extent of age sensitivity or decline with normal aging appears to be less, on average, for automatic memory than that found when effort is needed to register information in the long-term store.

Episodic memory is also distinguishable in terms of whether it concerns the content of events (for instance, the content of a specific beer commercial you watched on television) or some noncontent characteristic of the event, such as "When was it you last saw the commercial?" The age sensitivity of noncontent memory varies greatly with the characteristic involved, and is especially large for temporal memory (knowledge of the time of an event; *see* Temporal Memory) and very modest for memory of the frequency with which events occurred (for example, "How many times in the past week did you see the beer commercial in question?"; *see* Frequency-of-Occurrence Memory).

There are many other important questions that have been asked (and answered to some degree) by memory researchers. For example, does physical exercise of the right kind slow any age-related declines in memory proficiency? Yes, but perhaps only if it has been practiced regularly for a number of years (*see* Exercise [Relationship to Physical/Mental Performances]). Does intensive mental activity during late adulthood relate to the magnitude of age-related declines in memory proficiency? Here, the evidence is somewhat conflicting (*see* Activity [Mental] and Mental Performance). However, elderly people should take the position that mental activity cannot possible hurt them. Can memory training programs improve the memory proficiency of elderly adults? Perhaps not, at least for programs in use (*see* Memory Training).

Memory Span

Your memory span for a given type of item is the longest series of items that you can read or listen to and then recall without an error. It is a form of short-term memory or memory over a brief interval that is sometimes used to determine the amount of information that can be held in short-term memory (*see* Short-Term Memory). The most familiar tests of memory span are those for digits and for words. To test digit span, a participant starts by receiving a short series of randomly selected digits (for instance, 5, 2). Assuming this series is recalled correctly, another series is given that is one greater in length than the first series (8, 4, 7). This procedure (adding one digit to the series) continues until the participant no longer has an errorless recall of the series. The average digit span has been found to be about 7 digits for young adults and about 6.5 digits for elderly adults (sixty-five to seventy-five years of age). The age-related decline in span length is thus only about 7 percent (that is, the difference between the two averages divided by the average score made by young adults—0.5 divided by 7). A similar procedure is used to test for word span, only now common words are used instead of digits. The average word span is about six words for young adults and about five for elderly adults, again a modest age difference. Interestingly, older participants have been found to score best on word-span tests when given in the morning and worst when given in the evening. By contrast, the reverse is true for younger participants.

Memory Training

Can memory proficiency be improved? Memory training programs attempt to teach people ways of improving their episodic memory proficiency. Typically, such programs train the participant in the use of what are called *mnemonics* as a means of increasing proficiency of encoding information for registration in the long-term store. A mnemonic is a device or procedure for changing in some way the information you wish to remember in order to make it more memorable.

Most mnemonic procedures make use of translating verbal information into images. They are most likely to be applied when the material to be memorized consists of a series of words, such as *car* and *dog*. These are words that can be represented by images of the objects they represent.

Participants in a memory training program may be taught to use the *method of loci*. Here the trick is to make use of a well-traveled pathway with visually distinctive locations along the way. A participant's own house usually offers such a pathway. As you open the front door, you enter a hallway. Now the participant is urged to form an image of a *car* stuffed inside the hallway. Next comes the living room. Now form an image of a large *dog* sleeping on the sofa in the living room. This continues throughout the trip through the house, with an image of a word to be remembered in each location. To recall the words, you make the trip again, this time capturing the image of each word as you encounter it.

An alternative procedure is called the *peg-word method*. Here the participant is first taught a rhyme that begins with "One is a bun," "two is a shoe," and so on. Now the trick is to form an image of each word to be remembered with the object named in the rhyme. Thus, you might form an image of a Detroit (or Tokyo) sandwich in which a *car* (the first word in the list) is stuffed in a bun and dripping with mustard and other goodies, then an image of a *dog* wearing highly polished shoes, and so on. To recall the words, you simply say each number in the rhyme to yourself (for instance, "one"), recover the object named with it (a bun) and the image of the word to be remembered (a car).

Elderly adults can learn to use either the method of loci or the peg-word method. However, they are likely to discover that these methods have little usefulness in the everyday world. It is not often necessary to memorize a list of words, even a shopping list—why not write down the items and take the shopping list with you? Moreover, the methods rely on imagery, and elderly people are less proficient in the use of imagery than younger people (*see* Imagery). Even memory researchers report they rarely, if ever, use these mnemonic procedures in their daily lives.

A somewhat more useful mnemonic is the *key-word method.* It may be used to learn either face-name pairings or foreign-language equivalents of English words. In either case, imagery again is a basic ingredient of the mnemonic. Consider meeting Mr. Whalen at a party. The first step in associating his name with his face is to identify a prominent feature of Mr. Whalen's face (say, a large mouth). The next step is to translate the person's name into a word that is easily imagined ("a whale" in the case of Mr. Whalen). The final step is to imagine the imagined object in interaction with the prominent facial feature (a whale stuffed inside a large mouth). The idea is that on your next encounter with Mr. Whalen, you will notice the prominent mouth, recover the image of a whale, and come up with "Hi there, Mr. Whalen."

As with other mnemonics, elderly adults can be taught to use the key-word method to learn new face and name pairings. However, they are likely to abandon its use rather quickly. Again, the use of imagery decreases in proficiency with normal aging. Moreover, how often can you use a large mouth as the prominent feature? Surely, you will encounter other people with the same prominent feature, and confusion as to which image to retrieve for recalling the correct name will probably result.

The key-word method is probably most useful when you plan to visit a foreign country, and you would like to know a few words in that country's language. Suppose you plan to visit Russia, and for some reason you would like to remember that the Russian word for mountain is *gora.* To use the key-word method you would translate the Russian word to an English word that both sounds like a part (not necessarily all) of the foreign word and is very imaginable. In this case, the key word might be *garage.* Then form an image of a mountain stuffed inside a garage. When you next encounter *gora,* the image you receive should help you to remember that it means "a mountain."

Researchers at Washington University in St. Louis have prepared a self-instructional manual that describes these mnemonics (and others as well, such as the use of organizational strategies to find relatedness among events to be remembered; *see* Episodic Memory) and practice exercises in their use. However, they have discovered that the greatest benefit from the use of the manual comes when the participants also meet in group sessions with a trainer and other participants to discuss their memory problems and how mnemonics may help to reduce them.

Most problems with remembering face-name pairings are not likely to be memory problems at all. They are more likely to be attentional problems.

You probably were not paying sufficient attention to hear fully the person's name when he or she was introduced to you. When you hear the name, repeat it several times to yourself while looking at the person's face. If you are introduced to several people at about the same time, an effective way of improving your later memory of their names is to wait fifteen or twenty seconds after the introductions and then recall their names while looking again at their faces. Elderly people, in general, do have long-term memory-retrieval problems. The short-term retrieval of people's names should enhance later retrievability. Prior retrieval of paired nouns has been found to enhance their later retrievability, and reviewing events shown on a videotape has been found to enhance their retrievability for elderly adults (*see also* Action Memory). Unfortunately, memory training programs usually offer little assistance in improving the retrieval of information. The probable emphasis is on getting information into memory, and with most seniors their main problem is retrieving information.

There is an important (and perhaps the most important) further potential use of memory training. Depressed elderly people frequently express great concern about their memory problems. Researchers have discovered that a number of these depressed individuals have a significant reduction in their memory concerns after completion of a memory training program. Most important, many of them also appear to have a reduction in the intensity of their depressive symptoms.

Menopause and Ovulation

Menopause is the end of menstruation. While in their forties, women's menstrual cycles tend to become irregular, and they usually stop by the age of fifty to fifty-five years. The transition period during which ovulation stops is called the climacteric. Until recently, the end of ovulation was viewed as the end of a woman's childbearing years. This has changed drastically with the in vitro fertilization of women in their sixties.

With menopause there is a decrease in the levels of the sex hormones (estrogen and progesterone produced by the ovaries). The walls of the vagina become thinner and less elastic, and the production of vaginal lubricants decreases. The changes in the vagina may cause it to become irritated and lead to dyspareunia (painful intercourse). However, not every woman experiences these changes. For some they may last for years after menopause; for others they may occur only early in menopause.

The decrease in hormonal levels often results in hot flashes, headaches, and various other symptoms. Hot flashes vary in their frequency and severity. They usually last for about a minute, and, in some cases, they may occur four or five times a day. Some women experience nervousness or a degree of depression or both. Irritability may occur because of sleep disturbances from hot flashes. The decrease in estrogen level may also lead to osteoporosis (*see* Osteoporosis). Estrogen supplements have been used to treat the symptoms of menopause and to prevent osteoporosis. However, they may lead to some other health problems (*see* Estrogen Replacement Therapy [Hormone Replacement Therapy]).

There are a number of excellent books on menopause and the changes accompanying it. Check them out at your local library or bookstore.

Some men experience a form of "male menopause." There is a decrease in the male sex hormone testosterone in the late sixties. During this period some men may display symptoms similar to those found in female menopause, such as hot flashes. However, the decline in testosterone production is much less than the decline in sex hormone production for most older women.

Mental Health and Mental Health Services

Satisfactory mental health usually means that an individual is satisfied with his or her life; is adapting adequately to everyday pressures and stressors; is free of intense negative emotions such as anxiety, depression, and hostility; is free of psychosis and neurosis; and is free of negative personality traits like neuroticism. There is no reason to believe that the mental health status of older adults, in general, differs greatly from that of younger adults. When asked to rate their life satisfaction, elderly adults express a degree of satisfaction that is about the same as that of younger adults (*see* Life Satisfaction). Most elderly adults are fairly successful in coping with problems and stresses in their lives (*see* Stress and Coping with Stress). Severe depression seems to be no more prevalent late in adulthood than in earlier adulthood (*see* Depression [Incidence, Symptoms, Causes]). The onset of psychosis and neurosis is rare in late adulthood (*see* Neurosis; Psychosis). Negative personality traits such as neuroticism show little increase from early to late adulthood (*see* Neuroticism; Personality Traits).

Nevertheless, a number of elderly adults do experience mental distress, just as many younger adults do, and they, like younger adults, may benefit from treatment by mental health professionals. Unfortunately, such treatment is less likely to be received by older adults than by younger adults.

Surveys have indicated that only around 6 percent of the services offered by community mental health centers are provided to older adults, and an even smaller percentage of private-practice mental health services is provided for older clients. Part of the problem is the fact that training programs for mental health professionals, including both clinical psychologists and psychiatrists, have often ignored training experiences with the unique mental problems of elderly people (for instance, stress from the death of a spouse).

Also part of the problem is the fact that Medicare has placed financial obstacles in the way of treating elderly clients with low incomes. In the past, there has been a bias in the Medicare program against the long-term treatment of chronic mental and emotional problems. Inpatient services under Part A of Medicare were limited to a total of 190 days, and outpatient services under Part B to 50 percent to 60 percent copayment rate in contrast to the 20 percent copayment rate for physical health services. The bias also is evident in limitation of the services offered by a clinical psychologist to elderly clients. Diagnostic testing was reimbursed only if it had been requested by a physician, and psychotherapy only if it was supervised by a physician. Fortunately, these restrictions are gradually changing through the efforts of mental health professionals to influence Congress to modify the provisions of Medicare. For example, a bill passed in 1988 enabled psychologists to be paid by Medicare for services provided independently of physicians at rural health clinics and community mental health centers.

A further problem remains, namely, the reluctance of many older people to seek help for their mental and emotional problems, a reluctance much greater than that found for younger adults. This problem should diminish in the future as currently younger adults reach late adulthood. They will bring with them a greater knowledge of mental health services and a greater knowledge of what may be accomplished by such services.

It is estimated that fifteen million elderly people will suffer from a psychiatric illness by the year 2030. This number includes those suffering from mental illnesses associated with late adulthood as well as those who had mental illness earlier in life and continued to have it as they grew older. Mental health professionals and managed care facilities are not likely to be prepared for this. More training programs in geriatric mental health for primary care physicians will be greatly needed.

Mental Status Questionnaire

The Mental Status Questionnaire is widely used as part of the diagnostic procedure used to identify individuals likely to have true dementia, as distinguished from memory problems related to normal aging or depression-induced mental problems. The questionnaire is a ten-item inventory designed to determine the effectiveness of an individual's orientation with regard to time and place. Included are questions such as: "What is today's date?" "What is the month now?" "How old are you now?" and "Who is president now?"

Metamemory

"My memory is terrible—I can't even remember what I had for dinner last night." "I have trouble remembering the names of new people I meet." "My memory at age seventy is as good as it was thirty years ago." The people making these statements are, in effect, evaluating the proficiency of their own memory capabilities. Knowledge of our own memory system is termed *meta-memory*. Metamemory includes more than knowledge (correct or incorrect) about your own memory proficiency. It also includes your knowledge of how to improve your memory through the use of effective strategies.

One method used to determine age differences in the knowledge people have (or believe they have) of their own memory proficiencies is completion of a questionnaire in which respondents rate their proficiency on various forms and tasks of everyday memory functioning (*see* Metamemory in Adulthood [MIA] Questionnaire and Metamemory Functioning Questionnaire [MFQ]). In general, these ratings reveal that older adults have a lower regard for and less confidence in their memory abilities than do younger adults.

However, the scores of elderly participants on laboratory memory tasks have been found to be only slightly related to their proficiency ratings, and older adults with memory complaints often perform as well on these tasks as do noncomplainers (*see* Memory Complaints). In addition, there is evidence to indicate that individuals may not be the best evaluators of their own memory abilities. The ratings given by spouses of older people tend to relate more closely to scores earned on laboratory memory tasks than do the ratings given by the task performers themselves.

Another way to evaluate age differences in the knowledge (or lack of knowledge) people have about their memory abilities is to have them predict how well they will do on a memory task they are about to receive. Suppose, for example, that you know you will have three minutes to study a list of twenty common words (such as *apple* and *table*), and that you will then be asked to recall as many of the words as possible in whatever order you wish. How many words would you predict that you would recall? Five? You don't have much confidence in your memory ability. Fifteen? Overconfident, perhaps?

When faced with making this prediction, elderly participants tend to make the same prediction, on average, as young adult participants (usually a prediction of about ten words). The actual number of words recalled is likely to be closer to the predicted number for the young participants than for the older participants. In other words, elderly participants tend to be somewhat overconfident in their memory ability despite the lower ratings they usually assign to their memory functioning.

Overconfidence by older participants is revealed further when the situation with a word list is changed. This time the participants are told to study the list until they are ready to recall all of the words. Elderly participants, on the average, spend less time studying the list than do young adult participants, and therefore recall fewer words than do the young participants. Interestingly, when older participants are required to spend as much time studying as the average time spent studying by young participants, their recall scores more closely approximate those of the young participants.

Knowledge of how to use memory strategies effectively is especially important for proficient memory performances. Suppose you have been given a list of seven common words to learn in a specific order, that is, serial learning (*see* Verbal Learning) and without error. You have as much time as you need to master the list. An effective strategy for making certain of an observable errorless recall would be to study the list for a while and then monitor yourself to recall the words. If you found you made an error, you should study more and then test yourself again. This cycle of study and self-testing should continue until you no longer make an error. Researchers at the University of Akron discovered that this self-monitoring or self-testing strategy was used by most of their young adult participants, but by few of the older participants. When other elderly participants were instructed regarding the value of self-testing and encouraged to use this strategy, they approached the level of performance of young adults who spontaneously engaged in self-testing.

The effective use of memory strategies is likely to be part of the content in a memory training course (if not, it should be). For this reason alone, it is probably worthwhile for elderly people who seem to have a memory problem to participate in such a course.

Metamemory in Adulthood (MIA) Questionnaire and Metamemory Functioning Questionnaire (MFQ)

The Metamemory in Adulthood (MIA) Questionnaire and Metamemory Functioning Questionnaire (MFQ) are the two most widely used tests for assessing a person's view about how well his or her memory system is functioning in the everyday world (*see* Metamemory). The MIA has 120 items that measure eight dimensions of memory functioning. For example, one of the dimensions is labeled "Capacity," and it is measured by such questions as "I am good at remembering names (yes or no)." Another dimension is labeled "Strategy," and it is measured by such questions as "Do you write appointments on a calendar to help you remember them (yes or no)?"

The MFQ has 64 items that evaluate memory functioning in terms of seven different scales. One of these scales is labeled "Frequency of Forgetting," and it is measured by questions such as "How often do these present a memory problem to you? . . . names" (then other sources of potential problems are given). Another scale is labeled "Retrospective Functioning." It is measured by questions such as "How is your memory compared to the way it was . . . one year ago?" Other time references are also given.

Metaphors

Metaphors are frequently used in both literature and everyday communication. A metaphor is a figure of speech in which a word or phrase indicating one kind of idea or object is used in place of another through the use of a comparison (analogy) between the substitute and the idea or object it replaces. A familiar example is "The ship plows the sea." Here the ship replaces farm equipment that plows the land. Thus, the ship moves through the sea much the same as the farm equipment moves through the land. When given novel metaphors to interpret ("Man is a wolf"), older adults have been found to be just as insightful, if not more so, than young adults in their interpretations. This is to be expected, given the fact that verbal abilities, in general, are largely unaffected by normal aging (*see* Verbal Ability).

Midlife Crisis

Do most people go through a major crisis when they are in their forties and fifties in which they feel their lives are in turmoil, and they feel the need to make important changes in their lives? Actually, there is little evidence to support the existence of a midlife crisis in the lives of most Americans (often fictionalized as a middle-age man buying a sporty convertible automobile). In a survey of Americans between the ages of forty and sixty-five, only about 10 percent said they had lived through anything approximating a midlife crisis.

Migration (Moving)

Older persons have been moving less in recent years than they did earlier. According to the U.S. Census Bureau, only 4.5 percent of people age sixty-five and older change locations annually, compared to 31.8 percent for those people in the twenty-to-twenty-nine-year age range.

Most adults age sixty and older do not move to another state until after they have retired. This is especially true of moving within one's own county. However, interstate migration (moving from one state to another state) has been increasing, largely because of the better financial resources of many elderly people. Researchers at the University of Florida compared relocators with residents in three age groups: thirty-four to forty-six (young middle-aged), fifty-four to sixty-six (young-old), and sixty-nine to ninety-three (old-old). Relocators did not differ from residents in age, income, health, or marital status. Why moving? The young middle-aged adults moved mainly for job reasons, the young-old for retirement reasons, and the old-old to be closer to family members.

From 1955–1960 to 1990–1995, 60 percent of older immigrants settled in the ten most popular states. However, the percentage dropped to 54.4 percent in the 1995–2000 interval. This is an indication of a gradual trend in decentration of immigrants to what had long been favorite locations.

In 2000 the ten states receiving the most immigrants, in order, were

Florida, Arizona, California, Texas, North Carolina, Nevada, Pennsylvania, Virginia, Georgia, and New Jersey. Florida has long been ranked first. However, it had the greatest reduction in its share of immigrants (from 23.8 percent in 1990 to 19.0 percent in 2000). Southern Atlantic states and desert states gained the most in the number of immigrants they received.

Mild Cognitive Dementia

See Age-Associated Memory Impairment; Senile Dementia.

Mini-Mental State Exam

The Mini-Mental State Exam is one of the several tests used in the diagnosis of dementia. It contains eleven items dealing with the orientation, concentration, and language functioning of the client. For example, temporal orientation is tested by asking the year, season, month, date, and day when the testing occurs. Language functioning is tested by such requests as asking the client to write a sentence and to repeat the phrase, "No ifs, ands, or buts." Individuals with true dementia are likely to score very low on these questions. For example, they are unlikely to know what year or day it is. Researchers at the University of California at Davis have constructed a shorter version of the test in which items that bias against either Hispanics or other minority groups have been eliminated. Researchers in Colorado discovered that young-old Hispanics tend to be categorized as being more severely impaired than non-Hispanic whites of the same age. However, old-old Hispanics and non-Hispanic whites tend to perform similarly on the test after adjusting for educational differences between the two.

Some evidence of the value of the test was obtained by researchers at the University of Alabama at Birmingham. They found that scores on the test obtained by dementia patients were related highly and positively to the proficiency of performing both the physical activities of daily living (for instance, bathing) and the instrumental activities of daily living (using the telephone) (*see* Activities of Daily Living). This outcome was equally true for whites and African Americans.

Modifying Negative Health Behaviors

Among the behaviors considered to promote poor health are a sedentary lifestyle, smoking, excessive drinking of alcoholic beverages, and consuming unhealthy foods. Older adults are often neglected as possible targets for modifying these behaviors, given the common belief that they cannot or will not change their behaviors.

Researchers at Portland State University in Oregon discovered that there is, unfortunately, some truth to this belief. The participants in their study were more than seventeen thousand Canadian adults, age sixty and older. Many of them reported having risky health behaviors and that they made no effort to change them and improve their health. The main reason they gave for the failure to change their behaviors is that they simply lacked willpower. Clearly, health professionals need to discover interventions to improve the motivation for many seniors to overcome their lack of willpower.

Motion Perception

Sensitivity to the motion of objects takes several forms. One involves the ability to detect whether two slightly moving objects are moving in the same direction or in opposite directions. Elderly adults generally show moderately poorer discrimination of direction than do younger adults.

Another form involves the ability to detect motion for a previously stationary object. Researchers at Case Western Reserve University have discovered that older women tend to have higher motion thresholds (that is, it takes more movement before being detected) than elderly men and that elderly men are about as proficient as young men in detecting motion. They have also discovered that patients with Alzheimer's disease have significantly less sensitivity than normally aging individuals in detecting motion and that their sensitivity becomes progressively worse as dementia progresses.

Motor Behavior

Motor behavior refers to muscular actions performed to fulfill some objective of the performer. Examples of everyday motor behaviors are braking a car, pushing a lawn mower, shifting gears of a car, and hitting a golf ball. Although normally aging people are perfectly capable of performing most motor behaviors, nevertheless, some attributes of motor behaviors are expected to be affected by aging.

Most apparent is the slower reaction time in initiating motor behaviors and the longer time to complete many motor behaviors (for instance, locomotion). For example, it is expected that elderly people generally will be slower in braking their cars than younger people when some external event signals the need for braking.

Some simple motor behaviors are used to test the functional limitations of frail elderly people. The behaviors include stair climbing, standing up after sitting in a chair, and an eight-foot walk. Researchers in Massachusetts found that consistency of performance over several weeks varies greatly among such tasks, being especially low for standing after sitting and high for walking.

Laboratory research has revealed that there are also more subtle age differences in motor behaviors. For example, age differences have been found by researchers at the University of Wisconsin at Madison in the use of advance information to aid selection of a specific required behavior. Their participants performed simple movements of their arms that varied over trials in terms of which arm to move, the direction of the movement, and the extent of the movement.

Different amounts of advance information were given over many trials. On some trials, no advance information was given as to which arm would be signaled to move, which direction would be signaled, and the extent of the movement. On other trials, only one bit of advance information was given (which arm would be signaled to move). On still other trials, two bits of information would be given (which arm to move and in which direction). On the remaining trials, all three bits of advance information were given (which arm, what direction, and how far).

The researchers found that the speed of movement in response to the investigator's signal was, as expected, slower for elderly participants than for younger participants, regardless of the amount of advance information given. However, younger participants benefited less from advance information than did older participants. That is, their speed in responding was nearly as fast when no advance information was given as when all three bits of advance information were given. By contrast, the response speed of elderly participants was much slower without advance information than with all three bits of information. It does take older people longer to prepare for a movement than it does younger people. Therefore, any early start in preparing for that movement (as in the use of advance information) provides a greater advantage for older people than for younger people.

For example, a yellow light on a traffic signal tells you in advance that a red light is about to go on and you should be preparing to brake your car. This is information of greater value to older drivers than to younger drivers who are so fast in their behaviors that there is little room for advance information to facilitate their behaviors (unfortunately, a yellow light is an advance signal to some younger drivers to speed up and make it through the intersection before the red light comes on).

The Wisconsin researchers also found that elderly participants have greater difficulty than younger participants in coordinating movements of the two hands.

Motor Skill Learning

We learn many motor skills during the course of our lives and at different times in our lives. We learn to ride a bicycle, to play the piano, to drive a car, to type, to play golf, and so on. In each case, learning requires coordination between perception and muscular actions. For this reason, motor skill learning is often called *perceptual-motor learning*. Of interest is the effect of aging on both the retention of motor skills learned years ago and the acquisition of new motor skills.

Many motor skills learned years ago are retained remarkably well with considerable practice of those skills. For example, professional golfers, musicians, and typists practice their respective skills virtually daily throughout their adult lives. Tom Watson continues to be a great golfer even though he is now past age fifty. Great musicians like Pablo Casals and Arthur Rubenstein gave many excellent performances at very advanced ages. Skilled typists continue to do well into late adulthood.

But what about skills that have not been practiced during the intervening years? A familiar observation is that after years of not riding a bicycle, most people are able to regain their earlier skill with little practice. There is a large savings in terms of the amount of practice needed to regain the skill relative to the amount of practice needed to acquire the skill originally. There is evidence to indicate that the savings is also large for typing after some years of not doing any typing.

Of course, motor skill learning does not cease for older people. They may decide to take up golf when they are in their sixties or seventies, or they may have the need to acquire computer skills. Unfortunately, some may have to learn how to maneuver a wheelchair.

Age differences in motor skill learning have been investigated in the laboratory largely through the use of two different tasks. The first is called the pursuit-rotor task. A disk rotates fairly rapidly while a participant tries to maintain contact with a stylus on a designated part of the disk. Participants are given many trials of a set duration (for instance, thirty seconds). A number of studies have indicated that both young adults and older adults steadily improve the amount of time spent maintaining appropriate contact with the stylus as practice progresses. Learning occurs as participants acquire the visual-hand coordination needed to perform the task. However, the rate of learning is considerably slower for elderly participants than for younger participants.

The second task involves mirror-image tracking in which participants move a stylus through a six-pointed star cut through a metal plate while viewing the star in a mirror, that is, what the participants see is the reverse of the actual movements. Both young adults and elderly adults improve with practice on this task. The time needed to move through the star decreases regardless of age, as does the accuracy of movement. However, as with the pursuit-rotor task, the rate of learning the visual-hand coordination needed to perform the task is much slower for older adults.

The same age difference is present even when an everyday kind of task is brought into the laboratory. In particular, elderly participants have been found to learn word processing skills, but at a much slower rate than young adult participants. However, the rate of learning differs little between young adults and middle-aged adults. Learning of new motor skills is clearly well within the capabilities of most elderly people, but, as with other forms of learning, it is likely to be at a slower rate of progress. This is true for learning other computer skills as well as word processing. Not only do the elderly take longer to learn those computer skills, but they also make more errors while learning than do younger participants (*see also* Computers).

Multifactorial Memory Questionnaire (MMQ)

The Multifactorial Memory Questionnaire (MMQ) has separate scales for contentment (affect regarding your memory), ability (self-appraisal of your memory's capabilities), and Strategy (reported frequency of strategy use). Sample questions are "I am generally pleased with my memory" (contentment), "How often do you forget to pay a bill on time?" (ability), and "How often do you use a timer or alarm to remind you to do something?" (strategy).

Multi-Infarct Dementia

Multi-infarct dementia (formerly called cerebral arteriosclerosis) accounts for 10 percent to 20 percent of the cases of adult dementia. The incidence of this vascular dementia increases exponentially with age after age seventy. It consists of mental impairment caused by a stroke in which the flow of blood in the brain is disrupted (called an *infarct*) and areas of the brain are damaged. A series of strokes may produce pronounced dementia in the form of memory loss and disorientation and, in some cases, losses in the ability to understand language or to produce appropriate language (an aphasia; *see* Aphasia) or to recognize objects (agnosia) or both. Hypertension is a predisposing factor leading to the dementia. Antihypertensive drugs seem to be effective in reducing the risk of vascular dementia.

Multi-infarct dementia differs from that found in Alzheimer's diseases in several ways. The onset is sudden, rather than gradual (as in Alzheimer's disease), and the progression in severity occurs in stages or steps rather than continuously (as in Alzheimer's disease). The extent of dementia tends to stabilize (and improvement may occur with speech therapy and other forms of therapy, and even without the intervention of therapy) until another stroke occurs. If another stroke occurs, the severity of impairment is likely to increase.

Multi-infarct dementia is more common in men than in women; the reverse is true for Alzheimer's disease. Multi-infarct disease often occurs earlier in life than Alzheimer's disease. Neurologically, patients with multi-infarct dementia tend to have fewer senile plaques and neurofibrillary tangles in neurons than patients with Alzheimer's disease (*see* Alzheimer's Disease). Perhaps the most important difference between the two diseases is that multi-infarct disease may be prevented in many cases by medications for hypertension (high blood pressure), changes in diet and exercise habits, treatment of diabetes, and the cessation of smoking and alcohol consumption. Currently, there is no known method of preventing Alzheimer's disease.

Myths about Aging

A myth is a widely held false belief, usually resulting from hearsay evidence and casual and inaccurate evidence. For example, many people believe that there have been individuals who have lived 130 and even more years. There is no carefully documented evidence to indicate that this is true (*see* Life Span). Another biological myth about aging is that most people age sixty-five and older are so physically incapacitated that they cannot function on their own. In truth, nearly 90 percent of people in that age range manage to function adequately in their daily living. Perhaps the most prevalent myth about aging is that most older people become asexual, both in the sense of losing interest in sexual behavior and in the sense of losing the ability to perform sexually (*see* Sexual Behavior).

Myths are also widespread regarding the mental functioning of elderly people, including the belief that they are incapable of new learning (the "you can't teach old dogs new tricks" falsehood) and the belief that memory overall deteriorates greatly in late adulthood. Older people are indeed capable of new learning, even though it may progress a bit more slowly than it does in younger people (*see* Learning [Overview]; Motor Skill Learning; Verbal Learning). Memory is a complex system made up of a number of components, some of which show modest declines in proficiency for many people as they age, but other components are remarkably resistant to declines in proficiency in late adulthood (*see* Memory [Overview]).

Unfortunately, myths about aging are held not only by many young adults but also by many older people. Such beliefs could have serious negative consequences. For example, those elderly people who believe that new learning is beyond their present capabilities are unlikely to make an effort to participate in new learning experiences.

One of the major objectives of gerontological research is to replace myths about aging with facts based on scientific evidence. Fortunately, research is being conducted at a rate that is increasing exponentially annually. Eventually, there will be little room left for myths about aging, and, we hope, few individuals will remain who believe in such myths.

N

Nails

Fingernails and toenails do not grow as rapidly for elderly people as they do for younger people, and they therefore require less frequent trimming in later adulthood than in earlier adulthood. On the other hand, elderly adults' nails become dry and brittle, and they are more difficult to trim than they are for younger adults. Consequently, the need for assistance in trimming nails, especially toenails, tends to be greater for elderly adults than for younger adults.

There is no evidence to indicate that calcium supplements strengthen or improve the appearance of fingernails or toenails of postmenopausal women. Protein in their diet is more likely to affect the quality of their nails.

There are some abnormalities of fingernails that could be indicators of a serious health problem. One is nails that look like the back of a teaspoon. If they are curved that way and are white or pale, you could have anemia (*see* Anemia). A black streak that runs the length of a nail and is wider at the base could be a sign of a potential melanoma.

National Heart, Lung, and Blood Institute

Call 800-WELL for information on cholesterol and high blood pressure. Leave your name and address to receive written information.

National Institute on Aging

In 1974, the United States Congress passed the Research on Aging Act. The act noted the absence of any American institution devoted to intensive studies of the biomedical and behavioral aspects of aging. To remedy this problem, the act created the National Institute on Aging as the eleventh component of the National Institutes of Health. Operation of the institute began in 1976, with Dr. Robert Butler as the first permanent director.

One of the first steps taken by the institute was the incorporation into its programs of the Baltimore Longitudinal Study that had been undergoing planning since 1958. Initially, the study was a collaborative effort between the National Institute on Aging and the Baltimore City Hospitals. The first testing occurred in 1961 with 260 healthy men ranging in age from the twenties to age ninety-six. Eventually, thousands of additional men were added to the study, with women included as participants in 1978. All participants agreed to return a number of times for retesting. The study has been for years a major source of longitudinal information about aging's effects on physical health, sensory functioning, and cognitive functioning. This information was possible because participants received retesting on a number of diverse physical and cognitive functions.

Other programs soon became part of the institute's operations. They included the Biomedical and Clinical Medicine Program, the Behavioral Sciences Research Program, and the Epidemiology, Demography, and Biometry Program.

Some of the programs fund research by highly qualified scientists at universities and medical centers. Other programs are conducted by scientists who work directly in laboratories operated by the institute. Throughout the institute's history, Alzheimer's disease and geriatric medicine have been its major priorities. The institute is generally considered to be the premier institute on aging in the world. For further information, write to the National Institute on Aging, Building 31, Room 5C27, Center Drive, MSC 2292, Bethesda, MD 20892, or contact the Institute's Web site at http://www.nih.gov/nia.

Natural Disasters (Distress Experiences)

Both cross-sectional and longitudinal studies indicate that older adults experience less emotional distress after natural disasters (such as earthquakes or hurricanes) than do younger adults. Perhaps this is attributable to older adults having lived through more such disasters than younger adults.

Of course, not all disasters are natural. Perhaps the most famous man-made disaster was that of September 11, 2001. Here too resilience in recovering from posttraumatic stress disorder (PTSD) was found to be greatest for older adults. Dr. George A. Bonanno of Teachers College, Columbia University, and his associates contacted nearly three thousand adults ranging in age from eighteen to sixty-five and older living in the New York City area six months after the disaster. Resilience was defined as having either no or only one symptom of PTSD. For adults in the age ranges of eighteen to twenty-four, twenty-five to thirty-four, thirty-five to forty-four, forty-five to fifty-four, fifty-five to sixty-four, and sixty-five and over, the percentages were 62.2, 57.7, 68.4, 62.2, 69.4, and 79.5, respectively.

Not surprising, the least resilience was for those adults who were most closely exposed to the disaster.

Negative Stereotype and Memory

Many seniors accept the negative stereotype of aging, including the belief that it is a time of pronounced declines in memory ability (*see* Ageism). They are therefore likely to have a low level of confidence in their own memory capability.

There is evidence indicating that seniors with this negative view of their own memory ability perform more poorly on laboratory memory tests than do seniors who are void of this stereotyped attitude.

Researchers at Simon Fraser University in British Columbia, Canada, found that the attitude some seniors have about their own memory can be changed through appropriate training. They presumably leave the training program better prepared to handle the challenges of everyday memory performances (as well as laboratory performances).

Neurosis

A neurosis is a less severe psychological disorder than is a psychosis (*see* Psychosis), although neurotic symptoms may certainly make everyday functioning difficult. It is unusual for a neurotic person to become psychotic as the symptoms worsen. Individuals who are neurotic simply become more intensely neurotic. There are various forms of neuroses that differ in their symptoms. These include anxiety neurosis and obsessive-compulsive neurosis. Anxiety neurosis is characterized by an enduring, persistent feeling of uneasiness. Obsessive-compulsive disorder is characterized either by obsession with some trend of thought or by some ritualistic compulsive act (such as repeated hand washing to avoid contact with germs). Other neuroses are hypochondria in which a person believes he or she suffers from or may contract a particular disease and anorexia nervosa (in which individuals starve themselves). The onset of neurosis in late adulthood is rare. Well-adjusted younger people tend to become well-adjusted elderly people. However, young neurotics who remain uncured are likely to become elderly neurotics with the continuation of their symptoms.

A myth of aging is that the proportion of hypochondriacs among elderly people is greater than it is among younger adults. The incidence of hypochondria is no greater in late adulthood than in earlier adulthood. A true hypochondriac is likely to regard physical symptoms such as irregular bowel movements as an indication of a serious disease when medical evidence shows that none exists. When many elderly adults report various physical symptoms, they are likely to be manifestations of normal aging and not hypochondria. *See also* Self-Rated Functioning.

Neuroticism

Neuroticism is one of the basic personality traits identified by psychologists (*see* Personality Traits). At the low extreme of this trait are individuals who are well adjusted and emotionally stable, while at the high extreme are individuals who show maladaptive behavior (that is, self-defeating behavior that interferes with daily living) and negative emotions (such as anxiety and depression). Those individuals with neurosis score very high on this trait. However, neuroticism in varying degrees is one of the dimensions of normal personality. Most individuals fall in the middle between the two extremes of the trait.

Of those individuals who score high in neuroticism, most are not considered to be true neurotics who possess clinically significant symptoms. As is true for most personality traits, there is considerable evidence to indicate that neuroticism is remarkably stable with normal aging. That is, current elderly people who score low, average, or high in neuroticism were likely to have scored similarly as low, average, or high when they were young adults. One's level of neuroticism at any age level is an important determinant of life satisfaction and psychological well-being. A high level of neuroticism at any age level is a likely reason for medical complaints that have no apparent physical cause.

Nightmares

A nightmare is a frightening dream, usually so intense that it awakens the sleeper. Adults of all ages are susceptible to occasional nightmares. Of interest is whether they are especially likely to occur among older adults. The results from a study by researchers at the University of Arizona suggest that the frequency of nightmares is actually lower among healthy older adults than among college students. The participants in their study kept a log for two weeks in which they recorded each morning the number of nightmares they had during the previous night. Only about 25 percent of the elderly participants reported having at least one nightmare during the two-week period, in contrast to the nearly 50 percent of the college students. The overall number of nightmares reported during the interval was nearly twice as high for the college students as for the elderly adults.

Nocturia

Nocturia is a nocturnal diuresis (an increase in the secretion of urine) usually reported by elderly men who have a benign enlarged prostate gland. It may also occur with sleep apnea (*see* Sleep Disorders). Once the apnea is cured, the nocturia is usually eliminated.

Norms

One of the uses of the term *norms* is in the description of the standing of individuals with respect to others of their own age. Familiar to parents is the news that their child is at the 50th percentile rank in weight. This means that their child is average in weight, in the sense that the child has a "score" corresponding to the average score (that is, weight) for children of his or her own age. If the parents heard that their child is at the 25th percentile, then they would know that he or she is somewhat below average in weight.

Elderly adults may similarly discover their standing in weight with respect to other elderly people. Students taking college admission tests are similarly identified in terms of where they rank relative to other students on the same test. A score of 500 usually means that they have a score at the 50th percentile.

To be useful in knowing where an individual ranks with respect to others his or her own age, norms must be derived from a representative sample of individuals that age. Thus, to gather norms for weight, a large sample of children of a given age must be selected so that they are representative of all children of that age in terms of race, rural or urban residence, socioeconomic status of their parents, and so on. Based on the average weight and the variability of weights around that average for this representative sample, norms in the form of percentiles may be established.

Norms for mental performances and characteristics are, unfortunately, uncommon, especially after childhood. The major exception is for intelligence tests, particularly the Wechsler Adult Intelligence Scale (*see* Wechsler Intelligence Tests). Large and fairly representative samples of adults at a number of different age ranges were tested in the standardization of this test. For a given age range, say sixty to sixty-four, the average test score for the representative sample of people was assigned the intelligence quotient (IQ) value of 100. The score that was one standard deviation above average (a standard deviation is the score that when added to and subtracted from the average score gives the range of scores within which the middle two-thirds of the distribution of scores may be found; *see* Variability of Behavior) was assigned the value of 115.

Intelligence test scores tend to follow a normal probability (bell-shaped) curve or distribution; this means that roughly 34 percent of the sample had scores that corresponded to IQs between 100 and 115, and 16 percent had scores corresponding to IQs greater than 115. Similarly, a score that was two standard deviations above average was assigned the IQ value of 130. The norms based on this sample may then be used to identify the rank of any individual aged sixty to sixty-four who takes the test relative to the original representative sample. If that individual scores an IQ of 100, then he or she is at the 50th percentile (average). If the person scores 115 or 130, then he or she would be at the 84th or 97.5th percentile, respectively. Thus, the norms for this test are age-appropriate norms that take into account the decline in test scores that may occur with normal aging. That is, your normative score is based on others your own age, and not on the performance of only young adults.

Unfortunately, there are few other mental tests or tasks that are normatively age based in the same way as the Wechsler Adult Intelligence Scale. The selection of large and representative samples is a very difficult, expensive, and tedious process. The Wechsler Memory Scale that is widely used in memory dysfunction diagnosis does have norms of a kind, but they are generally considered by experts to be inadequate. Patient (and compulsive—and well-funded) researchers of gerontology are needed to provide the kinds of norms needed to interpret the performances of elderly adults on various mental tasks.

The term norm is used in another way as well, namely, in terms of incidence rates for such events as diseases, deaths, divorces, life crises, and dementia. Surveys or examinations of large samples of people are needed to determine what percentage in each age group is characterized by the event. Thus, for a particular disease we may discover that the national incidence rate for people age fifty-five to sixty-four years is 10 percent, and for people age sixty-five or older it is 35 percent. We would know immediately that the event in question is especially related to late adulthood.

If we knew the incidence rate in a particular part of the country is well above the national norm (for example, 55 percent when the national norm for people age sixty-five or older is 35 percent), we would have reason to examine what is causing the disparity. Or when we know the normative incidence rates for thyroid disorders, and discover that both husband and wife have the disorder, we are bewildered by the seeming defiance of the laws of probability. Naturally, we begin to wonder if the correspondence is indeed only a coincidence. Similarly, when we know that divorce is more the norm for younger people than for older people, we have a better understanding of why it is often more stressful for an elderly person—it is less expected.

Nun Study

The participants in the Nun Study joined the School Sisters of Notre Dame religious congregation when they were about age twenty. Of 1,027 eligible sisters, 678 have been participants in a study in which they receive annual assessments of physical and cognitive functions. They ranged in age from 75 to 102 at the time of the first assessment in 1991–1992.

The nuns are a very important source of information about various conditions that affect aging. They have had similar lifestyles and environments throughout their adult lives, and they have had minimal exposure to many variables known to affect health and mental functioning adversely in late adulthood (for example, they have had no smoking and no drinking of alcoholic beverages throughout their adult lives). Evidence from their assessments provides valuable information about how positive health conditions affect the incidence of Alzheimer's disease, brain infarcts, and functional disabilities (*see* Alzheimer's Disease; Self-Rated Functioning).

Nursing Home Admissions

More than one million elderly people are institutionalized in nursing homes annually. Married elderly people have about half the risk of admission as unmarried elderly people. Having at least one daughter or sibling reduces the likelihood of admission by about one-fourth. Researchers at the University of Florida found that the admission rate is 25 percent higher for elderly people living in sparsely populated areas than in cities, probably because rural areas have fewer alternatives to nursing homes, such as adult day care centers, that help partially independent elderly people avoid a nursing home. In addition, African Americans with Alzheimer's disease spend a considerably longer time in the community before being admitted to a nursing home than do whites.

Interestingly, researchers in Illinois found that older Medicaid recipients who live alone are admitted to a nursing home with better physical functioning than others who live with someone. Caregivers are much less likely to have their cognitively impaired relatives placed in a nursing home when family members give overnight help and assist the patients with the activities of daily living (*see* Activities of Daily Living).

There are some Alzheimer's disease patients whose functional health status permits living in assisted-living facilities (*see* Assisted-Living Facilities; Home Care). It is estimated that between 23 percent and 65 percent of nursing home residents with Alzheimer's disease could be served in assisted-living facilities. The potential savings from their placement in these facilities could be $1 to $2.7 billion annually.

Of interest are the reasons caregivers place their patients in a nursing home. Researchers at Duke University Medical Center asked twenty-two hundred caregivers who had placed their patients in a nursing home to identify the reasons they did so. The most frequent reason was the patient's need for more skilled care (65 percent). Other reasons were the caregiver's own health (49 percent), the patient's behavior (46 percent), and the need for more assistance (23 percent).

Nursing Home Deficiencies

Nursing homes are evaluated for their quality and their deficiencies once a year under the federal nursing home certification regulations. Deficiencies fall into three main categories: quality of care, quality of life, and other deficiencies. Quality of care includes nursing services, dietary services, physician services, rehabilitative services, dental services, and control of infections. Quality of life includes transfer and discharge rights and the physical environment. Other deficiencies include items on administration and medical records.

Researchers in San Francisco and Wisconsin analyzed data from all certified nursing homes in the United States. They found that fewer registered nurse hours and nursing assistant hours related to total deficiencies and quality-of-care deficiencies. In addition, homes that had more depressed and demented residents were smaller, were nonprofit or government owned, and had fewer deficiencies. Facilities with higher percentages of Medicaid residents had more deficiencies after controlling for staff size.

Nursing Home Discharge Outcomes

Discharge outcomes of elderly residents who are stroke sufferers or hip fracture sufferers without serious cognitive or behavioral problems have been found to be positively related to the amount of therapy they received as well as being of a younger age and having lower levels of functional impairment at admission.

Stroke victims have had more favorable outcomes for discharge when treated in rehabilitation centers. However, site (center or nursing home) seems to make little difference in discharge outcome for hip-fracture patients. Therapy received in the nursing home (physical, occupational, speech) is positively related to discharge and negatively related to mortality when controlling for age.

Nursing Home Infections

Annually, more than 25 percent of patients in nursing homes are transferred to a hospital or emergency room for evaluation and treatment. Many have recurring transfers. Most transfers are the result of infections, especially of respiratory and urinary tracts. Unfortunately, physicians usually prescribe antibiotics for these patients in the nursing home without seeing them. That is, evaluation and treatment are conducted over the telephone. Nursing homes could be the site for care, but most physicians avoid organizing their schedules to make visits there. By contrast, patients in the hospital are seen regularly by physicians.

Nursing Home Residents (Contact with Family and Friends)

According to the U.S. Department of Health and Human Services there were 1.5 million persons age sixty-five and older living in nursing homes in 1999. After people are admitted to a nursing home, how often do they have contact (visits or phone calls) with family members and friends? In a more recent study of more than 1,400 new admissions, it was found that contact decreased by nearly half following admission compared to reported readmission contact. Contact was found to be positively related to closeness with the resident, support-network proximity, nondemented status of the resident, and white race of the resident. Interventions need to be found that increase involvement with nursing home residents.

Nursing Home Residents (Number)

According to the 2000 U.S. Census, the percentage of people age sixty-five and older living in a nursing home was 4.5 percent. This is a decrease from the 5.1 percent in 1990. The decline was especially pronounced for those age eighty-five and older—from 24.5 percent in 1990 to 18.2 percent in 2000.

Nursing Home Residents (Their Rights)

Nursing home residents cannot be transferred or discharged unless one of the following conditions occurs: the resident has had a change in condition that requires a different level of care, the resident is in danger to his or herself or to other residents, no pay has been made for care, or the home goes out of business. The resident or his or her representative must receive written notice thirty days in advance. The written notice must include the reason for transfer or discharge. The resident has the right to appeal.

The rights of residents are determined by state and federal laws. These rights include voicing grievances, freedom from abuse and constraints, privacy and respect, free communication, keeping their own possessions, marital privileges, and purchasing goods and services.

Nursing Home Staff (Resident Dependency)

Many nursing home residents become almost completely dependent on staff members to perform everyday behaviors they are perfectly capable of doing themselves (such as washing their faces or feeding themselves). Staff members often expect residents to be dependent on them, and they therefore fail to encourage the residents to be as behaviorally independent as possible. Residents, in turn, are often rewarded for their dependency on staff members by the attention given to them by the staff. The danger is that residents may lose skills they possess if they are not practiced regularly, thus making them increasingly more dependent on others to help them.

Gerontologists in Germany have developed a training program for staff members in nursing homes that enables at least some staff members to change their caregiving style in a way that encourages more independence on the part of the residents under their care—and without risk to the well-being of the residents. Nursing homes should be encouraged to train their personnel to behave in ways that are suited to the skill levels of their elderly residents. Residents who are able to perform basic behaviors without assistance should be encouraged to do so.

Nutrition and Diet

Guidelines for good nutrition and a healthy diet in late adulthood closely resemble those in earlier adulthood—plenty of green vegetables and fresh fruits, protein sources that offer balanced amino acids, whole grains, and so on. However, more proteins may be needed in very late adulthood because protein metabolism may decline in efficiency. An increase in protein intake is often recommended for people with various diseases, and the proportion of elderly people with these diseases is greater than it is for younger people.

One problem facing elderly people with a low income is the high cost of meat, the common source of much of our protein intake. Poor chewing ability may also limit the amount of meat consumed by many elderly people. Dairy products and eggs may serve as a substitute, but they may, in some cases, present their own dietary problems, especially by increasing "bad" cholesterol levels. Fish and poultry are also substitutes. In one study it was found that women who eat seafood five times a week have a 50 percent lower risk of a stroke. A protein balance of the essential amino acids may be approximated by casseroles of beans and rice. Such casseroles have the advantage of being both inexpensive and easy to chew.

Carbohydrates make up the major portion of traditional diets at all ages. Aging is associated with a delay in the return of blood glucose levels to basal values after the consumption of glucose substances. It is estimated that 20 percent of older people have difficulty regulating glucose in their blood and have impaired glucose tolerance that is associated with an increased mortality rate from cardiovascular diseases. Such substances as nondietary candies and soft drinks should probably be avoided as much as possible by many elderly people.

The vitamin and mineral needs of elderly people are about the same as they are for younger people. Vitamin supplements should not be needed for most elderly people who consume a balanced diet. When supplements are needed, they should be at the recommendation of one's physician and a professional dietitian. According to a researcher at Boston University Medical Center, elderly people with a vitamin D deficiency should compensate for the deficiency by soaking up sunshine in small daily amounts on their hands, arms, and face rather than by consuming extra amounts of milk or by taking vitamin D supplements (*see* Vitamin D Supplements). Perhaps worth taking up with your physician is folic acid (a form of a B vitamin) if you feel your cognitive abilities need a boost. Researchers in the Netherlands found that adults age fifty to seventy who took it for three years outscored others of the same age range who took a placebo on several cognitive tests.

Fad diets have existed for years. A recent fad diet is the "Atkins Diet" that stresses low carbohydrates and a lot of protein. Followers of the diet peaked in early 2004 and then began to decline. The majority of dieticians and physicians seem to be suspicious of this diet. They favor a traditional balanced diet with a reduction in calories and ample amounts of physical exercise. Many believe that seniors should replace much of the meat and dairy products in their diets with more vegetables, fruit, and whole grains. In general, vitamin supplements are less effective in promoting good health than are the foods that contain the vitamins.

Other popular recent diets are the Weight Watcher's Diet and the South Beach Diet. The former has been around for years. It offers two different food plans for dieters. The latter has more than three hundred thousand online subscribers. The diet features fabulous foods and taste sensations.

Unfortunately, there are apparently a number of older adults who have an inadequate diet. A survey by researchers at the Ross Laboratories in Ohio of the food intake of nearly five hundred normally aging adults age sixty-five to ninety-eight revealed that 40 percent of these people had energy intakes from food that were well below the recommended amount. A number of these individuals also had deficiencies in their mineral intake. Alarmingly, more than 20 percent of the participants reported that they ordinarily did not eat lunch. In another study of a large sample of women over age seventy, 16 percent were underweight and nearly 30 percent failed to consume adequate amounts of the basic nutrients. Researchers in Georgia found no relationship between nutritional risks, that is, inadequate diets, and either occupational level or educational level.

Proper nutrition and diet for elderly people may be impaired by conditions that interfere with normal eating behavior. Eating commonly occurs in the presence of others at the same time, and it therefore serves as a source of (usually) pleasant social interactions. Perhaps the most serious negative condition is widowhood. A study by researchers at Georgia State University of fifty recently widowed elderly women revealed that the loss of their spouses had negative effects on their motivation to cook and to eat. Only 24 percent of the widows reported their appetites to be good or excellent, compared with 92 percent of the elderly women in a control group whose husbands were still living. Moreover, only 18 percent of the widows selected foods for their good nutritional content compared with 62 percent of the women in the control group.

It is important that elderly people realize the many health benefits obtained from consuming certain foods. Perhaps the greatest benefit is that obtained from eating tomatoes and tomato-based products. Men who eat cooked tomato products (for instance, pasta sauce) tend to reduce their rates of prostate cancer by as much as 40 percent. The ingredient responsible for these effects is a substance called lycopene. Other food substances that have a positive effect on health include red grapes, blueberries, spinach, nuts, salmon (and other fatty fish, such as sardines, herring, and tuna), and garlic. If your potassium level is low and is causing fatigue and other problems, you should add sweet potatoes, orange juice, bananas, spinach, and skim milk to your diet. Your physician may also recommend taking a potassium pill supplement.

On the other hand, foods that contain trans fats may raise the level of LDL (the bad cholesterol), leading to heart disease. They include butter, shortening, margarine, and lard, substances commonly found in crackers, cakes, and cookies. In 2006 the Food and Drug Administration required food manufacturers to list grams of trans fat on the nutrition facts panel.

Should you stick to a low-fat diet to maintain your physical health? For years dieticians have emphasized the health benefits of a low-fat diet. However, these benefits have been challenged by the results obtained in a component of the Women's Health Initiative Study (*see* Women's Health Initiative) that involved thousands of women aged fifty to seventy-nine. Women who limited the amount of low-fat foods in their diets were no healthier than women in a control group who had no restrictions on eating high-fat foods. Nevertheless, to be on the safe side, you should probably consume only moderate amounts of high-fat foods (such as cheeseburgers).

Perhaps you should add the daily consumption of grape juice and pomegranate juice to your diet. Among the health benefits of grape juice is the lowering of your level of bad cholesterol (*see* Grape Juice). Pomegranate juice appears to improve the flow of blood to the heart for men and women who have coronary heart disease.

To make certain they consume a healthy diet, elderly people should consult their physician and a dietician at a local hospital. *See also* Antioxidants; Bladder Cancer; Cholesterol; Prostate Cancer.

O

Obesity

Nearly half of adult Americans are overweight, and about 30 percent are considered to be obese. The frequency of obesity increases progressively from early adulthood to middle age. It then begins to decline. Seniors over age eighty are 92 percent less likely to be obese than seniors age sixty-five to sixty-nine. This is the case for both men and women.

Health problems associated with obesity do not disappear in late adulthood despite the declining incidence. However, there is evidence indicating that the health risk is much less after age seventy-five. Obesity is associated with such debilitating and life-threatening diseases as Type 2 diabetes, hypertension, and coronary artery disease. It is also associated with an increased risk of depression and a lowering of the quality of life. Similarly, in another study, nearly 50 percent of women in the fifty-five-to-sixty-four age range were seriously overweight.

Both male and female spouse caregivers of patients with Alzheimer's disease tend to gain significant weight. Sleep apnea (*see* Sleep Disorders) may also cause weight gain, and older men who snore are more likely to gain weight than those who do not snore. A higher risk of obesity is also associated with lower educational level, being unmarried, having limited ability to perform the activities of daily living, having several chronic diseases, and poor self-rated health.

To rid themselves of obesity many individuals have stomach shrinking surgery. This surgery is dangerous for the elderly, especially those with heart disease. Nearly one in twenty Medicare cases have been found to die within the first year after the surgery. The risk appears to be greater for men than for women. *See also* Obesity (Childhood Obesity Predicts Adult Obesity); Obesity (Effects on Longevity and Disability)

Obesity (Childhood Obesity Predicts Adult Obesity)

Researchers at Purdue University surveyed nearly seven thousand adults ranging in age from twenty-five to seventy-four at the time of their first assessment. The survivors were then surveyed again three more times at five-year intervals.

Participants who reported being overweight in childhood were likely to continue to be overweight in adulthood. This was true for both men and women, but especially so for men, even though the overall incidence of obesity in adulthood is higher for women than for men. More than 14 percent of the overweight children became seriously obese as adults, compared to 4 percent of normal weight children. Severe obesity was highest for participants between the ages of forty-five and sixty-four. It was also higher for African American participants than for white participants.

Obesity (Effects on Longevity and Disability)

Obesity appears to have little effect on life expectancy for both community-dwelling adults and long-term residents of nursing homes aged seventy and older. However, community-dwelling obese elders are more likely to become disabled than nonobese elders. Thus, obese elders live as long as nonobese elders, but the former have a greater likelihood of disability in their remaining lives.

Old (Defining Late Adulthood)

All researchers in gerontology share the problem of defining what is meant by "old." Phrased somewhat differently, the question becomes "What defines the onset of old age?" A firm definition is virtually impossible to attain. The difficulty rests in the fact that *old age* is a relative term. The aging process actually begins at birth and continues throughout the remainder of the life span.

The onset of "oldness" has no set physical marker, and the definition of *old* becomes arbitrary. In an important way, "old" depends on what physical ability or psychological ability is of concern. An Olympic-class gymnast is "old" at age twenty-five, whereas a professional baseball player is not "old" until past age thirty-five. By contrast, an Olympic-class yachting participant is "young" at age forty-five, as is a presidential candidate (Sir Eyre Massey Shaw won a gold medal in the 1900 Games for yachting at the age of seventy, and a presidential candidate in 1996 was in his seventies).

Clearly, aging affects various abilities at different rates. Moreover, there is a wide range of ages along the adult life span at which the onset of aging for specific abilities and functions becomes apparent. That range occurs later for the ability to hit successfully against a major league pitcher than for the ability to perform complex gymnastic exercises, and still later for the ability to maneuver a yacht.

Similarly, physiological functions age at different rates. Relative to young adults, the basal metabolic rate shows little change even at age seventy, whereas the maximum breathing capacity shows considerable decline by age sixty and younger. Such variability among different abilities and functions and among individuals at different ages has led to the concept of *functional age* as a way of defining old. The concept, however, has many problems, and it has not been widely used (*see* Functional Age).

In the absence of a firm biological or psychological criterion for defining the onset of old age, most people and gerontologists have turned to an arbitrary criterion. That criterion is the setting of a specific chronological age, that is, years since birth, as being the onset of old age. In recent years that age has been sixty-five years. Why age sixty-five? Until 1979, attainment of this age signaled forced vocational retirement for most people. Retirement at age sixty-five is a relatively recent event. It originated in Germany in 1889. Otto von Bismarck's statisticians determined, on an actuarial basis, that sixty-five was the ideal age for establishing a not-too-costly retirement pension plan. Retirement at age sixty-five eventually reached the United States and became the standard practice in 1935.

Now that the retirement age has been advanced to seventy years for many people by an amendment to the Age Discrimination in Employment Act, an interesting possibility is that old age will eventually be redefined as having its onset at age seventy. In practice, however, gerontological researchers usually set their own criteria for selecting samples of elderly participants in their studies. It is not unusual to discover studies in which membership in the "old" group is set at age sixty or even in the fifties.

When do you and other people think "oldness" begins? In a telephone survey, more than two thousand adults were asked "When does old age start?" The average age given was sixty-three years. Those in the survey who were already over age sixty generally placed the start of old age in the seventies. Interestingly, the more affluent the respondents were, the later they believed old age begins.

Older Americans Research and Services Questionnaire

The Older Americans Research and Services Questionnaire (OARS) is used to gather information about the functional status and service needs and uses of adults age eighteen and older. Its major use, however, has been with older adults. OARS has two main parts. The first assesses functional status in five areas, including physical health and the activities of daily living (*see* Activities of Daily Living). The second part assesses the need for and use of twenty-four services (for instance, transportation, financial assistance, and meal preparation). OARS is widely used in national health surveys and in assessing the functional status and service needs of older people with diseases such as arthritis.

Operant Conditioning

The basic principle of operant conditioning (or operant learning) is that the event following a response determines either the frequency or the speed of that response's future occurrences. If the event is something positive (for example, food to a hungry rat, candy to a child, money to an adult), then positive reinforcement occurs, and the consequence is an increase in the frequency or the speed of the behavior. If the event is negative (electric shock to a rat, spanking to a child, loss of money to an adult), then punishment occurs, and the consequence is a decrease in the frequency or the speed of the behavior.

B. F. Skinner, the famous American psychologist who discovered the principle in the 1930s, found that both human beings and animals are susceptible to behavior modification by either positive reinforcement or punishment. Older adults are no exception. For example, positive reinforcement has been found to increase their speed of performing various tasks (for example, memory scanning and digit symbol substitution; *see* Short-Term Memory; Wechsler Intelligence Tests).

Ethical issues limit research on the use of punishment to affect the behavior of older adults. However, when money is used for positive reinforcement of a fast response, then taking away that money may be used as a mild punishment for a slow response. This form of punishment after a slow response on a task has been found to decrease future occurrences of slow responses for both older and younger adults.

Positive reinforcement has been found to be effective with some patients with Alzheimer's disease in increasing the frequency of behaviors relevant to their own grooming and caretaking. Positive reinforcement has also been demonstrated to decrease the frequency of excessively aggressive behaviors of institutionalized elderly people. Here the treatment consists of positively reinforcing nonaggressive behaviors.

Operant conditioning is also frequently used as a form of therapy (called behavior modification) to promote greater occurrences of behaviors that are advantageous to the individuals receiving the therapy, such as quitting smoking and managing pain. *See also* Pain Management; Psychotherapy; Psychotherapy with Nursing Home Residents; Smoking.

Originality

If you were asked to list six uses for a newspaper other than its main use (for reading, of course), what would you say? "To start a fire" is highly likely—and it would be an answer given not only by you but by many others as well. Would you have included "To provide the words for constructing a kidnap ransom note"? This is the type of question included on an "Unusual Uses" test. The purpose of this test is to measure individual differences in *originality*. Originality calls on what psychologists term *divergent* or *productive thinking* in which the objective is to give a unique solution to a problem (such as what to do with a newspaper).

By contrast, most of our everyday problem solving calls on *convergent thinking* in which the objective is simply to find the most appropriate solution to a problem, regardless of the originality of that solution. Starting a fire with a newspaper would not be very original, whereas constructing a ransom note from it would be quite original (that is, given by very few people) and dependent on divergent thinking. The more such unique (but rational) answers you give on the Unusual Uses test, the higher your originality score.

Research with the Unusual Uses test, along with other tests of originality, has revealed that older adults display moderately less originality than do younger adults. The most comprehensive study was conducted with participants in the Baltimore Longitudinal Study (*see* Longitudinal Studies of Aging's Effects on Health and Cognition). More than eight hundred men ranging in age from 17 to 101 received a battery of six tests, each designed to measure originality in some form.

For example, one of the tests required imagining the consequences of unusual situations. The correlation between age and scores on this test was negative (there was a trend for scores on the test to be lower for older than for younger participants) and statistically significant (unlikely to be related to chance). However, the magnitude of the correlation was modest. The implication is that originality is by no means the exclusive province of young adults. Many elderly adults show as great, if not greater, degrees of originality than do many much younger adults.

Osteopenia

Osteopenia is a bone mass that is significantly below the average (defined as two standard deviations below the mean, for those who know statistics) bone mass for young normal women at either the lumbar spine, the proximal femur, or the radius. By age eighty, nearly 50 percent of women have osteopenia. Osteopenia is a critical cause of osteoporosis (*see* Osteoporosis).

Osteoporosis

Bone loss and an increase in the porosity of bone mass are part of the aging process. These processes (known as osteopenia; *see* Osteopenia) begin in the thirties and increase in the fifties. The rate and amount of loss are greater, on average, for women than for men. If the loss is severe enough, osteoporosis is the result. It is found more often in older women, especially small-boned women, than in older men.

It is estimated that ten million Americans, mostly women (about four-to-one ratio to men, although two million men do have osteoporosis), have osteoporosis, and another thirty-four million are at risk of having it. The risk factors include age (risk increases in late adulthood), body size (small, thin-boned women have a greater risk than other women), race (African American women have a lower risk than white women or women of Asian descent), and family history of the disease. The risk is also increased by excessive alcohol consumption, cigarette smoking, and an inactive lifestyle.

Only 30 percent of physicians discuss bone health with female patients. Fewer than 25 percent of older female patients ask their physician for information about osteoporosis. The most visible sign of the disease is likely to be a stooped posture resulting from a curved spine.

In its early stages osteoporosis can be detected by scanning for bone density. Estrogen-replacement therapy may slow the progression of the disease in some postmenstrual women, but it may be associated with an increased risk of breast cancer, stroke, and heart disease (see Estrogen-Replacement Therapy [Hormone-Replacement Therapy]). Bone density may be maintained, at least to some degree, by supplements of calcium and vitamin D, (see Fractures [Hip]) combined with regular exercise, absence of smoking, and the drug Actonel for bone resorption.

Osteoporosis greatly increases the risk of fractures in elderly people. Hip fractures represent the greatest hazard, especially for people in their seventies and older (see Fractures [Hip]). It is estimated that osteoporosis is responsible for 300,000 hip fractures annually (of the 1.5 million fractures annually attributable to osteoporosis). Researchers at Tufts University found that taking 500 milligrams of calcium citrate and 700IUS of vitamin D daily reduced the fracture rate in both men and women by half, but the reduction was found to be much less than that for women in the Women's Health Initiative Study (see Women's Health Initiative).

It is estimated that insufficient nutrition is related to about two-thirds of the cases of osteoporosis. However, it may also result from the surgical removal of the ovaries or from dysfunctioning of the ovaries as a result of chemotherapy or radiation therapy. Osteoporosis is irreversible, but there are steps that may be taken to slow down its progression, such as taking certain drugs (for instance, Alendronate, Evista, and Raloxifene) and possibly estrogen replacement, following a particular dietary regimen (especially green leafy vegetables and fruits, especially cantaloupe, which is rich in potassium) and exercises that do not put excessive strain on your bones. See also Paget's Disease.

Ovarian Cancer

Most ovarian cancers occur in women over the age of fifty. The highest risk is for women over age sixty. Besides age, the greatest risk factors of developing the disease are never having children and a family history of the disease. Ovarian cancer cells may spread to other tissues and organs of the body.

Ovarian cancer often shows no apparent symptoms until late in its development. Eventually, the symptoms that do appear are likely to include abdominal discomfort, nausea, loss of appetite, weight gain or loss without reason, and abnormal vaginal bleeding.

The usual initial treatment is surgery in which the ovaries, fallopian tubes, the uterus, and the cervix are removed. Abdominal lymph nodes and various abdominal tissues may also be removed. Surgery is then often followed by either chemotherapy or radiation therapy. There is evidence to indicate that some women who have advanced ovarian cancer increase their years of survival by having their chemotherapy medicines injected by a catheter into their abdomen as well as being injected intravenously (the prior standard method).

There is the danger of an increased risk of developing ovarian cancer for women who used estrogen therapy alone (that is, without progestin). The risk increases progressively with the number of years receiving the estrogen. After twenty years the risk is three times that of women who did not have estrogen.

Overmedication

One of the problems confronting many elderly people is their under-adherence to their medication regimen (*see* Medication Compliance and Comprehension). A different, but equally serious, problem is the risk of overmedication.

It is estimated that one-fourth of the more than one billion prescriptions issued annually are for elderly people. Moreover, about 25 percent of older adults are required to take at least three prescription medicines. This should not be surprising, given the incidence of various diseases in late adulthood. The health risk exists because medicines often interact with each other, and their interaction may produce memory problems, dizziness, and bladder problems, along with a number of other potential problems, as side effects.

P

Paget's Disease

Like osteoporosis (*see* Osteoporosis), Paget's disease is a disease of the bones in your body. The disease involves the breaking down of a bone, and when it grows again it is softer than normal. Soft bones tend to bend or break easily. The affected bone may become shorter, or it may become longer. The disease usually affects the skull and bones in the hips, pelvis, legs, or back. It often affects only one or two bones. The cause of the disease remains unknown. The disease usually affects people over age forty (estimated to be about 3 percent of them). It affects more men than it does women.

Warning signs of the disease include pain in or above a bone, and the area around it may feel warm. If it affects your skull, your head may get bigger. If it affects a leg, the leg may bend or bow.

Treatment is likely to include medicines that help to rebuild bones (bisphosphonates, such as Fosamax). You would need to make certain that you have enough calcium in your body. This may be accomplished eating foods that are sources of calcium, such as milk and milk products, mustard greens and kale, and canned sardines and salmon. Supplements of calcium may also be required. Exercise of the right kind is recommended (consult with your physician).

Pain

Pain is a major source of discomfort regardless of one's age. Of course, it may also play an important role in alerting a person to the presence of life-threatening circumstances. What happens to the sense of pain as we age is poorly understood. A number of researchers have examined age differences in pain sensitivity by determining age differences in the pain threshold (that is, the minimal intensity of a pain-provoking condition that is felt as being painful). A variety of conditions have been used, with a variety of body parts receiving the conditions. For example, in some studies radiant heat has been applied to the arm, and in other studies electrical stimulation has been applied to an unfilled tooth. Several of these studies have reported sensitivity to decrease with increasing age, whereas others have reported either increasing sensitivity with increasing age or no age difference in sensitivity. It seems probable that the extent of change in sensitivity is likely to be modest.

On the other hand, clinical evidence from patients with real-life pain-provoking injuries and diseases suggests that older people may feel pain less intensely than do younger people. Conditions, such as appendicitis, that produce intense pain in younger adults often produce little pain in elderly adults. This, of course, is a mixed blessing in that some elderly adults may be unaware of an impending illness. Tolerance of pain is only partly a physiological function. It also depends on a person's attitude toward pain and whether an event is expected to increase or decrease the pain.

Pain (Chronic)

Chronic pain is usually defined as pain from an illness or injury that persists for one month or longer and has not responded to treatment. It tends to peak in occurrence between sixty and seventy years of age. Elderly adults are more likely than younger adults to experience chronic pain associated with such diseases as osteoarthritis and gout. The most frequent pain complaints by older adults are for back, joint, and muscle pains. There is evidence indicating that seniors who rate the intensity of pain the lowest are those whose brains produce natural painkillers (opioids) the fastest,

The frequency of chronic pain is estimated to range from 25 percent to 75 percent of the elderly population. The frequency is difficult to determine precisely because many older adults do not report their chronic pain to physicians. They tend to regard it as simply part of normal aging.

Pain Management

Health practitioners are finally realizing that chronic pain (*see* Pain; Pain [Chronic]) need not necessarily be tolerated—it can be managed or controlled. Pain treatment centers that offer a number of ways for managing pain are now located in many hospitals (usually affiliated with universities) around the country. Unfortunately, people over age seventy tend to be underrepresented as clients at these centers. Many elderly people seem to accept pain as simply being part of being old. In addition, too many physicians fail to medicate their elderly patients adequately for pain relief.

A number of approaches to minimize pain are now available. For example, much of pain comes from muscles. It may be largely relieved by training the patient to relax through the use of *biofeedback* (*see* Psychotherapy) or to perform certain exercises. Exercise has been found to be a critical means of managing pain for many people with arthritic pain. Appropriate exercise keeps their joints flexible and protects them from undue stress.

Patients with cancer or postsurgical patients with intense pain can have narcotics delivered to their bodies by a computerized pump that administers *patient-controlled analgesics*. Patients may administer pain-relieving drugs to themselves whenever they experience pain. Postsurgical patients have been found to administer less of these drugs than physicians would have prescribed for them.

Another approach involves the injection of a nerve-deadening solution (called a *nerve block*) into the spinal cord. It blocks pain from traveling by spinal nerves to the brain. Behavior modification (*see* Operant Conditioning; Psychotherapy) has also been used effectively to manage some types of pain. Patients are reinforced during periods of pain for visualizing pleasant images and repeating positive words.

For more information on pain management, write to the National Chronic Pain Outreach, 7979 Old Georgetown Road, Suite 100, Bethesda, MD 20814, or to the International Pain Foundation, 909 Northeast Forty-third Street, Suite 306, Seattle, WA 98105. Informative books about pain management include the *Handbook of Chronic Pain Management* by Dr. C. David Tollison and *Management of Pain* by P. P. Raj.

Pain Medications (Analgesics)

An *analgesic* is a pain-relieving medication. Americans take more than twenty-six billion pain medications daily, including everything from aspirin to prescription pain relievers. Nearly 20 percent of Americans over age sixty regularly take medications for pain. One-fourth of those who take these medications suffer from such side effects as drowsiness, dizziness, and stomach problems.

A wide variety of pain-killing medications are available without prescription to relieve mild to moderate pain. Many of these are of a general class known as NSAIDs (nonsteroidal anti-inflammatory drugs). They can be effective by decreasing the level of inflammation at the site of tissue injury. Among these drugs are aspirin (the original NSAID drug). For some older people aspirin may cause uncomfortable gastric side effects (*see* Aspirin for other effects). Both aspirin and ibuprofen may cause severe heartburn if used excessively. A noninflammatory alternative drug is acetaminophen (found, for example, in Tylenol: Extra Strength), but anyone suffering liver disease must be careful to avoid excessive use of this drug. It is also found in many other pain medications and cold remedies. You should not take more than four thousand milligrams of acetaminophen a day.

Opiate analgesics, used for moderate to severe pain, require a prescription. Included among these drugs are codeine, morphine, methadone, and demerol. One of the most potent pain relievers for chronic pain is

OxyContin. It requires a prescription, and it can become addictive. One of these drugs is likely to be the one used in a patient-controlled pain management program (*see* Pain Management).

One of the most widely used pain medications, Vioxx (a COX 2 inhibitor), was taken off the market by its manufacturer in 2004 when a long-term study showed it could double the risk of a heart attack or stroke if used for eighteen months or longer. A number of lawsuits have since been filed against the manufacturer. More recent evidence has indicated that regular use of the medication for periods much shorter than eighteen months could cause serious heart problems. The problem with this pain reliever has raised questions about the safety of other pain relievers, and whether they received adequate extensive clinical trials.

Interestingly, painkillers may be more effective if given before an operation and not just after. This supports what is called the "nerve wind-up theory." According to this theory, pain activates spinal pathways, and this makes a patient more sensitive to it. Painkillers before an operation are needed to prevent pain, and not just to reduce it when it is already present.

Pancreatic Cancer

The pancreas is an organ located in the back of the abdomen behind the stomach. It manufactures both enzymes that aid in the digestion of food in the small intestine and insulin that controls the amount of sugar in the blood. *Pancreatic cancer* is often called a silent killer because there are no obvious symptoms in its early stages, and it is difficult to detect until it is in an advanced stage. The highly lethal disease occurs mainly in older people, rarely occurring before age fifty and with an average age at diagnosis of fifty-five. It occurs nearly twice as often in men as in women, and slightly more often in African Americans than in whites. It is the fourth leading cause of deaths from cancer. There are about thirty-two thousand cases of the disease in the United States each year.

As the cancer grows and spreads, there is often pain in the upper abdomen and sometimes in the back. Symptoms at more advanced stages may include nausea, weight loss, loss of appetite, and a general feeling of weakness. A biopsy seems to be the only reliable diagnostic test. The five-year survival rate, even following surgery, is low. If it has spread, palliative treatment can improve patients' quality of life by controlling the symptoms of the disease.

Parent-Child Conflicts

Conflicts do occur between aging parents and their adult children. Are these conflicts perceived by the parent and the adult child to occur for the same reasons or for different reasons? The results obtained in a survey by researchers in California indicate that they indeed do differ. About two-thirds of both the parents and the adult children expressed having con-flicts. However, the two differed in what they perceived to be the nature of the conflict. The cause of conflict most often listed by parents (38 percent) was habits of the adult children (for instance, style of dress) and their lifestyle (such as sexual activity). The conflict most often listed by the adult children (34 percent) was failure of communication and the parents' style of interacting (yelling too much or being too critical). Conflicts over child-rearing practices were nearly equally listed by parents (14 percent) and their adult children (16 percent).

Parenthood in Later Life

This entry deals only with parenthood at middle age and beyond. By then most women have passed the childbearing years. By contrast, more middle-aged men do become fathers, perhaps for the first time. There is evidence to indicate that men who become fathers in middle age are likely to expe-rience more companionship with their children than men who become fathers at an earlier age.

Middle age, however, is most commonly associated with parents whose children have grown up and are independent, thus creating an "empty nest." The consequences of an "empty nest" are varied. Long of interest to family researchers has been the development of "empty nest" symptoms in some mothers who have lost their role as a caregiver to a child or adoles-cent. They perceive their lives as now having little purpose. The most com-mon symptom for these mothers is depression.

However, many other mothers react to the independence of their chil-dren quite differently; they experience relief and satisfaction. They now see themselves as having more time for travel and pursuit of other leisure activi-ties than was previously possible. This is especially likely for mothers who have worked. Unfortunately, the impact of an "empty nest" on fathers has not been widely investigated.

Of course, in recent years a number of middle-aged parents (and some elderly parents) have seen "empty nest" become a "refilled nest" as unmar-ried adult children and even married children return to live in their parental home, thus creating an "extended family." This is especially likely to happen when the "child" has lost his or her job or has to accept a very low-paying job.

A survey in 1990 revealed that 16 percent of young adults age twenty-five to twenty-nine were living with their parents—and the percentage is proba-bly even higher today. A study conducted by researchers at Brown Uni-versity revealed that unmarried children were much more likely than married children to live with their parents. They also found that it is the children in the extended family who are most likely to benefit from the shared living, especially in terms of the parents being the main contributors to living expenses.

Middle age also presents the danger of divorce for parents whose main roles in life centered on their children. Now that they no longer share the responsibility of child rearing, they may discover that they have little else in common.

Older women are likely to have a closer relationship with their daughters than with their sons. After a divorce or the death of their husbands, they are more likely to share a residence with a daughter than with a son.

During late adulthood, parents usually assume a new role as grandparents (*see* Grandparenting), as well as continuing in their roles as parents to their adult children. In most cases, contact and mutual help between older parents and their adult children are at a high level, even when they live far apart. The positive relationships may be strained, however, by a number of factors. Included are the high time and resource demands placed on the adult children as they raise their own families and the reliance of some older parents on their adult children for financial aid and health care.

Parkinson's Disease

Patients with Parkinson's disease have a deficit in one of the chemical transmitters, dopamine (*see* Brain and Aging), found in the area of the brain controlling motor or muscular behaviors. Among the symptoms of the disease are the presence of tremors, difficulty initiating movement, and loss of postural reflexes. Depression, amnesia, and mental confusion occur in a fairly large proportion of patients with Parkinson's disease as the disease progresses in severity. Neurological examinations given to nearly five hundred residents of Boston who were age sixty-five and older indicated that 15 percent had the disease, with the incidence being a striking 30 percent for those age seventy-five and older. Parkinson's disease is an age-associated neurological disease in that its incidence below age forty is very low (actor Michael J. Fox is a prominent exception—he was age thirty when diagnosed with the disease). Symptoms may appear by age fifty-five, but the average age of onset is believed to be in the late sixties.

The four main symptoms of the disease are trembling in the hands, arms, legs, jaw, and face; rigidity or stiffness of the limbs; slowness of movement; and postural instability. As the disease progresses, shaking may interfere with performing the normal activities of daily living (*see* Activities of Daily Living). Other symptoms may include depression; difficulty in chewing, swallowing, and speaking; and sleep problems. In some advance cases dementia may occur.

There is no cure for the disease. However, the drug levodopa combined with other drugs enables nerve cells to make dopamine and replenish the brain's supply of dopamine. Levodopa helps control to some degree many of the symptoms of the disease for at least three-fourths of those with the disease. Other drugs such as Requip (ropinirole; *see also* Sleep Disorders) imitate the role of dopamine and cause neurons to react as they would to dopamine. The disease is also commonly treated by the drugs Sinemet and Mirapex (*see also* Sleep Disorders).

For advanced cases in which the disease does not respond to drugs there is a therapy called deep brain stimulation (DBS). Electrodes are implanted into the brain and connected to a small electrical device called a pulse generator that can be programmed carefully for when stimulation is needed. DBS can reduce the need for levodopa and other drugs and may decrease tremors, slow movements, and gait problems.

Recent research with mice and rats has indicated that extra amounts of exercise cause the animals to have less dopamine than animals without the extra exercise. Conceivably, this could lead to some form of an intervention for human beings with Parkinson's disease.

Participant Selection for Research Studies

An important question to ask about aging research is "Do volunteer elderly participants differ from those selected randomly?" Researchers at the University of Pittsburgh compared a random sample of more than 1,400 community-dwelling elderly adults (age sixty-five and older) with a sample of 259 volunteers recruited by advertisements. Volunteers consisted of significantly more women, better-educated persons, and people less likely to have used health and human services in the recent past than those selected randomly. The volunteers also had higher Mini-Mental State Exam scores (*see* Mini-Mental State Exam) and higher levels of ability on the instrumental activities of daily living (*see* Activities of Daily Living). After a six-to-eight-year follow-up, the volunteers also had a significantly lower mortality rate than the randomly selected participants.

Participation in Research

An advancement in gerontological research necessarily requires the participation of older people in biological, psychological, and sociological studies. A major problem confronting gerontological researchers is the reluctance of many elderly people to serve as participants in research studies. The National Center for Health Statistics reports a participation rate of 75 percent for adults age twenty-one to sixty but less than 60 percent for adults over age sixty. Obviously, many older people view such participation negatively.

The participation rate is usually higher when potential participants perceive their participation in a study as being personally beneficial (for example, taking part in a study on urinary incontinence) than when they see no personal benefit (such as taking an intelligence test). Payment for participation is a common method used to recruit older participants for their part in a study.

Participation in a research study usually involves consent in which potential participants are fully informed in advance of what will happen to them during their participation and what potential risks may be involved in their participation. They are also offered the opportunity to withdraw from the study at any time without receiving punitive action (that is, nonpayment for their service).

Participation in Voluntary Organizations and Volunteer Work

Millions of Americans belong to seemingly countless numbers of voluntary organizations and clubs. Memberships and active involvement in these organizations are low for adults in their twenties but quite high for adults in the age range of thirty-five to forty-four. Of great interest to gerontologists is the degree to which older adults withdraw from participation in voluntary organizations. A significant reduction relative to middle-aged adults could be taken as a sign of the preference for many elders to withdraw from active lives.

Evidence from a survey of two hundred people age sixty-five and older in an Ohio community indicates that participation in organizations remains high in late adulthood. Of those surveyed, 87 percent reported belonging to one or more organizations, and 74 percent reported attending meetings at least once a month. Moreover, 69 percent stated that they were very involved in the activities of their organizations. Men were as likely as women to be members of organizations. However, women were more likely to be actively involved than men. There was only a slight tendency for those age seventy-five and older to be less involved than those in the sixty-five-to-seventy-two-year age range. The modest decline in very late adulthood is probably due to the greater incidence of poorer health than in earlier late adulthood.

Volunteerism may also involve working in some capacity (usually unpaid, such as staffing an information desk at a hospital). It is estimated that more than 40 percent of elderly people participate in volunteer work. This percentage is considerably higher today than it was twenty-five years ago (about 11 percent). Moreover, the percentage of volunteer workers is likely to increase in the future as the educational level and the health status of new generations of elderly people increase.

Researchers at the University of Michigan found that volunteering may be beneficial for elderly people in terms of their mortality. However, their evidence indicated that this is true only for moderate amounts of volunteering (forty hours or less over half a year). Volunteering in greater amounts was found to have neither a positive nor a negative effect on mortality. The positive effect of moderate amounts of volunteering was strongest for eld-erly people with low levels of social interaction and who do not live alone.

There is evidence indicating that caregiving does not reduce the fre-quency of participation in voluntary activities. Caregivers seem to use out-side activities as a way of relieving the stress of caregiving.

To help find volunteer work, write to AARP Volunteer Talent Bank, 601 E Street Northwest, Washington, DC 20049. Also, the Points of Light Foun-dation has five hundred centers with information on local volunteer needs. To find the nearest center, call 1-800-59LIGHT.

Partners in Caregiving: The Dementia Services Program

The Partners in Caregiving program provides technical assistance and some funding to adult day-care centers. It has supported fifty centers in twenty-eight states and the District of Columbia, and it has provided models and advice for other centers. The program is sponsored by the Robert Wood Johnson Foundation. Its national office is located at the Bowman Gray School of Medicine at Wake Forest University. For further information, write to the Dementia Services Program, Department of Psychiatry and Behavioral Medicine, Bowman Gray School of Medicine, Wake Forest University, Winston-Salem, NC 27157-1087 (telephone 910-716-4941).

Patronizing Communication

Patronizing communication is speech that resembles baby talk or elder-speak (*see* Baby Talk [Elderspeak]). Like elderspeak the speaker uses simple grammar, short utterances, and exaggerated prosody (rhythm). However, it also includes exaggerated gestures and the inclusion of such terms of endearment as *honey* and *sweetie*. What do elderly people think of such speech? Some like it, but many do not. Much depends on their level of self-esteem (the higher the self-esteem, the less unfavorable the reaction to it).

Peripheral Arterial Disease and Claudication

Poor blood flow in the arteries of the muscles in the legs is called periph-eral arterial disease (PAD). The poor flow is usually caused by arteries that are narrowed or blocked by the accumulation of fatty deposits. It is caused by such factors as high blood pressure, diabetes, high cholesterol level, and smoking. It is most frequently found in older adults.

The fact that not enough blood flows to leg muscles often results in a painful leg condition known as claudication. The pain is usually noticed when you are walking. It tends to diminish or even disappear when you are resting. Claudication occurs more often for seniors who have blocking in arteries other than the legs, such as the heart or brain, than for seniors without this blocking. Those suffering from claudication may have had a heart attack or stroke.

PAD may be suspected when your physician listens with a stethoscope to the blood flow in your legs. If there is a suspected problem, the physician will have you take a more rigorous test involving sound equipment.

PAD and claudication may be treated by diet and exercise, and sometimes medicine (for instance, Pentoxil). If the blockage is not too severe, walking at least three times a week for thirty to forty-five minutes each time is recommended, taking rests when the pain becomes intense. If the blockage is severe, you may need angioplasty in the afflicted artery (*see* Cardiovascular Diseases). If the blocked area of the artery is very long, surgery may be needed. The surgeon will remove a vein from another part of your body and attach it above and below the blocked artery to allow blood to flow around the blockage.

Personality and Mortality

Is there an association between personality and mortality in late adulthood? For years gerontologists believed there is. Although early studies were inconsistent in finding evidence to support this belief, more recent evidence gathered by researchers of the Rush Institute for Healthy Aging and Rush Alzheimer Disease Center in Chicago has been more supportive.

The participants in their study were nearly nine hundred Catholic clergy members who averaged seventy-five years of age at the beginning of the study and were followed over five years. They were assessed on five different personality traits: neuroticism (being nervous), extroversion (outgoing and energetic), agreeableness (altruistic and helpful), conscientiousness (reliable and moral), and openness (intellectually curious and independent in judgment).

Participants who scored high on neuroticism were nearly twice as likely to have died during the five years than those who scored low on the trait (*see* Neuroticism). Presumably, neuroticism adversely affects the body's immune system. The only other trait to be related significantly was conscientiousness. Participants who scored high on this trait had a risk of death that was nearly half that found for those who scored low. High scorers may have better health-promoting behaviors (for example, more frequent exercise) than low scorers.

Personality (Overview)

"Sally has a sparkling personality." "Joe's personality really turns me off." These statements show how people usually refer to personality in their everyday lives. They are referring to how one person perceives another person. Sally is perceived by the person who made the statement as someone who is lively and perhaps even bubbly, whereas Joe is perceived as someone who is irritating and boorish.

To psychologists, however, personality has a different meaning. It refers to the collection of traits, beliefs, motives, values, styles of behavior, and so on that characterize any given individual. It is the unique organization of these attributes that defines the individual's personality. Every individual seemingly has a different organization than everyone else. Nevertheless, the different components of personality may be separated and studied independently of other components.

Traits may be measured as one component of personality. This is accomplished by the use of questionnaires in which respondents answer questions about themselves (often true-false questions). From the answers given, the respondents are scored on a continuum on such traits as introversion-extroversion.

Interest in gerontology centers largely on the question of age comparisons on the different components of personality. For example, how do adults at different ages compare on the trait of introversion-extroversion? These age comparisons are usually directed at answering the question of whether personality remains stable (that is, basically unchanged) or altered in some significant ways from early to late adulthood. In terms of the trait of introversion-extroversion, do young adults become increasingly introverted as they grow older? Alternatively, do those individuals who are extroverted when they are young remain basically extroverted when they become old? (*see also* Control of Life's Events; Personality Stages; Personality Style; Personality Traits).

Personality Stages

A stage theory is one that views life-span development in terms of a series of major transitions that everyone undergoes and in the same order of stages. A successful transition from one stage to the next means that the individual has moved from one level of functioning to another qualitatively different level of functioning. The ease of making a transition from one stage to the next depends on how successfully an individual has made earlier transitions. Stage theories have been applied to both cognitive (mental) life-span development (*see* Cognitive [Mental] Stages of Development) and personality. The most prominent stage theories of personality are those of Erik Erikson, whose theory dates back to the late 1950s, and of Daniel Levinson, whose theory was developed in the late 1970s.

Erikson's theory states that personality development over the course of the life span is determined by the interaction between biological and psychological forces within an individual and the external demands of society. There are eight stages assumed to be encountered during the entire life span, beginning in infancy and ending with old age. Each is characterized by a struggle between two opposing tendencies that create a crisis for the individual.

Erikson is perhaps best known for giving us the term *identity crisis* in reference to the stage and crisis confronting adolescence (the fifth stage in his theory). Here, the issue is whether the adolescent will find an identity for himself or herself. If not, the presumed consequence is that of identify confusion. Failure to resolve this crisis successfully is likely to affect negatively the resolution of crises at later stages of development.

Our interest rests in the seventh and eighth stages of Erikson's theory. The seventh stage is found in middle age and is characterized by the crisis between *generativity* and *stagnation*. Generativity refers to the caring for the young and working to improve the living conditions for future generations (*see also* Generativity). Failure to achieve generativity (that is, stagnation) should result in the individual becoming directed only at self-interests with little concern about society's future. Successful resolution of the generativity-versus-stagnation crisis is deemed necessary if an individual is to adjust satisfactorily to old age and to avoid dwelling on a meaningless life.

The eighth and final stage is characterized by the crisis between *integrity* and *despair.* The crisis begins with awareness of an old person that death is near. Integrity refers to the evaluation of one's own life and finding that it had meaning. Without such meaning, one faces impending death with despair.

Levinson's theory is based on the concept of a life structure that is created by an individual. This structure defined the individual's goal at a particular period of life and the various roles that the individual must assume in regard to family, work, and society at large in order to attain that goal. This life structure must experience transitions as the individual progresses through life and the roles expected of him or her are altered. For example, during midlife the individual evaluates past accomplishments within earlier life structures. If these accomplishments are not viewed satisfactorily, then a midlife crisis is likely to occur, and the individual feels the need for creating a very different life structure (*see also* Midlife Crisis).

Personality Style

Personality style refers to the manner in which individuals perceive the events occurring in their environments. For example, how sensitive are individuals to the context (that is, things going on in the background and where they are taking place) that surrounds the events important enough to attract their attention? To what extent do individuals perceive irrelevant events (events not related to their immediate objective) while attending to relevant events (events directly related to their immediate objective)? Psychologists view individual differences in sensitivity to contextual events and irrelevant events in terms of a broad personality-style dimension called *field dependence–field independence.*

In general, people classified as field-dependent are believed to rely primarily on external stimuli and events in making perceptual judgments and to experience their environments in a global, relatively undifferentiated way. By contrast, people classified as field-independent are believed to rely largely on internal stimuli (for example, their own thoughts about events) in making perceptual judgments and to experience their environments in a relatively differentiated way. Field-dependent people are, therefore, more likely than field-independent people to be distracted by irrelevant events and to have attentional problems when confronted by multiple stimuli.

A standard test for measuring a person's dependent-independent dimension is the rod-and-frame test. The person is tested in a darkened room with an apparatus composed of a luminescent rod surrounded by a luminescent square. The person's task is to move the rod until, on some trials, it is vertical with respect to the floor or, on other trials, it is horizontal with the floor. The task is made difficult by tilting the square background, thus making accuracy, as measured by deviation from verticality or horizontality, contingent on the person's ability to ignore the distorting background offered by the square.

Several cross-sectional studies have compared the performances of young adults and older adults on the rod-and-frame test. Accuracy scores are greater for young adults than for elderly adults. The implication is that elderly adults are, on average, more field-dependent than are younger adults.

Comparable outcomes have been found in other cross-sectional studies employing different tests for field dependency and field independency. This evidence is consistent with laboratory evidence indicating that older participants have greater difficulty than younger participants in ignoring irrelevant information (see Selective Attention). Unknown, however, is the extent to which this age difference is the consequence of a true age change; that is, do people really become more field-dependent as they progress from early to late adulthood? Conceivably, these cross-sectional age differences reflect a difference among generations. That is, members of earlier generations may be more field-dependent throughout their lives than are members of later generations.

Researchers at Duke University found that elderly men and women who are open and trusting in their personality style had better health and a greater sense of well-being than those who had a more cynical and suspicious personality style. They also found that those with an optimistic style of thinking had greater life satisfaction than those with a pessimistic style of thinking.

Personality Traits

Personality psychologists view a *trait* as a component of personality that accounts for relatively permanent dispositions and consistencies in an individual's behavior over time. Each trait is regarded as being defined by bipolar opposites, such as introversion and extroversion. A trait is therefore a dimension that ranges between two extremes, with different individuals scoring at different points on that dimension. Thus, individuals may be characterized as being highly introverted, mildly introverted, moderately introverted, and so on, through being highly extroverted. Individuals who are highly introverted are likely to behave in a withdrawn manner across a wide range of situations and circumstances. Similarly, individuals who are highly extroverted are likely to behave in an excited, somewhat boisterous manner across the same situations and circumstances in which the introverted person behaves in a withdrawn manner.

Traits are identified by psychologists through the use of personality tests and questionnaires in which people answer questions about themselves and their behaviors. On the basis of answers to different questions, the respondents are scored on the traits believed to be measured by the specific tests. The number of personality traits measured may vary from several to more than a hundred, depending on the specific personality test. The personality test currently of interest in gerontology is called the NEO Inventory, a test containing 144 items. The test measures three broad traits and a number of specific traits.

The first broad trait is neuroticism, which is defined by the extremes of emotional stability and instability. The specific traits included under neuroticism are traits expressing feelings of anxiety, hostility, self-consciousness, impulsiveness, and vulnerability. The second broad trait is extroversion, defined along the introversion and extroversion dimension. The specific traits included here are the three interpersonal traits of warmth, gregariousness, and assertiveness, and the three temperamental traits of activity, excitement seeking, and positive emotions. The third broad trait is openness, which is defined by the extremes of openness and closedness in feelings and ideas. Specific traits are openness to fantasy (for example, having a vivid imagination), openness to aesthetics (for example, appreciation of art and beauty), openness to actions (for example, willingness to try something new), and openness to ideas (for example, valuing knowledge for the sake of knowing).

Considerable research, both cross-sectional and longitudinal, has indicated that these traits show little change from early to late adulthood. That is, older adults differ little from younger adults in their trait scores, and scores on each trait remain about the same when respondents are retested after a period of years.

A number of other studies with other personality tests measuring a greater number of traits have provided similar evidence. For example, researchers in California measured age differences for adults ranging in age from eighteen to sixty. Assertiveness was found to be about the same at each age represented in their study. Dependability was found to increase up to about age thirty, and then remain stable. Thus, personality traits do seem to remain relatively stable from early to late adulthood.

The traits you have as a young adult are likely to be the same as you grow older. It should be noted that some early studies on age differences in personality indicated that elderly people did differ from younger adults on such traits as introversion-extroversion, with older people scoring as being more introverted than younger people. We know now that the cross-sectional age differences found in these studies were the result of cohort or generational effects (*see* Cohort [Generational] Effect) and were not the result of people changing from extroversion to introversion as they grow old. People from earlier generations appear to have been more introverted than people of later generations. It is members of these earlier generations who served as the participants in the early studies on adult age differences in personality traits. *See also* Caregivers (Family and Friends); Centenarians; Control over Life's Events; Neuroticism.

Pessimism about Your Physical Health and Depression

How do you rate your physical health—excellent, good, fair, poor, very bad? If you rate it as poor or very bad when physical evidence indicates your health is actually good or excellent, you are considered to be a pessimist. Older adults are more likely than middle-aged adults to be pessimists. Older adults who are pessimists about their health are more likely to suffer from depression than older adults who are optimists about their health (that is, they rate their physical health as good or excellent when physical evidence indicates it is not).

Pet Therapy

The relationships between human beings and their pets have long been recognized as providing many benefits for the human beings, such as unconditional love and companionship. It has been only in the past twenty-five years, however, that the potential therapeutic value of pets on nursing home residents has received attention. Residents of geriatric nursing homes are frequently adversely affected by institutionalization. They tend to become increasingly emotionally flat, socially withdrawn, and solitary in their behavior as their stay in the nursing home becomes prolonged. The hope is that the presence of a pet, either a dog or a cat, in the nursing home will delay the occurrence of these negative symptoms of institutionalization. In effect, resident interactions with a pet are hoped to provide a kind of therapy.

Two kinds of pet-therapy programs have been introduced for elderly nursing home residents. For the first, residents are permitted to have brief, occasional visitations with a dog or cat. The available evidence indicates that this type of program has little benefit for the residents. The other kind of program requires the dog or cat to become a permanent resident of the nursing home, with freedom to visit individual rooms, dining halls, meeting rooms, and so on. In this situation, the therapeutic value of the pet is likely to be greater. The most comprehensive study of the impact of a resident pet on the behavior of the human residents was conducted in an Australian nursing home. It was found that a dog did increase social interactions and decrease solitary behaviors among residents, but only for a month or two after the dog entered the home. After five months or longer the residents had largely reverted to the behaviors characteristic of them before the dog's arrival. Part of the problem in retaining the improved functioning of the residents over a longer period was related to the dog herself. She spent more time with staff members, and less time with residents, during the five-month period. To ensure maximum benefit from pet therapy, some way of avoiding the "staff drift" must be implemented in the nursing home.

Pet therapy is not restricted to geriatric nursing homes. The University of Alabama at Birmingham Hospital has had what administrators call the Canine Ambassador Program. The program intends to enhance the healing of patients and improve their experience with the hospital. The program is not limited to older adults, but many of the patients are seniors. Dogs visit patients for five minutes, with visits scheduled in advance. Patients, physicians, and program coordinators all believe that the results of the visit have been very positive.

Nor are interactions with pets limited to residents of nursing homes or hospitals. Many older community-dwelling adults have a pet in their homes with whom they have many pleasant interactions. A reasonable belief is that such interactions should enhance the psychological well-being of the older adults and thereby enhance their physical health as well. This seems to be the case for older adults who have been experiencing severe stress in their lives. For most older adults, however, the evidence indicates that pleasant interactions with a pet at home have little effect on physical health and little effect on longevity.

Physical Attractiveness

At what age is physical attractiveness at its peak? The results of a national survey indicate that this age depends on the age of the beholder. For those under age thirty-five in the survey, the peak was at age thirty; for those age sixty-five and older, it was age forty-six.

Physicians (Communication with)

One problem confronting health care for older people is the barrier many elderly patients face in communication with a physician. Physicians realize the importance of effective communication with their elderly patients, but they often complain that their busy schedules do not permit much time to discuss the problems of their patients in any great detail.

The total time spent in communication during an office visit is not the only important element in aiding elderly patients. Perhaps more important is how the available time is spent. Researchers at the City University of New York–Brooklyn College examined the flow of communication for a group of elderly patients making their first visit to a specific physician. The physicians tended to dominate the conversations. Responses to patients' questions were more likely to be effective if the questions were related to topics raised by the patients themselves. In addition, the physicians were likely to communicate better with elderly patients who expressed less concern about control of their own health than with elderly patients who expressed more concern about the control of their own health.

Elderly patients should stick to the point in talking with their physicians. They should give a brief description of their symptoms, including their frequency and when they started. They should not be afraid to ask questions seeking clarification of words or phrases used by the physician that they do not understand (for example, *aneurysm*). If they have a problem hearing, they should let their physician know about it. They should not lie to their physicians. For example, if they still smoke, they should not deny it to their physician. They should consider asking for permission to tape-record their sessions with their physicians. This way they could later review the information conveyed to them by their physicians, information that may not have been clearly understood at the time of the visit.

Interestingly, the average time of seniors' visits with their physicians in their offices increased from 16.3 minutes in 1989 to 20.4 minutes in 1998. Apparently, the increase in managed health care has not been associated with less time per office visit. Perhaps seniors are becoming increasingly aware of their health concerns and of the need to share those concerns with their physicians.

Older adults often fail to remember an appointment they have with their physicians. Their memory for date, time, and purposes of the appointment is likely to be increased if they have a telephone message that they can repeat or if they take down notes during the telephone conversation.

Physiological Functions

One way of expressing age-related changes in physiological function of some organ or system of the body is in terms of the percentage of proficiency of average functioning in a given age range, relative to the functional level at age twenty. These percentages reveal both the magnitude of the declines in functioning with age and the considerable variability in magnitude for different functions.

For example, the velocity of nerve-signal transmission is about 95 percent (of what it is at age twenty) at age sixty and about 90 percent at age eighty. The kidney filtration rate is about 85 percent at age sixty and about 75 percent at age eighty, and the maximum breathing capacity is about 62 percent at age sixty and 42 percent at age eighty. These are average figures, and there is considerable variability or dispersion about these averages at each age level (*see* Functional Age).

Maximum breathing capacity is the maximum amount of air taken into the lungs with a single breath. The decline in capacity results in the frequent shortness of breath (a condition called dyspnea) experienced more by older people than by younger people and in the greater fatigue likely to be experienced during exercise by older than by younger people.

Digestion is usually not greatly impaired by aging, but many elderly people do experience irritable bowel syndrome, diverticulitis (pouches in the walls of the intestines), and constipation (*see* Bowels). Laxatives are often used by elderly people, but they often reduce the efficiency of digestion and lead to nutritional deficiencies. Constipation and diverticulitis are most effectively treated by a controlled diet, certain drugs, and exercise. Older people with these digestive dysfunctions should consult their physicians regularly for the treatment likely to benefit them.

Kidney function declines in efficiency in late adulthood as the number of nephrons (the kidney's functional units) declines to about half the number present at birth. As a consequence, stress is more likely to produce kidney failure in elderly people than in younger people. Normally aging elderly people are likely to have an increase in the frequency of urination, relative to younger people, and a larger residual amount of urine after urinating, as a result of age-related changes in the elasticity and responsiveness of the bladder. Kidney stones are composed of a chemical called calcium oxalate. Patients with kidney stones should drink a number of glasses of water daily, avoid drinking grapefruit juice and eating foods rich in oxalate (for example, chocolate and nuts), and cut down on their salt consumption. Calcium stones may recur within ten years for about half of the people who have them.

Picture Memory

When young adults have their memories tested for pictures of scenes or pictures of common objects that are presented in a lengthy series, their accuracy of identifying old pictures (that is, they were included in the series) as old and their accuracy of identifying new pictures (that is, they were not in the series) as new are both quite high. In fact, their accuracy is much higher than it is for similar identifications of words seen in a lengthy series. The difference in accuracy between recognizing pictures and recognizing words is known as the *picture superiority effect*. Older adults also show the picture superiority effect. However, the accuracy of picture memory has generally been found to be less for elderly participants than for younger participants. Nevertheless, the age difference in memory proficiency favoring younger adults has generally been found to be less for pictures than it is for words.

Plasticity Theory

Some degeneration of the brain occurs with normal aging. Some neurons are lost, while others decline in their functioning. However, positive changes also occur in the brain; for example, the number of dendrites connecting neurons with other neurons may increase, as may the complexity of the connections. Of great interest is the discovery of means of increasing the plasticity of the brain, that is, its capability of compensating via positive changes for the negative changes. Research with rats has discovered that old animals given an enriched environment (for example, placing colorful and manipulable objects in their environments) show greater plasticity of their brains than do other old animals who remain restricted to their colorless and sterile environments. Most important, old rats in enriched environments display greater learning proficiency than old rats without such enrichment.

Plasticity theory suggests that comparable effects should occur for the older human brain. Stimulating environments and stimulating mental experiences and activities should increase the amount of plasticity occurring in the brain. To date, the evidence indicating that high levels of mental activity relate positively to higher levels of performances on various mental tasks is somewhat ambiguous (*see* Activity [Mental] and Mental Performance), but research in this area is in its infancy. More supportive of plasticity theory is evidence that practice and training on some mental tasks lead to improvement in performance on those tasks for elderly people. Such experiences may be regarded as stimulating the brain's plasticity.

Pneumonia

Pneumonia is an infection of the lungs that affects either a section of a lobe of the lungs (*lobar pneumonia*) or patches scattered throughout both lobes (*bronchial pneumonia*). There are more than thirty different causes of pneumonia, but the three main causes are bacteria, viruses, and mycoplasmas. Pneumococcus pneumonia is the most common form of bacterial pneumonia (accounting for about one-fourth of all cases of pneumonia). Pneumonia-producing bacteria are present in some healthy throats. When a person's resistance to disease is low, as it may be in many elderly people, the bacteria may work their way to the lungs, causing part of a lobe or even an entire lobe or several lobes to fill with liquid. The infection may then spread through the body by way of the bloodstream. Symptoms of bacterial pneumonia may include chills, severe chest pain, a cough that produces rust-colored or greenish sputum, lips and nails with a bluish cast, and fever (as high as 105 degrees).

Viral pneumonia account for nearly half of all pneumonia. Early symptoms may include a dry cough, fever, and muscle aches. Primary influenza virus pneumonia is especially severe and may be fatal. Most cases of viral pneumonia occur in people with preexisting heart or pulmonary disease, which makes older adults especially vulnerable. There are no known medicines for treating viral pneumonia. Time usually will produce a cure on its own, but medicines can treat the cough. You may want to consider eating yogurt. It has been found to help fight off pneumonia by strengthening your immune system.

Mycoplasma pneumonia is caused by small organisms with characteristics of both bacteria and viruses. The disease occurs mainly in older children and young adults, and it is usually mild and rarely fatal. Mycoplasma pneumonia usually begins suddenly with severe chills, followed by a fever, chills, and a cough. Bed rest is required for the state of exhaustion accompanying the disease.

Prompt treatment with antibiotics may cure bacterial and mycoplasma pneumonia. The specific antibiotic is determined by the nature of the organism causing the pneumonia. In the year 2000 the U.S. Food and Drug Administration approved a new antibiotic called tequin for the treatment of pneumonia and other respiratory-tract infections, such as bronchitis. The drug has been demonstrated to have a success rate greater than 90 percent in treating these infections. Possible side effects found in clinical trials were gastrointestinal in nature (for example, nausea and diarrhea).

It is important to continue taking whatever medication you need as instructed by the physician after the fever has subsided, or the pneumonia may recur in a more severe form than the original form. Full recovery from the disease may take a number of weeks for older adults. They should make certain they have adequate rest during this period, but usually they may perform their normal daily activities.

A vaccine is available for pneumococcal pneumonia, and it should be given to those with the greatest risk of pneumococcal pneumonia, including people age sixty-five and older. It is estimated that the vaccine is effective in preventing pneumococcal pneumonia for about 40 percent to 60 percent of older adults who receive it. The vaccine is especially useful in reducing the severity of the symptoms and decreasing the risk of death for elderly people who do contract the disease. Elderly adults should have a revaccination five years after receiving the original vaccination. It was once thought that a booster vaccination had bad side effects. However, a study at Fitzsimmons Army Hospital found the side effects to be no different from those encountered after the first vaccination (soreness at the site of the vaccination) and perhaps a mild fever. It is unfortunate that fewer than 20 percent of people age sixty-five and older receive the vaccination.

Portion Size and Heart Health

Surprisingly, the mortality rate from heart disease is less for elders in France than it is for older Americans. It is surprising because the diet for French elders is high in both bad cholesterol and fats—factors that seemingly should increase and not decrease deaths from heart disease. This has become known as the *French paradox.*

The French paradox has been explained in part by the large amounts of red wine consumed by most French adults. Red wine contains antioxidants that may help preserve the health of French seniors.

However, there may be another reason as well. Adults in France, including elders, eat less than Americans, and therefore actually consume less cholesterol and fats than their American counterparts.

One reason French adults eat less is that the portions served in restaurant chains are smaller than portions served in the United States. In addition, the size of portions served in French homes is smaller than those served in this country. The number of people served in France from meat and starch recipes is significantly greater than in the United States.

Posttraumatic Stress Disorder

It is not unusual for individuals who have survived a traumatic event in their lives to experience a form of long-lasting anxiety known as posttraumatic stress disorder (PTSD). There are three main symptoms: reexperiencing the traumatic event, avoiding situations that are reminders of the event, or diminished responsiveness.

The event may be a natural disaster or military combat. A natural disaster, such as a severe earthquake, may be experienced by individuals at any age. In terms of military combat, PTSD is most commonly associated with combat veterans of the Vietnam War, veterans who have yet to reach late adulthood. Of particular concern in gerontology is the possibility that some combat veterans of World War II and the Korean War may still have PTSD. These veterans are now members of our elderly population.

According to a 1987 survey by the Department of Veterans Affairs, nearly 65 percent of men over age fifty at the time of the survey served either in World War II or the Korean War. More than half of those in World War II and more than a third of those in the Korean War experienced combat. Several studies have revealed that the presence of PTSD in elderly combat veterans is relatively low, but somewhat higher in veterans of the Korean War than in veterans of World War II. A probable reason for the difference is the greater unpopularity of the Korean War and the general lack of recognition given to veterans of that war, relative to veterans of World War II (and even the Vietnam War).

PTSD is treatable with appropriate psychological and medical therapies.

The drug propranolol has been tested as a means of reducing the stress symptoms of memories of traumatic events. Early studies with a small number of participants with PTSD have been encouraging.

A related issue concerns the effects of the disruption of an individual's life by entry into military service. Unique to World War II was the upper age limit of the draft (the upper thirties) than in other wars. Researchers at the Carolina Population Center found that older men in their study's sample have had a greater risk of physical health problems than men who entered military service at a much younger age. The researchers attributed the effect of age at entry to the greater disruption of their social and occupational lives for the older men than for the younger men. Consequently, distress and its negative effects on health after service were likely to be greater for the men who were older at the time of entry. *See also* Natural Disasters (Distress Experiences).

Postural Change and Orthostasis

Orthostasis refers to the rapid decline in blood pressure that occurs when there is a rapid change in body position from a supine (lying) to an erect posture or even from a sitting to an erect position. Most people have experienced one of the possible consequences of orthostasis, at least occasionally, in the form of light-headedness when they stand up rapidly from a sitting or reclining position.

Normal changes with aging in arterial flexibility and in the nervous system make the reflexive raising of blood pressure during a position shift especially difficult for older people. The risk of fainting from orthostasis is therefore greater than it is among younger people. Physicians commonly recommend that elderly people who are prone to more severe declines in blood pressure after standing avoid diuretics as much as possible and wear support hose. Researchers at the University of California at Los Angeles discovered that some elderly people may be trained to use behavioral techniques as a means of preventing severe blood pressure declines during orthostasis. The techniques involved in their study were either squeezing a handgrip device or performing a mental arithmetic task (summing numbers). The mental arithmetic task was found to be somewhat more effective than the handgrip task. As noted by the researchers, physicians should be alerted to the potential positive effects of these behavioral techniques and be prepared to train their elderly patients to use them, especially those patients who are vulnerable to orthostatic hypotension.

Fainting may also occur among older adults for reasons other than simple orthostasis, particularly for nervous system dysfunctions of unknown origin. Such dysfunctions are fairly common and are considered benign. Usually recovery from fainting begins quickly after the person falls to the floor, and consciousness is regained after a brief period. Elderly persons are advised by physicians to sit or recline at the first sign of dizziness. They may avoid the loss of consciousness by doing so. Frequent changes of body positions are believed to reduce the chances of fainting. Of course, elderly people who experience episodes of fainting should seek medical evaluation to determine whether a more serious medical problem is causing the fainting. *See also* Dizziness.

Posture

The control of body posture, as revealed by swaying while standing up, decreases with aging. The decline in postural control is sufficient to be a contributing factor to the high incidence of falls experienced by elderly people (*see* Falls). Researchers in Australia demonstrated that the degree of swaying while standing on a firm surface is associated with the amount of sensory information received by the brain from the lower legs (proprioceptive stimulation), especially the ankles. The age-related decline in visual functioning and inner ear (vestibular) functioning appears to play only a minor role in determining the degree of swaying.

It is a different matter, however, if the elderly person is standing on a less firm surface. In such cases, the amount of sensory information from the lower legs is reduced, and the degree of swaying is associated largely with the elderly person's visual proficiency and muscular strength in the lower legs. Canadian researchers found that elderly people require a greater amount of attention directed to balance needed for different postural tasks than do younger people. In addition, British researchers found that postural stability for elderly people is adversely affected when they are performing tasks that place a heavy demand on their working memory (*see* Working Memory). Elderly people should seek physical support of some kind when standing on less than firm surfaces (and to be on the safe side, even when standing on firm surfaces). This is especially true for those with poor vision and diminished muscular strength.

Try balancing on one foot for a minute or two. It is not easy. Now try doing it while you are reciting the alphabet. The difficulty has increased somewhat. Finally, try it while again reciting the alphabet, but this time backward. Now the difficulty increases considerably, especially if you are an older adult.

Cognitive or mental processes play an important role in controlling our posture and balance. Our cognitive resources, however, diminish somewhat as we grow older. The processes needed for controlling standing on one foot are challenged somewhat when you perform another cognitive task at the same time. The challenge increases as the complexity of the concurrent task increases. In this case, the concurrent task is reciting the alphabet either forward or backward. Older adults should not be thinking of some complex event while trying to walk on an icy sidewalk.

There is a new method of teaching postural control that is called the

Alexander Technique (AT). It employs a repatterning of coordination to improve the body's mechanics. Researchers at the University of Georgia found that eight 1-hour biweekly sessions of AT instruction improved balance and reduced the risk of falls for normally aging older women.

Practical Intelligence

Practical intelligence refers to the ability to solve everyday problems, and thus differs from the traditional view of intelligence as a set of abilities largely related to academic success. An important component of practical intelligence is what Dr. Robert J. Sternberg, a leading researcher in the area of practical intelligence, calls tacit knowledge. It is the kind of practical know-how that one acquires on the job or in everyday kinds of situations, and not from academic instruction. Once tacit knowledge is applied to skilled performance on a job, it is commonly called expertise (*see* Expertise). Unlike traditional intelligence, practical intelligence may be expected to grow with age, as experiences increase with age.

An example of evidence for the importance of practical intelligence comes from a study of Brazilian bank managers. They were given both traditional tests of intelligence and a test of tacit knowledge (for example, knowledge of how to motivate employees to increase their productivity). Older managers had lower scores than younger managers on standard intelligence tests, but higher scores on the tacit knowledge test. The highest scores on the tacit knowledge test were earned by older managers who also had the highest job-performance ratings.

Primary Mental Abilities (PMA) Test

The Primary Mental Abilities (PMA) Test is a widely used group intelligence test in research on adult age differences in intelligence. It is the test used in the Seattle Longitudinal Study (*see* Longitudinal Studies of Aging's Effects on Health and Cognition), and it has been the major source of information about longitudinal changes in intelligence as measured by a standardized test.

The PMA was introduced in 1941 as a test of seven different factors or primary components of intelligence. The original seven factors were number, word fluency, verbal meaning, memory, reasoning, space, and perceptual speed. Eventually the test was reduced to measuring only five factors: number (numerical ability), word fluency, verbal meaning (vocabulary), reasoning, and space (spatial ability). A total score may be obtained from all five separate tests, as may separate scores for each of the five components. Cross-sectional studies generally indicate substantial decline in total test scores from early to late adulthood. The decline has been much less when the longitudinal method has been used. However, the extent of the decline varies greatly across the five separate abilities being measured. The age-related decline is slight for the number, verbal-meaning, and word-fluency components, and, in general, is found only after age sixty. The decline is fairly large for the reasoning and space components and occurs before age sixty.

Prisoners (Elderly)

All parts of the United States are graying, including its prisons. As you probably realize, many of the older prisoners (age fifty and older) are people who committed serious crimes years ago and are serving either a life sentence or a very long-term sentence. However, 45 percent of the prisoners age fifty and older are in prison for recent serious crimes, such as rape and murder. The fact that health problems increase with age creates a financial problem for prisons. Especially a problem is those prisoners who have reached late adulthood. They receive health care that is better than the health care received by elderly people who are not in prison. As a result, it costs about three times more to keep them in prison than it does to keep younger people in prison (about sixty-five thousand dollars a year).

Problem Solving

Your car will not start, and you are trying to figure out why. This is an example of a problem (the car will not start) and *problem-solving behavior* (figuring out why). The problem solver has a goal in mind: coming up with a solution to some situation for which there is no immediate correct behavior.

Laboratory research with rather abstract problems, such as problems involving a variation of the old "twenty questions" game, has typically revealed that older participants have greater difficulty in finding appropriate solutions than do younger participants. On the twenty-questions task, the participant's goal is to discover the object the investigator has in mind among a series of pictures of objects in plain view (for example, a picture of a hammer, a cup, a cow, a child, and so on). The participant is allowed to ask questions that may be answered only by a yes or a no. On average, elderly participants tend to ask fewer constraining questions of the kind "Is it living?" than do younger participants. A constraining question is one that by its yes or no answer immediately eliminates a number of objects from consideration as the one to discover. As a result, older participants generally average more questions to find the solution than do younger participants. However, with practice and training, elderly participants are found to approximate the level of performance of younger participants.

Of greater importance to our understanding of age differences in problem-solving proficiency are those studies by Dr. Nancy Denney in which participants are presented with everyday problems and are asked what they would do in these situations. For example, "You come home late at night and discover that your front door is unlocked and opened somewhat. You are surprised because you know you locked the door when you left home. What should you do?" The quality of solutions to problems of this kind has been found to be the highest for people in their forties. Older participants typically score only moderately below the level of middle-aged participants and as well as young adult participants.

Moderate age differences favoring younger participants have been found on a test of practical problem solving devised by Dr. Sherry Willis and her colleagues at Pennsylvania State University. The test asks for solutions to problems in three different domains: food preparation, medication intake, and telephone use. Interestingly, elderly adults who score high on traditional intelligence tests also tend to score high on this practical problem-solving test.

Moreover, when the problems given to participants are ones dealing with interpersonal relations, problem-solving proficiency has been found to increase progressively from early to late adulthood. That is, the most effective solutions are those offered by elderly adults. This is the kind of problem solving generally associated with the concept of wisdom (*see* Wisdom).

For normally aging individuals, there is no reason to believe that their everyday problem-solving ability decreases markedly from what it was earlier in life. In fact, with the experience they accumulate during a lifetime of confronting problems, they may even gain in proficiency for some kinds of everyday problems.

It is a different matter, however, when very unique solutions or highly creative solutions to problems are required. Here, there is evidence of declining ability with normal aging (*see* Creativity; Originality). *See also* Practical Intelligence.

Problems Perceived by Elderly People

Americans in the eighteen-to-sixty-four age range are more likely to overestimate the frequency and seriousness of the problems facing people age sixty-five and older than are elderly people themselves. For example, in a major survey 64 percent of those in the eighteen-to-sixty-four age range perceived insufficient money to be a serious problem for people age sixty-five and older, compared to 55 percent of those age sixty-five and older. Similarly, 61 percent in the younger age range, compared to 43 percent in the older age range, perceived insufficient medical care to be a serious problem for those people age sixty-five and older. The percentages perceiving not feeling needed to be a serious problem for people age sixty-five and older were 57 percent and 43 percent for participants in the two age ranges.

Problems Physicians Have with Older Patients

Older adults (age sixty-five and older) account for 30 percent to 40 percent of the visits to primary care physicians. However, many internists and family physicians are unwilling or unable to serve older patients. There are several reasons many primary care physicians are reluctant to take on older adults as patients. Well recognized is the frustration they often experience in dealing with the fees and documentation requirements established by Medicare. However, this is only the tip of the iceberg, as revealed by researchers at the University of Nebraska Medical Center.

They conducted in-depth interviews with ten internists and ten family physicians who ranged in age from thirty-two to seventy. The physicians were asked to describe the frustrating experiences they had with older patients. A major problem was simply the fact that older patients are more difficult to care for than are younger patients. Many older patients have chronic health problems that cannot be cured. Added to the problem was the fear that the medications the physicians prescribed could have adverse side effects.

Another problem the physicians had was communicating with many older patients. Some older patients have hearing impairments that make it difficult for them to understand instructions and advice. Older patients should bring with them friends or relatives who can participate in discussions with their physicians.

The physicians also reported that their Medicare claims are often denied for trivial reasons. They also questioned the practice of Medicare in reimbursing them.

Progeria

Progeria is a rare, fatal childhood disease that is characterized by a precocious senility of a severe degree. An eight-year-old child with the disease is likely to have the physical appearance and the bodily functioning of an eighty-year-old person. The child is likely to be susceptible to heart attacks and arthritis as the disease progresses. However, other diseases associated with aging, such as cancer, are usually absent. The cause of the disease is unknown, and there is presently no known cure. Werner syndrome is also a disease characterized by premature aging and early death,

Prospective Memory

Memory research has typically concentrated on what may be called *retrospective memory* (memory for past things and events). Consequently, we know a great deal about what happens to retrospective memory as people age (*see* Episodic Memory and other memory-related entries). In the everyday world, however, there is another form of memory that plays an important role in our everyday lives. Our failure in executing this form of memory is often referred to as "absentmindedness." To psychologists, however, the failures involve what they term *prospective memory*.

Prospective memory requires performing some action at an appropriate time. For example, we intend to stop at the market on the way home from work, to drop a letter in the mailbox as we pass it on the street, to take prescribed medicine at designated times, and so on. However, we often discover that we forgot to stop at the market and must do without coffee the next morning, that the letter to be mailed is still at home, and that the night has gone by without our having taken the medicine. One of the more famous lapses of prospective memory occurred some years ago when a prominent professional golfer forgot to sign his card after completing a round at a major tournament, a lapse that cost him winning the tournament (and much money). Prospective memory, like retrospective memory, is obviously imperfect. Our interest is in the extent to which its imperfection increases during late adulthood.

Testing for age differences in the proficiency of prospective memory requires giving young and older adults a series of tasks to perform, each at some designated time. One way of accomplishing this is to send research participants home from the laboratory with a number of postcards. The first card is to be mailed to the investigator on the following Tuesday, the second on the next Friday, the third on the following Monday, and so on. How many times will they remember to mail the card at the right time? Alternatively, participants may be asked to call the investigator at designated times over several weeks. With either procedure, the results have been rather surprising. Elderly adults return the cards or make the calls at the right times more often than do young adults.

Researchers in Australia compared young adult, young-old (sixty to sixty-nine years), and old-old (eighty to ninety-two years) on several different naturalistic prospective memory tasks (for example, pressing a button on a time-logging device at set regular times over a week). On each task the older participants at each level demonstrated superior prospective memory relative to the young participants.

There is a problem, however, in concluding from this evidence that prospective memory proficiency, unlike proficiency for most forms of retrospective memory, actually increases from early to late adulthood. The problem stems from the possibility that elderly adults are more motivated to conform to the request of the investigator than are young adults (typically college students) in research of this kind. In fact, the evidence indicates that when young adults fail to perform the action it is not always because they did not remember to do it. Instead, when they remembered, they were often preoccupied with some other activity and did not want to interrupt it. However, the Australian researchers concluded from their evidence that age difference in motivation was an unlikely contributor to the age difference in prospective memory proficiency favoring older adults (the two older groups did not differ from one another in prospective memory proficiency).

There is laboratory evidence to support further the possibility that one form of prospective memory, called *event-based prospective memory* by memory researchers, does not decline greatly with normal aging (that is, the number of their prospective memory failures for seniors is no greater than that for the young adults). The implication is that prospective memory proficiency is not greatly affected by normal aging. However, if there is a delay before the requested action is to be performed, older participants show a greater failure to remember to perform the action than do the younger participants.

This form of prospective memory occurs when there is some kind of external event present to serve as a reminder to perform the designated activity. There is another form of prospective memory, *time-based prospective memory*, in which the designated activity is not cued by some physically present event. Here, the activity is to be performed at some designated time, such as keeping a ten o'clock appointment with a physician or taking a medication at the correct time. Laboratory evidence indicates a moderate decline with normal aging for this form of prospective memory. Here, the requested action is to be performed at a certain time while performing on a task of some kind. The magnitude of the age-related deficit is greater while performing complex tasks than while performing simpler tasks.

Adults of all ages should be aware of the imperfection of prospective memory and take steps to avoid its failures. One obvious way is to make external cues available to help you remember what you need to do. This is the technique represented by the old gimmick of tying a string on your finger. The problem, however, is that you may no longer remember what action is to be performed.

A more effective technique is to make clearly visible a cue that is more directly related to the action itself. Thus, why not place the empty instant coffee jar on the front seat of your car when you need to buy more coffee? The sight of the jar on the way home from work that evening should remind you of the need to stop at the store. Such reminding cues are especially important for older adults. They are more likely to need prescribed medicines than are younger adults. Failure to conform to a prescribed regimen could have a serious outcome; thus, it is very important that they should not be forced to rely on their prospective memories without environmental support. Fortunately, pharmaceutical companies are becoming increasingly aware of this problem, and they are introducing aids to ensure conformity to a prescribed schedule (*see* Medication Compliance and Comprehension).

Prostate Cancer

Cancer of the *prostate gland* (*see* Prostate Gland), of course, is found only in men. It is the most frequently diagnosed cancer among men (230,000 North American men are diagnosed annually with the disease) and the second-leading cause of death from cancer (30,000 deaths annually; lung cancer is first). It usually occurs after age sixty-five. About two-thirds of the deaths from the disease are for men age seventy-five and older. Prominent older men who died from it recently include Don Ameche and Telly Savalas. Among those treated recently for it is Joe Torre of the New York Yankees. African Americans are two times more likely to die from it than are other American men.

Possible signs of prostate cancer include weak or interrupted flow of urine, frequent urination (especially at night), difficulty urinating, painful urinating, blood in the urine or semen, and pain in the back, hips, or pelvis that does not go away.

Initial diagnosis of the disease is by a digital rectal exam feeling for lumps or an abnormal area on the prostate gland and by a blood test for a protein known as PSA (prostate-specific antigen). The PSA has been found to be more effective in early detection than the digital rectal examination alone. About 30 percent of men who have a biopsy after a mildly elevated PSA test are found to have prostate cancer. However, many men who tested positively do not have prostate cancer, and many men who tested negatively do have the cancer. The continued use of the test for early diagnosis of prostate cancer is a hotly debated topic among health experts.

An elevated PSA level in the blood may be the result of an infection or inflammation of the prostate gland rather than the result of cancer. An elevated PSA level may call for the use of a transrectal ultrasound endoscope. It is a thin, lighted tube that is inserted into the rectum that bounces high energy sound waves off the internal tissues of the gland. The echoes make a picture (called a sonogram) of the tissues to aid in identifying cancerous cells.

For men who have the disease in an early low-grade stage, no treatment seems to be nearly as effective as treatment by surgical removal or radiation. In a study reported in the *New England Journal of Medicine* men in the early stage who had no treatment, but whose disease was carefully monitored, were nearly as likely to be alive after ten years (about 87 percent) as were other men who received treatment in the early stage (about 93 percent).

When the cancer is in an advanced or late stage, treatment by surgery or radiation is likely. One form of surgery is a radical prostatectomy in which the entire prostate gland and surrounding tissue are removed. Advances made in this procedure have made it possible for some men to have penile erections after the surgery. A survey of more than twelve hundred men who had the surgery within six months of being diagnosed with prostate cancer revealed that those over age seventy, 42 percent recovered sexual functioning if only a few nerves were destroyed in the surgery. Incontinence for several weeks is likely to occur following the surgery, and it may last for a much longer period for some patients.

Another form of surgery is a transurethral resection in which the cancer is removed from the prostate, but the entire prostate is not removed. Radiation is usually used when the cancer is in more than one area of the body. Impotence may be a consequence of the therapy. Hormone therapy may be used when the cancer has become widespread.

For men who have had surgery, a rising PSA level indicates some tumor cells remain and are growing. However, prostate cancer grows so slowly that the patient may die from something else before the prostate cancer causes his death. Undoubtedly, men who have had surgery or radiation therapy for prostate cancer should have regular PSA tests and regular visits to their oncologist.

There is evidence to indicate that diet may slow or possibly stop the growth of early prostate cancer (*see also* Nutrition and Diet; Tomatoes). Men who eat cooked tomato-based products tend to have lower rates of prostate cancer than men who do not. The benefit comes from pasta sauces, tomato juice, raw tomatoes, canned tomatoes, and tomatoes baked in pizza. A study by researchers at the Harvard School of Public Health found that men who had ten or more servings a week had a 45 percent reduction in the incidence of prostate cancer. Those who ate only four to seven servings had a 20 percent reduction. Tomatoes are rich in an antioxidant called lycopene. Daily doses of lycopene may have the same protection value as the consumption of tomato-based foods.

Especially important is that high-fat diets should be avoided. There is also evidence that exercising more frequently, even in moderation, may help to slow down growth of an early cancer. Interestingly, there is evidence indicating that men who have a high exposure to the sun have half the risk of prostate cancer than men who spend most of their time indoors. The vitamin D that the body makes with exposure to the sun helps prostate cells remain normal.

Prostate Gland

The prostate gland is a walnut-sized structure that is located just below the urinary bladder and through which the urethra passes. The prostate gland secretes a substance that aids the flow of sperm. The gland increases in size in older men (known as *benign prostatic hyperplasia [BPH]*), and it may eventually press against the urethra, hindering the passage of urine. About two-thirds of American men suffer from enlargement of the prostate gland by the time they reach their sixties. Men with an enlarged gland may not be aware of it for ten to fifteen years. A more serious problem is the risk of prostate cancer, especially in older men.

Men often seek treatment for BPH at age sixty to sixty-five after experiencing problems with urination. The two most troublesome symptoms are nocturia (getting up at night to urinate) and inability to stop urinating when desired. About 80 percent of men with BPH either do not need treatment or their symptoms are relieved by drugs. Prescription drugs include Flomax and Cardura. The drug Proscar inhibits the sex hormone testosterone and may shrink the prostate gland.

Surgery, if needed, consists of cutting away excess tissue. A less invasive procedure is laser treatment in which the laser goes through the urethra to the inside of the prostate gland, destroying an area of the gland. A new treatment is Targis microwave therapy that does not require anesthesia or sutures. It may be used on men who are at high risk for surgery (for example, those with lung disease). *See also* Prostate Cancer; Sexual Behavior.

Proverbs (Interpretation)

"Don't cry over spilt milk." "A stitch in time saves nine." These are examples of familiar proverbs. A proverb offers a concrete analogy for a more general set of circumstances that the interpreter attempts to describe (for example, "Once something is over, there is nothing you can do to change things" as an interpretation of the "Don't cry over spilt milk" proverb). Interpreting the meaning of a proverb requires a form of reasoning (*see* Reasoning).

A test of adult age differences in the ability to reason through the analogy between a proverb and its meaning in everyday life requires the use of proverbs that are unfamiliar to participants of all ages. There is only limited evidence of age differences in this reasoning ability. The results of several studies indicated a moderate age difference in the ability to interpret such proverbs, with older adults giving more literal interpretations than younger adults.

This outcome is surprising in that older adults are usually found to be at least as proficient as younger adults in the adequacy of the interpretations of metaphors. Interpreting a metaphor seemingly requires the same kind of reasoning through analogy required in interpreting proverbs (*see* Metaphors). However, the evidence on age difference in proverb interpretation comes only from cross-sectional studies. The extent to which the age difference is the result of a cohort or generational effect (*see* Cohort [Generational] Effect) is unknown. It is possible that members of earlier generations simply give more literal interpretations of proverbs than do members of later generations.

Psychosis

A psychosis is a severe mental disorder that greatly impairs the individual affected by it. The two most common psychoses are schizophrenia and clinical depression.

The major symptom of schizophrenia is a thought disturbance characterized by intrusions of irrelevant, and often bizarre, thoughts when the disorder is in an active state. There are other symptoms that are present in different forms of schizophrenia. They include a flattened emotional state in one form and a heightened "silly" state in another form and hallucinations in still another form. Schizophrenia, regardless of its specific form and symptoms, usually has its onset in early adulthood. The incidence of its onset in late adulthood is quite low.

Of great interest is what happens to long-term schizophrenics as they age. It is estimated that there are about three hundred thousand people age sixty-five and older in the United States who have schizophrenia. In general, the symptoms found earlier in the lives of schizophrenics become less pronounced during late adulthood.

There is, however, a form of schizophrenia known as late-onset schizophrenia. The onset is usually between the ages of forty-five and sixty, and more often for women than for men. The symptoms are more likely to be paranoid delusions than hallucinations. There is usually less apathy and cognitive impairment than in earlier-onset schizophrenia. There may also be reclusiveness and social isolation.

Clinical depression is an intense and persistent state that greatly hinders everyday functioning (*see* Depression [Incidence, Symptoms, Causes]). Like schizophrenia, it is uncommon for clinical depression to have its onset in late adulthood. In general, when clinical depression does occur in late adulthood, its symptoms differ somewhat from the symptoms present earlier in adulthood. Affective symptoms (feelings of sadness, despair, and hopelessness) are likely to be less intense for elderly depressed individuals than for younger individuals, whereas the reverse is true for somatic symptoms (complaints about physical functioning, such as sleep disturbances). Clinical depression may occur along with mania (excessive exaggerated behaviors) in what is known as a *bipolar psychosis.*

A less frequent form of psychosis is paranoia. It is characterized by a persisting and dominating false belief, often one in which the affected individual believes he or she is being persecuted and that other people are "out to get me." The delusion is likely to lead to very bizarre behaviors and suspicious attitudes about events and persons in the individual's world. As is true of schizophrenia, the onset of paranoia among elderly people who are aging normally is rare (less than 1 percent). However, it is not unusual to find individuals with Alzheimer's disease who have major symptoms of paranoia.

Milder forms of paranoic symptoms may be a bit more common. According to a survey conducted in North Carolina, they are present in about 10 percent of the elderly population. The symptoms include the belief that people are unfriendly and that they dislike the individual affected by the belief. The researchers in North Carolina found the symptoms to be associated with being African American, having a low income, having less education, and being depressed. For African Americans, the symptoms may represent an appropriate response to a hostile environment rather than to any kind of psychopathology.

Psychotherapy

Emotional and behavioral problems occur for adults of all ages. One form of treatment of these problems for aging adults is psychotherapy. Psychotherapy has many different forms, and the appropriate form depends on the nature of the problem to be treated.

One form of psychotherapy is called *behavior modification*. It consists of the application of either classical-conditioning learning principles or operant-conditioning learning principles (*see* Classical Conditioning; Operant Conditioning) to modify a specific or habitual behavior of an individual.

Classical conditioning enters into several specific forms of behavior modification. One form is called *aversion therapy;* another is *systematic desensitization.* Aversion therapy has been used to treat bad health practices such as excessive drinking of alcoholic beverages and smoking. The objective of the treatment is to condition an aversive reaction to what had been previously a regular behavior of the client (that is, drinking or smoking). For drinking, tasting an alcoholic beverage is accompanied by the intake of a drug to induce severe nausea. The idea is to form a conditioned reaction of nausea to the taste of the beverage. For smoking, the client is forced to smoke one cigarette after another until nausea results. The idea is to associate smoking with nausea.

Systematic desensitization is used in the treatment of phobias (intense fears provoked by specific objects, such as a snake, or conditions, such as being in an enclosed area [claustrophobia]). During the treatment the client is first taught to relax as much as possible. In later sessions with the therapist, the client is gradually introduced to the phobic object or condition while in a relaxed state. The objective is to condition a feeling of relaxation to the phobic object or condition to replace the feeling of intense fear.

Classical conditioning has also been used in some cases of intense hypertension. The client is placed under physical conditions (for example, listening to soft music in a darkened room) that lead to lowering of blood pressure. At the same time a conditioned stimulus (for example, the sounding of a bell) is present. There is evidence of successful treatment of at least some younger adults with these forms of behavior modification. However, evidence regarding successful treatment with older adults is sparse. Such methods may not work well with elderly clients. Elderly people are much slower in acquiring conditioned responses in the laboratory than are younger people (*see* Classical Conditioning), and in each of these forms of behavior modification the acquisition of a conditioned response is essential to the success of the therapy.

Operant conditioning is often used in behavior management to aid an individual to rid himself or herself of an unwanted and unhealthy habit, such as excessive eating or smoking. The objective of behavior modification with obese individuals is to help them control their weight through changes in basic eating habits. For example, they are trained to avoid eating while engaged in some other activity, such as watching television, when eating has become automatic for most obese people. The objective of behavior modification with smokers is to help them control their smoking through changes in their smoking habits. For example, they may be trained to reinforce or reward themselves (for example, a trip to a mall) whenever they go through a period of nonsmoking or to find substitutes for smoking (for example, taking a walk instead of smoking). These methods work for some individuals, but not for all. In addition, relapses (returning to the old habits) do occur. Nevertheless, the success rate should be as high for older adults as it is for younger adults.

Unlike classical conditioning, operant conditioning has been found to be well within the capacity of elderly adults. A unique form of behavior modification is through the use of *biofeedback*. Biofeedback consists of information that informs a client that a change has taken place in some physiological function. For example, brain waves may be monitored, with the client receiving feedback every time their frequency has increased. Elderly adults have been found to increase their brain-wave frequencies through this method. Most important, those who have been successful often show an improvement in their reaction time or speed of responding.

Other forms of psychotherapy are designed to help clients handle their emotional problems and to enhance their feelings about themselves, rather than to change their observable behaviors. The oldest, and best-known form, is *psychoanalytic therapy*. The objective is to enable clients to discover and deal with their unconscious guilts, impulses, and conflicts. The therapy often takes years to complete, and it is expensive. Both of these factors usually make it unavailable to elderly adults. Sigmund Freud, the pioneer psychoanalyst, doubted the success of the therapy with elderly adults, and he himself treated few patients as old as the forties and fifties. Some later psychoanalysts have questioned the inapplicability of their therapy for older clients, but there is little evidence to indicate its successful application.

It is through their efforts, however, that the technique of allowing elderly clients to reminisce about their past lives and review their major life events has been incorporated into various other forms of psychotherapy (for example, group therapy; *see* Reminiscence).

One currently popular and more successful form of psychotherapy is called *cognitive therapy*. Cognitive therapists believe that the way an individual thinks largely determines how that person feels. The therapist then helps the client to alter his or her maladaptive thinking habits. The technique is frequently used to treat such emotional disturbances as depression, anxiety, and hostility. Like other forms of therapy, the treatment is not always successful, and even when it is, clients may return to their old maladaptive ways of thinking about themselves. However, the success rate does seem to be about as high for elderly clients as it is for younger clients.

Older adults often think of themselves in ways that are inaccurate (for example, that they have become totally incompetent), thus making them ideal clients for cognitive therapy. Researchers at Stanford University found that elderly adults have lower relapse rates following cognitive therapy than do younger adults. They also found that cognitive therapy may actually work about as well alone as it does combined with drugs. This is especially important for elderly adults who have serious side effects with drugs used to treat depression.

Another currently popular form of psychotherapy is *family therapy*. It is useful when one or more elderly people are members of a dysfunctional family. The family is regarded by family therapists as being a system in which the members mutually influence one another. If the behavior of one member of the system could be changed, then the behavior of other members should change as well.

The treatment is useful for families in which there is a conflict between elderly spouses (for example, over one spouse's physical disability) or a conflict between older parents and their adult children (for example, over the child-rearing practices of the adult children with their own children; *see* Parent-Child Conflicts). The treatment stresses more effective communication among family members so that each member may express more clearly his or her feelings and concerns. The therapy seems to be effective for many older adults. It is also a form of therapy that may greatly benefit caregivers of physically or mentally disabled elderly adults (see entries involving caregivers).

Group therapy has long been used with older clients. It may take several different forms. In life discussion groups, members discuss their own problems, enabling elderly people to discover that they are not alone in their problems. The groups are usually smaller in size, and the durations of the discussions are shorter than when the groups are composed of younger adults. Group therapy is especially valuable as an alternative to cognitive therapy in the treatment of depression. It may be given in various settings, including hospitals, community mental health centers, and even senior centers and retirement communities.

Unfortunately, elderly adults are less likely to benefit from psychotherapy than are younger adults, simply because they are less likely to seek help when they are confronted by behavioral and emotional problems than are younger adults (*see* Mental Health and Mental Health Services). Efforts have increased in recent years to familiarize elderly adults with mental health services through radio and television commercials. This effort would be even more successful if there were more television programs, both dramas and documentaries, that centered on the emotional problems of older adults and the ways they may be treated successfully.

Psychotherapy with Nursing Home Residents

Nursing home residents are commonly found to be apathetic and disoriented and to have feelings of isolation. Their behavioral and emotional problems have required psychotherapies that differ greatly from those used among community-dwelling elderly adults. A number of such therapies have been introduced in recent years, and they have generally been found to be fairly successful in increasing the well-being of nursing home residents.

One form of treatment is called *reality orientation*. Its objective is to keep residents in touch with the world. To accomplish this, numerous clocks are placed in the nursing home, and calendars are located in prominent places. Name cards are used to identify each other at meals, birthdays of residents are individually recognized, visiting hours are made as liberal as possible, and independence is stressed as much as possible. To aid in orientation, halls and residential rooms are often painted in different colors.

Remotivation therapy is intended for residents who seem understimulated in their current environments. Basically, it is a form of group therapy (*see* Psychotherapy) in which small groups of residents meet to discuss shared topics of interest, such as food and clothing. The idea is to create a climate in which the residents may appreciate the contributions of the other residents. Group therapy may also include activities performed in groups, such as singing, playing bingo, and so on, that help to decrease the feelings of social isolation.

Sensory training is a form of therapy for those older residents who are highly disoriented and unlikely to benefit from other forms of treatment. The residents are given body awareness exercises and sensory stimulation by observing, touching, smelling, and sometimes tasting common objects.

Some residents with mild mental impairment who are also affected by depression have benefited from some form of cognitive therapy for their depression (*see* Psychotherapy). The therapy does not alter the mental impairment, but it does enable the resident to make fuller use of his or her mental abilities. The resident's diminished mental functioning is otherwise limited to an even greater degree by the debilitating effects of depression.

Behavior modification through the use of positive reinforcement (that is, rewarding specific behaviors to increase their frequency of occurrence; *see* Operant Conditioning; Psychotherapy) has been found to be successful in some cases in increasing such behaviors as participation in rehabilitative and recreational behaviors and in increasing self-care and social behaviors. Some institutionalized older people exhibit excessive aggressive behavior that may be harmful to both themselves and other residents. The positive reinforcement of nonaggressive verbal behaviors by following their occurrences with praise has been found, in combination with other forms of treatment, to lead to a decrease in verbally aggressive behaviors for some patients (*see also* Agitative Behaviors).

Public Assistance

Public assistance, or welfare, is offered for older adults by various governmental agencies and programs or by other public or charitable organizations. It is intended to improve the lives of older people who are living on a substandard income.

Does it necessarily improve the lives of older people who receive welfare of some kind? To some older people there is a stigma associated with welfare. Receiving it could lower their self-esteem or feeling of self-worth. It could also be perceived as a detriment to their beloved independence. Researchers at the University of Michigan found that older men, but not older women, did indeed have lower self-esteem if they enrolled in a welfare program.

In addition, public assistance may reduce the informal social support the recipients receive from family and friends. The researchers at Michigan found that diminished informal support for older men, but not for older women, did tend to occur after receiving formal public support. Older women who received welfare benefits actually received more informal support from family and friends than did older women without welfare benefits. Thus, welfare programs have both benefits and costs, especially for older men.

Public School Support

Seniors have long had the reputation of opposing increases in public school taxes. This has been known as "the gray peril." However, in recent years seniors have, in general, been quite supportive of educational spending. In 1973, 51 percent of seniors believed that educational spending was too low. In 2002 the percentage had increased to 74 percent. Researchers at Pennsylvania State University discovered that their analyses of per-pupil spending revealed that communities with very high concentration of seniors do not spend appreciably less on schools than other communities. They actually spend slightly more.

Q

Quackery

Elderly adults are the most likely victims of medical quackery and fraud. It is estimated that they make up as much as 60 percent of such victims. Billions of dollars are spent every year on so-called remedies that not only are unhelpful to their users but may actually be harmful to their health. People with arthritis are among the most frequent victims; many bogus remedies have been introduced over the years. Patients should check with their physician before purchasing some advertised remedy.

R

Racial and Ethnic Differences in Aging

Although there is some disagreement as to what defines a race or an ethnic group, the term *race* is widely used in our society, especially in reference to what are considered to be minority races. Our concern is with the possibility that aging may have different effects on members of minority racial and ethnic groups than on whites. The reason for this possibility is one that has little, if anything, to do with inherent biological differences among races. Instead, the possibility arises from the fact that proportionally more members of minority groups live in impoverished neighborhoods, have lower economic resources, and have fewer cultural and educational opportunities than do the white members of our society. These factors expose many more minority members than majority members to high-risk health conditions and to less utilization of health care facilities.

Not surprisingly, life expectancy at birth is five years less for African Americans than for whites. This difference is related to the higher mortality rates for African Americans than for whites at all ages except very late adulthood. Even African Americans who are in good health earlier in life show greater decline in health with aging than do whites of equal early health. At about eighty or eighty-five years of age there is a crossover effect in mortality rates: African Americans at this age and older on average live as many, and perhaps more, additional years than do whites. This is true even though disability and morbidity are significantly greater for elderly African Americans than for elderly whites, as indicated, for example, by the greater number of average annual sick days experienced by elderly African Americans.

Most important, the incidence of heart disease is significantly higher among elderly African Americans than among elderly whites (although there has been a striking reduction in the presence of hypertension among elderly African Americans in recent years). Health statistics indicate that the crossover in mortality rates occurs at a much earlier age for Mexican Americans than it does for African Americans, but the incidence of morbidity or disease is, nevertheless, higher for elderly Mexican Americans than for elderly whites. By contrast, Native Americans have mortality rates comparable to those of whites, and Asian Americans appear to have even lower mortality rates than the general population of elderly people.

Even with similar medical conditions, disabled African Americans are less likely than disabled whites to use prescriptions and physician services. The race difference is unrelated to race differences in financial assets. Makers of public policy need to consider differences between disabled African Americans and whites in the accessibility of such services and in their acceptability.

There is little information about the health care needs of Asian Americans. A popular belief is that they have fewer needs because they tend to be better educated and are better off financially than members of other minority groups. However, their Westernization is likely to increase their health risks as brought about by such customs as eating high-fat fast foods.

The extent of the health problem facing racial and ethnic minorities is clearly visible in the fact that in January 2000 the United States Department of Health and Human Services released its *Healthy People 2010* report. In it this country's health goals for the next decade were identified. The first goal is to increase the years of good health for all people, and the second goal is to eliminate the racial and ethnic disparities in illnesses.

The overall poorer health of elderly African Americans and members of some other minority groups is an outcome predicted by what sociologists call the *double-jeopardy hypothesis*. According to this hypothesis, the negative effects of living for years in an impoverished environment and living under the burden of racism add to the negative effects that accompany normal biological aging for people of all races and therefore amplify the problems experienced by minority group members.

Seemingly in conflict with the double-jeopardy hypothesis is the fact that the incidence of elderly African Americans living in nursing homes is from one-half to three-fourths of that of elderly whites. However, there are reasons other than health that seemingly account for this disparity.

Elderly people who are forced to live alone are the most likely candidates for becoming nursing home residents. Elderly African Americans are less likely to live alone than are elderly whites, and they are therefore less likely to enter nursing homes. Moreover, elderly African American women are more likely to be heads of households than are elderly white women, meaning that they are also more likely to serve as caregivers of family members and less likely to be recipients of caregiving.

However, an analysis of a survey conducted in the late 1980s revealed that elderly African Americans are no more likely than elderly whites to receive instrumental support (for instance, for housekeeping and transportation) and social support from others. In addition, Hispanic elderly people are less likely than elderly white people to receive instrumental support.

The double-jeopardy hypothesis is strongly supported by evidence revealing, on average, a lower level of life satisfaction among elderly African Americans than among elderly whites (*see* Life Satisfaction). Dr. Neal Krause of the University of Michigan, a prominent researcher in the area of life satisfaction, has concluded that the lower level for elderly African Americans is the result of various factors. For example, elderly African Americans often experience a greater gap than do elderly whites between their earlier educational goals and their educational attainment and between their retirement plans and what their economic conditions permit after retirement. In addition, elderly African Americans usually are more dependent on financial assistance from family members than are elderly whites. These factors, combined with the overall poorer health status of elderly African Americans, inevitably lead to lower life satisfaction. Fortunately, these factors can be overcome by greater allocation of our country's health services and financial resources to the needs of elderly minority-group members.

There are other, less obvious, factors that are likely to contribute to the lower level of life satisfaction among elderly African Americans. For example, married elderly people tend to be in better health and to have a higher level of life satisfaction than unmarried elderly people. Elderly married African American women are in a minority (about 25 percent compared with about 41 percent of elderly white women), as are elderly married African American men (about 54 percent compared with about 76 percent of elderly white men). The probability of having a spouse to serve as a caregiver is therefore greater for elderly whites than for elderly African Americans. In addition, the quality of housing remains less satisfactory for elderly African Americans than for elderly whites, even though the quality of housing has increased during the past two decades for both whites and African Americans. A less livable home is likely to make daily living less satisfactory than does a safe and comfortable home.

With one exception, there has been little research on racial differences in mental abilities. The one exception is in the area of intelligence. There is no doubt that African Americans score lower than whites at all age levels, including late adulthood, on traditional academically oriented intelligence tests, such as the Wechsler Adult Intelligence Scale (*see* Wechsler Intelligence Tests). Hispanics tend to score somewhere between African Americans and whites, and Asian Americans often score above whites in late adulthood as well as at younger ages.

Please note that the lower scores by African Americans and Hispanics are exactly that—lower scores on tests that place them at a considerable disadvantage, and certainly not necessarily in intelligence as it concerns coping with problems in the everyday world. In fact, little is known about racial and ethnic differences, if any, in so-called practical intelligence, as distinguished from academically oriented intelligence (*see* Practical Intelligence). Traditional intelligence tests have typically been constructed to predict academic achievement in a white-oriented society. They may, therefore, have little validity for individuals who are outside that society.

Interestingly, the difference in average test scores between whites and African Americans on most traditional intelligence tests is lowest for people of relatively little formal education. It is here that African Americans are least disadvantaged relative to whites of the same educational level. That is, with increasing education, the advantage of whites over African Americans in average intelligence test scores increases progressively. The picture clearly indicates that African Americans receiving the same quantity of education as whites are also receiving less quality of education.

Do the races differ in such basic mental functions as learning and memory? Probably not. There is no reason to expect such differences, except for tasks in which the greater opportunities provided for whites in our society provide them with greater familiarity with the tasks to be mastered. There is, however, no scientific evidence to indicate whether there are real differences among the races in learning and memory abilities—or, for that matter, in reasoning and problem-solving abilities. Researchers rarely report information about the racial composition of participants in their studies of learning, memory, reasoning, and so on. If they did, it is doubtful that any significant racial differences would emerge.

Researchers at the Johns Hopkins School of Medicine found that older African Americans reported more anxiety, restlessness, and thoughts of death than did older whites. Depressive symptoms have been found to be higher for African American women in the age range of fifty-eight to sixty-four years than for white women in the same age range. Elderly African Americans tend to report fewer complaints about sleep than do elderly whites.

African Americans and Hispanics have a higher risk of Alzheimer's disease than do whites. However, African Americans with the disease are less likely than whites with the disease to become residents of nursing homes, with home care being more frequent for African Americans than for whites. In general, African American caregivers of patients with Alzheimer's disease report less depression and perceived burden than do white caregivers. African American caregivers are less likely than white caregivers to be the spouse of the patient, and more likely to be an adult child, friend, or other family member of the patient.

Racial Differences in Functional Decline

African Americans show a greater decline in functional health (the ability to perform basic activities of daily living, such as bathing and toileting) than whites with aging. Researchers at the San Francisco Veterans Affairs Medical Center found evidence linking the racial difference to greater cognitive decline, as measured by such tasks as counting backward from twenty and identifying who are the president and vice president of the United States, by their African American elderly participants than by their white elderly participants. The greater cognitive decline for the elderly African American, in turn, was attributed to the greater frequency of chronic health problems they had relative to the elderly white participants.

Reaction Time

You are the first one in line at a stoplight. As the light turns from red to green, you press down on the accelerator of your car to proceed. How much time elapsed between the appearance of the green light and the movement of your foot on the accelerator? That time is an example of a *reaction time.* Reaction time is the time separating the appearance of a signal and the initiation of a response to that signal. If you are an elderly driver, your reaction time in the stoplight situation is likely to be some seconds slower than if you are a younger driver. The slowing down of reaction time to various sources of stimulation does seem to be an inevitable consequence of normal aging, and it is part of a general slowing of physical and mental activities that accompanies normal aging (*see* Slowing-Down Principle).

Although slower reaction times may be characteristic of older people, in general, the amount of slowing does vary considerably among different elderly people. Reaction time, for example, is one of the abilities affected by long-term regular exercise. Elderly people who have been regular exercisers for many years have been found to have faster reaction times than elderly people who have had less physically active lives. In fact, many regular exercisers have been found to have reaction times that are as fast as many younger adults.

Age differences in reaction time are studied in the laboratory by having participants of various ages perform different kinds of reaction-time tasks. A simple reaction-time task is one in which participants execute a response, such as pressing a button, each time a signal (a tone or a light) occurs. Reaction time on this task increases progressively from young adulthood to late adulthood. The slowing with aging is more pronounced, however, on a choice reaction-time task. Here, two different signals are used, each requiring a different response. For example, when a low-frequency tone is sounded, the participant presses one button; when a high-frequency tone is sounded, the participant presses a different button.

Of great interest in gerontology is whether interventions of some kind (other than long-term physical exercise) can be found that will facilitate an older adult's response to signals (that is, reduce reaction time). There is some limited, but promising, evidence to indicate that such interventions may be possible. Extensive practice on a video game has been found to have a positive effect on reaction time. Elderly participants who played the game for two hours per week for seven weeks had faster choice reaction times on a laboratory task at the end of the practice period than other elderly participants who had received no prior practice on the video game.

Another possible intervention is based on a suspected relationship between the frequency of alpha brain waves and reaction time. Seniors trained through the use of biofeedback (*see* Psychotherapy) to increase the frequency of their alpha waves seem to enhance their reaction times as well.

Reading and Reading Skills

Do adults age sixty-five and older spend more time reading daily than do younger adults? In a recent survey, it was reported that older adults spend an average of seventy-seven minutes reading daily compared to sixty-two minutes for adults age fifty-five to sixty-four and twenty-three minutes for adults age twenty-five to twenty-nine.

Although the evidence is somewhat conflicting, elderly adults, in general, appear to be somewhat slower readers than younger adults. Nevertheless, their reading strategy seems to be similar to that of younger adults. For example, both younger and older readers increase their reading time when they encounter major and minor clauses in sentences.

There do seem to be some moderate adverse effects of aging on the comprehension of paragraphs, but only when the content is fairly complex and requires making inferences of some kind about the events being described. When reading material is of sufficient difficulty, the age difference in comprehension favoring younger adults is greatly decreased when the material is preceded by what are called *advance organizers*. In addition, elderly readers may compensate for whatever comprehension problem they have by breaking down the text into smaller units and by taking advantage of their general superiority in knowledge. However, most reading material is not of sufficient difficulty to present any real problem to older readers. *See also* Lexicon.

Reasoning

Through reasoning we are able to draw valid conclusions from facts that either are known to be true or are assumed to be true. A reasoning problem is one in which logical relationships between events are given and a solution based on these relationships is sought.

A common laboratory task used to study age differences in reasoning ability involves problems called syllogisms. A syllogism is an argument composed of two (or more) premises or assertions. From those premises, a logical conclusion is to be derived. Consider, for example, two premises: all psychologists are scientists, and all scientists are computer experts. Now consider the conclusion that "All psychologists are therefore computer experts." Is it true or false, based only on the information given in the two premises? (Assume the premises to be true, even though they are not.) A correct conclusion in this case is "true." In general, older participants perform at a lower level on syllogism problems than do younger participants.

Comparable outcomes (that is, lower scores by older than by younger participants) have been found for other tasks that evaluate other forms of reasoning, such as *functional reasoning* or reasoning through the use of analogy and *inferential reasoning*. Functional reasoning is the kind of reasoning needed to give interpretations of proverbs (*see* Proverbs [Interpretation]). It is also the kind of reasoning needed to solve this problem: Aa, Bb, C?. What should fill in the question mark? You need to discover what change occurred to the *A* and *B* in the series, and then apply that change analogously to the *C* to reach the solution of *c*.

Inferential reasoning is involved when participants receive a series of rule-based items and then must infer or deduce what should be next in the series. For example, the series might be 2 8 32—what number should be next? To respond with "128," you must discover the rule that relates the first three numbers to each other (namely, each successive number is four times the preceding number).

The decline in average scores found with normal aging on laboratory reasoning tasks may well exaggerate the extent to which everyday reasoning abilities decline. The laboratory tasks used in studies of age differences in reasoning ability are quite artificial, and likely to be quite different from the kinds of reasoning tasks encountered by older adults in the everyday world (for example, deducing what your partner meant by that last bid in playing bridge or deducing which stock purchase is best at this time; *see* Ecological Validity).

Moreover, the mental skills needed to solve laboratory reasoning problems are not necessarily beyond the capabilities of most normally aging elderly adults. There is convincing evidence to show that older adults improve their scores greatly on inferential reasoning tasks after they have had instructions on what kind of mental operations are needed to solve the problems and after they have had practice on similar problems (*see* Transfer of Learning/Training). Thus, elderly adults demonstrate considerable plasticity in their ability to overcome apparent deficits in mental skills (*see* Plasticity Theory).

In addition, many older adults continue to perform exceptionally well on jobs and hobbies that demand reasoning abilities as part of their expertise (for example, executive management and playing bridge and chess), despite the fact that they score well below the level of younger people on laboratory tests of reasoning ability (*see* Expertise).

Recognition Memory versus Recall Memory

Is the title of this entry (a) Recognition Memory, (b) Recall Memory, (c)

Recognition Memory versus Recall Memory, or (d) Recognition Memory and Recall Memory?

The correct answer, of course, is "c." This is an example of a question on a multiple-choice test, a testing format familiar to millions of students. Multiple-choice tests evaluate the students' memories for recently studied (and, one hopes, acquired) information. Instead of being asked to recall all of the information recently studied, students are asked simply to recognize it and discriminate that information from distractors (that is, information somewhat similar to the studied information, but not identical) that are present.

A multiple-choice test is one of the methods often used by memory researchers to test for age differences in recognition memory. The procedure consists of presenting younger and older participants with a series of items or episodic events, with each item presented individually for several seconds. The items may be familiar words, pictures of objects, or pictures of scenes. The participants then receive a series of test items in which each of the previously studied words or pictures is presented along with several distractors, and participants are asked to select from each test item the "old" (previously studied) word or picture.

An alternative testing procedure is to present in a random order a series of words or pictures in which half are "old" (previously studied) and half are "new" (distractors not previously studied). As each test item is encountered, the participants respond "old" or "new." Correct identification of old items as old and new items as new are called "hits." Incorrect identifications of new items as old are called "false alarms."

Regardless of the recognition testing procedure used, age differences in memory scores favoring younger participants are usually found to be much smaller than when participants are asked to recall the previously studied items. That is, older participants more closely match the performance of younger participants on a recognition memory test than on a recall memory test. In fact, in some instances the age difference found on a recall test all but disappear when a recognition test is used. This is the case, for example, when the episodic events are actions performed in the laboratory (*see* Action Memory).

Recognition and recall differ in an important way. To recall previously studied information, you have to conduct a vigorous search of your long-term memory store to find the memory traces of the previously studied items. Once a trace is found, then you need to recognize that it is indeed one for a just-studied item. Such a search is an effortful one that is more difficult to conduct, on average, for older adults than for younger adults. Older adults tend to have a greater retrieval problem than do younger adults.

The intensity of the search, and therefore the difficulty of retrieval, is reduced greatly when participants face a recognition memory test. The old items are reinstated at the time of the test, thereby directing the search to specific memory traces. The fact that the memory performance of elderly adults more closely approximates that of younger adults on a recognition test than on a recall test suggests that much of the difficulty experienced by older adults in episodic memory stems from their diminished retrieval proficiency. However, the fact that an age difference favoring younger adults often persists even on a recognition memory test suggests that at least part of the episodic memory problem of elderly adults is related to their less proficient encoding of the information studied.

Of great interest is a sixteen-year longitudinal study conducted by Dr. Elizabeth Zelinski of the University of Southern California. The participants were fifty-five to eighty-one years old at the time of initial testing. Later testing showed a decline in recall memory proficiency, but not in recognition memory proficiency.

There is another interesting outcome of research on age differences in recognition memory. Elderly participants typically have more false alarms (calling new test items old) than do younger participants. Cautious people would seemingly be more reluctant than less cautious people in identifying new test items as old. This is further evidence to indicate that older adults should not be viewed as possessing a general characteristic of cautiousness to a greater extent than do younger people (*see* Cautiousness).

The greater false-alarm rate for elderly participants is especially true when new words on the test list are related in some way to prior study-list words (for example, *pretty* as a study-list word, *beautiful* as a new test word). It is also true when a new word in a test list is thematically related to prior study-list words but was never included in the study list (for example, *thread, pin,* and *sew* as study-list words, *needle* as a new test-list word) (*see also* False Memory).

Relationship with Physician (Duration)

In a study of more than seven thousand people age sixty-five and older, researchers at Columbia University discovered that nearly 31 percent had been seeing their primary physician for at least ten years (the "long" group), whereas 11 percent had been seeing their physician for less than a year (the "short" group). The participants in the long group were slightly more likely to be white, have a higher income, have a better education, be in better health, and have fewer hospitalizations than the participants in the short group. However, the longer relationship did not result in increases in healthful behaviors, such as quitting smoking.

Religion and Meaning in Life

Older adults who are actively religious (for example, frequent praying) tend to have better physical and mental health than older adults who are less religious.

According to Dr. Neal Krause of the University of Michigan, the reason for the association between religion and health is that seniors who are actively religious have a greater sense of purpose, meaning, and direction in their lives than seniors who are not actively involved in religion. In support of his hypothesis, actively religious elders in his studies have been found to have stronger agreement with such statements as "My faith gives me a sense of direction in my life" than less religiously active elders.

Religion in Later Life

The results from four large national surveys indicate that nearly all older people have a religious affiliation of some kind. Elderly people are highly religious. It is estimated that from 60 percent to 95 percent of older adults pray daily, compared to about 50 percent of younger people. On a number of indices of religiosity (for example, frequency of prayer), elderly women are more religious than elderly men, and African Americans are more religious than whites.

Increasing religiosity in later life from what it had been earlier in life has been found to be associated with the loss of important relationships (for example, death of a family member) and other adverse life events, the need to encourage religious beliefs of their children, and awareness of approaching the end of life. Stable religiosity from early to later adulthood is prevalent either for those with great faith that never wavered or for those who always had a low level of religious beliefs. Decreasing religiosity with aging is often brought about by poor health or by changes in church doctrines over the years.

Older people frequently use prayer as a means of coping with stressful events in their lives. One common source of stress late in life is physical illness. A study conducted in North Carolina revealed that a large percentage of the older participants reported the use of prayer when they had symptoms of illness they believed to be serious.

Other researchers in North Carolina found that nearly half of the elderly people they surveyed reported using religious activities as a means of coping with other kinds of stressful events. In general, morale and satisfaction with one's life have been found to be greater for elderly people who report frequent religious activities than for elderly people who report less frequent activities. Dealing with the distress associated with financial problems has been found to benefit African American church members, but not white church members, who receive emotional support from their fellow church members.

Despite the apparent religiosity of older people, there is evidence indicating that they participate less frequently in organized religious practices compared either with themselves when they were younger or with current younger people. A study conducted some years ago in New York State revealed that only 43 percent of the older adults surveyed attended church (church here refers to any facility where people meet for a formal religious service, such as a cathedral, synagogue, or mosque) regularly. A more recent study of older adults living in central Missouri also indicated that fewer than 50 percent of those surveyed were regular church attenders. The percentage of younger people attending church regularly is considerably higher.

However, the decline in church attendance does not mean that there is a decline in religiosity with normal aging. The study in Missouri revealed the reasons that older people do not attend church regularly are poor health, bad weather, and lack of transportation, and not a declining interest in religion. Religiosity obviously needs to be measured at a more personal level, such as the regular use of private prayer. As noted above, when measured in this way, it is apparent that most older people do indeed keep their religious convictions; they simply have to express them less formally than in the past.

The positive benefits of religion in the lives of elderly adults are many. Researchers at Georgetown University reviewed more than two hundred studies on religion and health. They found that three-fourths of the studies revealed the positive effects of religion on drug abuse, depression, blood pressure, and heart disease. Other researchers have found that the greater the religious involvement of elderly people, the greater their self-esteem. Religious participation has a special significance in improving the quality of life for physically disabled elderly people. Caregivers of disabled elderly people who use religious beliefs in coping with the stress of caregiving have less depression and better relationships with the recipients of their care than do caregivers who do not use religious practices as a form of coping with their stress. Private prayer has also been found to be associated with less depression following coronary bypass surgery.

Does religion actually serve to improve the health of elderly people? More than ten years of studies at various university hospitals indicated that, regardless of the nature of a person's religious preference, people who have a deep religious faith seem to get sick less often and get better faster when they do get sick than people with much less religious faith. Those with a strong religious faith have also been found to have lower rates of heart disease, stroke, and cancer.

Perhaps the most striking finding comes from a study of nearly four thousand people in the 64-to-101-year age range in North Carolina. Over a six-year period, 37 percent of the participants who attended religious services once a week or more survived, compared to 23 percent of those who attended services less than once a week. The higher survival rate for frequent church attenders was especially characteristic of women, but it did apply to men as well. Most important, the difference in survival rates held up even after controlling for differences between frequent and less frequent attenders in health and health practices.

Seniors in North Carolina gave self-reports of their participation in private religious activities, such as prayer, meditation, and Bible study. They were then contacted again six years later. It was found that the seniors who participated in private religious activities suffered from fewer impairments in performing normal activities of daily living (for example, bathing or dressing) than those who did not participate in private religious activities.

Not surprisingly, a number of the 125 accredited medical schools in the United States have included religious or spiritual teaching in their curricula. For example, at Harvard Medical School students are taught how to obtain a patient's spiritual history and how to discuss spiritual concerns with a patient.

What about those elderly persons who have doubt about their former positive belief and faith in religion? In a study of nearly fifteen hundred elderly persons by researchers at the University of Michigan, it was found that doubt is associated with diminished feelings of well-being. However, they also found that younger people who have doubts about their former religious beliefs are more likely to experience negative emotional effects than are older people. *See also* Grandparenting; Religion and Meaning in Life; Widowhood and Widowerhood.

Reminiscence

Thinking and talking about the "good old days" and your life events at that time is a phenomenon known as reminiscence that is commonly associated with elderly people. A particular form of reminiscence in which a participant is asked to review his or her life is sometimes used as a component of psychotherapy for older people with depression and for nursing home residents to help them reduce their feelings of isolation. Reminiscence is also used in some senior centers to help participants cope with stress.

The therapeutic value of reminiscence has been questioned by some gerontologists. However, it does appear that some forms of reminiscence are more characteristic of elderly people who are aging successfully, defined in terms of both positive physical health and mental health status, than of those older people who are aging less successfully. Canadian researchers asked a number of elderly people to reminiscence about their lives. They found that most of the statements given by less successfully aging people were simple narrations about events in their lives without interpretation of their significance. Successfully aging participants gave fewer narrative statements and more integrative statements than less successfully aging participants. An integrative reminiscence is one indicating acceptance of one's life as having been worthwhile.

In a study of ten thousand older people in a number of communities, it was found that when older people share stories of their meaningful life experiences with other people, it improves their sense of psychological well-being and gives them a greater feeling of community and an awareness of their useful contributions to others. In another study, it was found that seniors age sixty-five and older who are functioning poorly psychologically (for example, have depression or death anxiety) frequently reminiscence about their bitter life experiences to escape boredom and to prepare for their deaths. Such seniors need counseling to restructure their reminiscences.

Other forms of reminiscence include escapist reminiscence (glorifying past achievements and yearning for the "good old days") and obsessive reminiscence (statements revealing guilt and bitterness about the past). Escapist reminiscence was found by the researchers to occur rarely for either successfully or less successfully aging participants. Obsessive reminiscence occurred moderately often for less successfully aging people.

It seems apparent that successfully aging people have succeeded in integrating life experiences positively and feel little despair about their current life status (*see* Personality Stages). The treatment of depression in some older adults may be successful to the extent that the clients are successful in reevaluating their lives and finding that they have been worthwhile. Reminiscence may not be therapeutic, but it may serve as a useful index for identifying those individuals who are aging successfully. As discovered by a researcher at the Medical University of South Carolina, a structured reminiscence of one's life history from birth on may increase one's self-esteem.

There does seem to be a "memoir fever" sweeping the United States. As noted by Dr. James Birren, a prominent gerontologist, looking back at your life makes you realize how much you have survived—there must be some true grit in you. *See also* Diary Keeping.

Residence

Many elderly people change their residence from time to time, while others show stability and permanence in where they live. For the young-old, the most stable living arrangement is living alone or with a spouse. For the oldest-old, the most stable arrangement is living with one of his or her adult children. An unstable and unpleasant residence is likely to yield considerable stress for an elderly occupant, stress that could exceed that person's capacity for resolving it satisfactorily (*see* Environmental Press).

Respect for Elderly People

Most people do believe that older people deserve special respect because of their age (even though they may also believe that older people are likely to be senile and grumpy). However, in a large-scale survey of people spanning the adult life span, more people (88 percent) in the eighteen-to-sixty-four age range reported believing in the respect principle than people age sixty-five and older (75 percent). Moreover, 72 percent of the younger ones surveyed strongly approved such respect compared to only 59 percent of the oldest ones. Perhaps ageism (*see* Ageism) is finally on its way out for future generations of younger people.

Respite Care

Respite care is intended to provide caregivers (usually relatives) of disabled elderly people (*see* Caregivers [Family and Friends]) periods of rest and relief away from the person receiving care. The objective is to reduce the strain and stress experienced by caregivers in prolonged service. By so doing, it is also hoped that admissions of persons to nursing homes may be delayed or even avoided completely, thereby reducing the heavy financial cost of nursing home residence.

Respite care may be accomplished in several ways. Disabled recipients of the care may spend part of their time away from their homes and caregivers. Such possibilities include periods of time spent in a day-care center or periods of time spent in a nursing home. Alternatively, a substitute caregiver may be contracted to serve on occasions in the recipient's home during the day or evening or during weekends. Such respites enable the family caregiver to recover from an illness, to attend an important function, or simply to have time for relaxation.

A yearlong study conducted at the Philadelphia Geriatric Center compared caregivers who received respite care with caregivers who did not receive the service. Respite care was found to delay admission of disabled recipients to a nursing home by an average of several weeks. Although the caregivers receiving the respite care expressed great satisfaction with it, at the end of the year there was little difference in their mental health status compared with caregivers who did not receive respite care. Researchers at the University of Nebraska at Omaha also have found that the greater the use of respite care by caregivers, the less the probability that the recipients will be placed in a nursing home.

Retirees and Reentry into the Workforce

It is not unusual for men in the sixty-to-sixty-five age range to go back to work after retiring. Researchers in New York surveyed a number of these men and discovered they were likely to have had unstable jobs throughout their adult lives, low pay, and no pension after retirement. In another survey, 20 percent of retirees reported having paying jobs. Of these people only 18 percent said they were doing it for the money. In the same survey, 42 percent of nonretirees indicated that they planned to work on a different job after their retirement. After age sixty-five the number returning to work following retirement decreases greatly as Social Security benefits change their situation.

Retirement (Adjustment to)

Retirement is usually defined as withdrawal from the paid workforce or from full time participation in a paid occupation of some kind. However, many retirees continue to work part-time for pay, and even more work as volunteers without pay for various nonprofit organizations.

Do life satisfaction and self-esteem increase after retirement? Do depressive symptoms decline? Higher life satisfaction after retirement has been found in some studies, but not in others. In general, retirees with higher postretirement incomes report greater life satisfaction after retirement than do retirees with lower incomes. White-collar workers tend to be more satisfied with their lives after retirement than are blue-collar workers. The better the physical health of a retiree, the better his or her self-esteem. Retirees with an internal locus of control over events in their lives (*see* Control over Life's Events) report less depression and less anxiety and greater happiness and life satisfaction than retirees with an external locus of control.

Older workers in North Carolina were followed for two years after retirement and compared with fellow workers who continued to work. The retirees had greater self-esteem and less depression than the continuing workers.

Retirement Communities

Retirement communities in the United States are either subsidized by a government agency, most frequently by the Department of Housing and Urban Development, or nonsubsidized and paid for by private incomes. The subsidized communities are for low-income retirees; the nonsubsidized communities are for those with larger incomes. The nonsubsidized housing varies from modest mobile homes to luxurious homes.

Retirement communities vary in their size, level and kinds of services offered, and profit or nonprofit governance. They comprise five basic categories. The first consists of new retirement towns. These are large communities (for example, Sun City in Arizona), usually constructed by private developers, that cater to younger and more active retirees and have large recreational facilities, health services, and commercial facilities. Retirement villages make up the second category. They are of medium size and are usually privately developed by an organization (for example, a union). They tend to have more limited recreational, health, and commercial services than does a new town. The third category consists of retirement subdivisions that are located in a section of a large city. They are essentially naturally occurring retirement communities. They, too, have limited services, and they cater largely to younger retirees who wish to be near a large city. Retirement residences, the fourth category, consist of clusters of apartments that are usually found in large-city, high-rise buildings. Their residents are likely to be older and less active people. Their facilities are limited, but they may include daily meals. The final category consists of continuing-care retirement communities that are small in size and are designed to offer comprehensive health care and sedentary leisure activities for older and more frail people.

Retirement communities offer retirees social interactions with other retirees, and they are an alternative to the age isolation often experienced by older people who remain in their original residences after retirement. There is evidence to indicate that people living in planned retirement communities express greater life satisfaction and have better health status than other older people living in communities that are more heterogeneous in regard to the ages of the residents. However, residents of some retirement communities should be prepared to conform somewhat to the rules and regulations of their community.

Elderly people who live alone and whose children do not live near them are more likely to move to retirement communities than are other elderly retirees. Elderly retirees who do move to a retirement community may be motivated to do so by their physical frailty and disability as well as by their need to have more social interactions. Movement of retirees to communities tends to increase as the physical disability of the retirees increases to moderate levels and then decrease as the severity of the disability continues to increase.

There are a number of guidelines to aid retirees in finding the right community for them. Retirees should decide what level of care they need and how independent they would like to be. If possible, they should spend several days in a guest apartment at the community, participate in activities there, and talk to residents who have lived there for a while. If this is not possible, they should at least visit the community several times and at different times of the day. A visit to the nearest town or city should be conducted. Does the community have a transportation service? Medical facilities? Entertainment options? Above all, they should check out the financial status of the community. These are all critical steps to take before deciding that "this community is the one for me."

In a study of residents of a continuing-care retirement community sixteen services were analyzed in terms of the frequency of their use. The most frequently used ones were those that are convenient to the residents. They include an on-site pharmacy, bank, swimming pool, health/wellness program, and fitness facility.

Retirement (Contact with Adult Children)

Does the retirement of parents affect contact (visits, letters, telephone calls) with adult children not living at home? A national survey of parents who were age fifty-five to seventy-five at the time of their retirement found that retirement had no significant effects on telephone contacts. For children living within ten miles, their mother's retirement was found to be associated with fewer visits and their father's retirement with more visits. For children living more than ten miles away, mothers were found to decrease their visits with their childless children, whereas fathers were found to increase their visits with their childless children.

Retirement (Involuntary)

Involuntary retirement could result from ill health or pressure from an employer. Whatever the reason, involuntary retirement does carry with it the risk of both physical and psychological problems. In general, people who retire involuntarily have been found to adjust to retirement more poorly than do people who retire voluntarily. Involuntary retirees also tend to have poorer physical health and more symptoms of depression than voluntary retirees.

Interestingly, involuntary retirement is reported more frequently by individuals classified as having a type-A behavior pattern than by individuals classified as having a type-B behavior pattern. A type-A individual is a person who attempts to control his or her environment and appears to be aggressive and ambitious in "getting ahead" on the job. Type-A individuals have been commonly viewed as people who are especially susceptible to coronary diseases. A type-B individual is a person who takes events more calmly and is not very assertive and ambitious in job-related situations.

Researchers at the Yale University School of Medicine found that involuntary retirees did not increase their daily alcohol consumption. However, they were more likely to start drinking alcoholic beverages when they had not been drinking before they were forced to retire.

Retirement (Life after)

A popular theory suggests that retirees are likely to progress through several stages after their retirement. The first stage is called the honeymoon stage, in which the retiree does the things that had been largely ruled out by full-time work (for example, extensive traveling). This stage may then be followed by one of disenchantment, in which the retiree must adjust to the realities of retirement, such as reduced income that may restrict many of the activities planned during retirement. During this stage the retiree needs to discover appropriate new activities. If successful, then the retiree enters the final, and satisfactory, reorientation stage, in which he or she accepts the limitations incumbent with aging and settles into a retirement routine.

Considerable research has indicated that these are not inevitable stages. Some retirees do not experience all of the stages, and others may encounter the stages in a different order than that proposed by the theory. Thus, some retirees may not have sufficient funds for a true honeymoon phase, whereas others pass from the honeymoon stage to the reorientation stage without experiencing disenchantment. In some cases, retirees have a period of relaxation, either immediately after retirement or after the honeymoon stage. This usually leads to boredom, and the retiree enters the reorientation stage and begins establishing a daily routine.

Evidence indicates that the enthusiasm of retirees is usually high immediately after retirement and that some emotional letdown occurs during the second and third postretirement years. Some retirees do experience a prolonged disenchantment stage, but many do not.

Studies indicate that individuals who had satisfying hobbies and recreational activities before retirement are most likely to enjoy their retirement years. A number of retirees who become bored and disenchanted attempt to solve the problem by joining a senior center or by either developing new interests or finding part-time work. Near retirement communities, such as those in Florida, it is not unusual to find elderly retirees working as gas station attendants, supermarket baggers, retail store clerks, and so on, usually for minimum- or near minimum-wage pay. It is estimated that more than 25 percent of retirees accept some type of employment within four years after retirement. Nearly half of the retirees in the United States have Social Security as the primary source of income, and Social Security is often their only income.

Most studies have indicated that there is no trend toward increased marital strife after a husband's retirement when his wife is not employed. In fact, in many cases the relationship between spouses is likely to improve as they find they now have time to pursue common recreational interests.

However, in a recent study in Florida, slight negative effects on marital satisfaction were found for wives who were still working after their husband's retirement. An apparent reason for this dissatisfaction is the failure of many retired husbands to assume a fair share of household duties. In general, women tend to perform three-fourths of the household chores, even after they continue to work, when their husbands have retired. Researchers at Old Dominion University found that employed wives were unable to elicit more household help from their retired husbands than they did before they retired. This is especially true for what are generally considered to be women's chores (for example, washing dishes).

A husband's adjustment to retirement depends largely on his morale. After retirement, men become more dependent on their marriage, often expecting it to fill the void after leaving work. When one spouse retires, both spouses need to rethink how household chores will be redistributed. They should also consider making changes in their house, such as adding a home office (and resolving the issue of who gives up space to have the office).

It is estimated that 20 percent to 30 percent of retirees in the United States cite ill health or disability as the reason for their retirement. However, it is likely that some retirees cite their health as the reason simply to justify their voluntary retirement. There is no apparent trend for retirement to result in diminished physical health, once preretirement health status is considered. On the other hand, there is some evidence to indicate that psychological symptoms, such as anxiety and depression, appear more frequently in retirees than in age-matched people still in the workforce. In addition, some evidence suggests that psychological symptoms may be present more frequently in both early and late retirees than in retirees who retire at the more standard age of sixty-five.

For past generations, retirement usually meant adjusting to a very low income. However, the number of retirees with incomes well above the government-defined poverty level has increased steadily. These financially advantaged individuals are ones who are likely to have income sources in addition to Social Security benefits (that is, private pensions and investments).

Financial planners say that retirees will need about 75 percent of their preretirement annual income to live comfortably. Unfortunately, many retirees are uninformed on how to manage their money. They may not know how to avoid paying taxes on Social Security income, and they may be afraid to change investments for fear of losing principal. It would be prudent for many retirees to consult with an experienced investment professional. They will learn how annual compounding makes their money grow faster, how to make a tax-deferred gift for a grandchild's future college tuition, how a living trust operates, and so on.

Many who are not yet retired believe that retirement is a chance for a new beginning, with more travel, new hobbies, and so on. However, surveys of those who are retired indicate that more than half believe retirement is either simply a continuation of their preretirement life or a step down.

Retirement (Locations)

Where do people live after they retire? According to a survey by a researcher at Wake Forest University, most people actually prefer not to move during their retirement years. At least that is what 84 percent of the participants (age fifty-five and older) in the survey indicated. According to the 1990 census, about 75 percent of retirees actually do not move after retirement. Of retirees who do move, 10 percent stay within their county, 10 percent move outside their county but stay within their state, and about 5 percent move to another state. For those retirees who do relocate in another state, Florida and California continue to be the most popular choices, although their popularity has been declining in recent years. States that have been gaining rapidly in popularity for relocation are Georgia, North Carolina, and Virginia (*see* Migration [Moving]).

Retirement (Planning)

For a satisfying life after retirement, workers should begin to plan for retirement long before they actually retire. This includes establishing a pension program of some kind so that Social Security payments will not be the only source of income. The fact that retirement may be forced on an individual earlier than planned makes it especially important to begin this financial program as early as possible. Savings in most individual retirement account (IRA) plans are untaxed. Consult with an accountant to determine if eventual conversion to a Roth IRA is to your advantage. Once in the plan your earnings and withdrawals will be tax free after five years in the plan.

Equally important is the preretirement development of interests, hobbies, and multiseasonal leisure activities that will sustain the retiree long after the likely honeymoon period of retirement has ended (*see* Retirement [Life after]).

An important issue concerning planning for retirement is how people in their fifties feel about their eventual retirement. Of interest are the results of a survey conducted in the Boston area of a number of professional people (physicians, lawyers, professors, and so on). The professionals who least looked forward to retirement were those who anticipated that their work agendas would be incomplete before retirement, those who had a high current level of job satisfaction, and those who believed that retirement would create a financial strain. Of the professors in the survey, only about 30 percent viewed their future retirement positively. About 20 percent of the professionals surveyed revealed that they had not even thought about retirement.

Workers with jobs that provide intrinsic rewards (that is, they work mainly because they like the job and not for the money) are generally unlikely to plan for their subsequent retirement. This is also the case for workers whose rewards are mainly positive social relations with coworkers. Thus, workers who have rewarding jobs tend to do less planning for retirement than workers with less rewarding jobs.

Of further interest are the results of a survey conducted on participants in the Normative Aging Study (*see* Longitudinal Studies of Aging's Effects on Health and Cognition). Two-thirds of the people surveyed predicted correctly (within one year) when they would retire. This means that one-third of the participants did not foresee their date of retirement and either had to extend their work life by some years or had to retire prematurely.

Especially important are the results of a large survey of workers in the age range of fifty to sixty-four. More than 60 percent of those surveyed stated that they had not planned sufficiently for retirement. In fact, about half of the people surveyed admitted that they had not thought about the income they would need after retirement, and that they did not even know what their Social Security and other pension payments would be. In general, living expenses are reduced after retirement, meaning that retirees need about 75 percent or 80 percent of their preretirement income to maintain their preretirement standard of living. However, the present average retiree has an income that is only about two-thirds of his or her preretirement income. Clearly, more early financial preretirement planning is needed for the majority of workers in the United States.

Some individual companies, businesses, and universities offer formal programs to assist their employees in planning for retirement. However, in a survey conducted in the 1980s fewer than 5 percent of retirees reported participating in such a program, and only 12 percent believed they had the opportunity for participation. It is primarily economically advantaged employees who have the opportunity to participate in a preretirement program, meaning that those employees who may most need assistance have little or no opportunity. Employees should be made more aware of the benefits to be gained from participation in a preretirement program (for example, financial planning), and they should urge their supervisors to introduce such programs, if they do not already exist.

Retirement (Racial Inequity)

African Americans live fewer years after retirement than do whites. This is because they spend a greater portion of their lives working and have a higher mortality rate than do whites (*see* Racial and Ethnic Differences in Aging). The difference in health between the races is a major contributor to the racial inequity in retirement. There will soon be more than three million African Americans over age sixty-five. Increasing incomes for African Americans will enable them to retire earlier in larger numbers. Unfortunately, white retirement communities are too expensive for them, or they discriminate subtly against African American residents. There are only a few predominantly African American retirement communities.

Retirement (Theories of Life Satisfaction)

There are two major theories regarding the determiners of retirees' satisfaction with their lives during their retirement years. Both theories focus on adapting to the loss of the role as a worker that accompanies retirement. *Crisis theory* states that successful adjustment to retirement depends on a retiree's ability to substitute meaningful activities for work. *Continuity theory* argues that retirees need to expand and develop new roles in their lives in order to achieve satisfaction within their lives. Both theories stress that retirement itself can provide its own path to higher self-esteem if either new activities or new roles can be introduced in the life of the retiree.

Retirement (Timing)

Over the years there has been a trend for both men and women to retire at an earlier age. In the period 1955–1960 the median age at retirement was 65.8 for white men, 64.7 for African American men, 66.1 for white women, and 66.3 for African American women. In the period 1985–1990 the median ages for the same groups were 62.6, 61.7, 63.0, and 61.7. As a result, the percentage of men age 65 to 69 in the labor force decreased from about 60 percent in 1950 to about 27 percent in 1990. There are several reasons for the trend toward earlier retirement. They include increased coverage of Social Security benefits, more private pensions, and more employers covering health insurance before Medicare takes over.

Men who expect to receive a defined benefit pension plan in which they receive 60 percent to 79 percent of their prior pay after retirement are more likely to expect to retire before age 62 than men without such a plan. Even many workers who expect to receive only a modest pension after retirement expect to retire before age 65. However, do these workers really retire before age 65? They may expect to do so, but few actually carry through with early retirement. They hate to give up their salaries and health insurance benefits before they reach age 65.

Companies often give a pension to workers who retire early. Workers often worry that they may lose their jobs or be transferred if they do not accept early retirement. General Motors had its first early retirement agreement in 1964. At that time there was mandatory retirement in the company at age 68. Workers with a minimum of ten years' service could retire with reduced benefits at age 60. Those with thirty years or more of service could retire at age 55. It was found that those with thirty or more years of service were generally healthy and received good financial benefits, but they were, nevertheless, still more dissatisfied after retirement than those workers who retired at the mandatory retirement age.

Retirement (Uncertainty)

A survey of nearly four thousand preretirees age fifty-one to sixty-one found that many, perhaps as many as 20 percent to 40 percent, were uncertain about their future retirement in terms of how they leave their jobs or when they would leave their jobs. Women and those not enrolled in a pension plan were the ones who were most likely to be unsure of form and time of retirement. Unmarried workers were less sure of form and time than married workers. Workers with less education and workers in smaller workplaces were also less sure. Part-time workers were especially uncertain about both form and time.

Rigidity

One of the commonly held beliefs about aging is that people tend to become more rigid and inflexible as they become older. One type of rigidity refers to the ability to make shifts and changes in one's behavior, especially when conditions seemingly call for such changes. Rigidity may be contrasted with its opposite, namely, flexibility of behavior.

The belief that rigidity in behavior increases with aging received support from studies conducted in the 1950s. Both younger and older participants received problems to solve that involved pouring water into various size jars to obtain a set amount of water. The first sets of problems all involved application of the same, rather complicated procedure in which several different pours between jars were required. The final problem could also be solved by this same complicated procedure. However, a simpler procedure to reach the same solution was also available. Younger participants made the switch to the new procedure more frequently than did older participants, thus suggesting greater rigidity on the part of the older participants.

Later research compared participants of various ages on paper-and-pencil tests of rigidity. These studies indicated that age itself is an unlikely determinant of age differences in rigidity. The more likely determinant is the cohort or generation to which one belongs. That is, members of earlier generations were found to demonstrate greater rigidity in their behaviors on the tests than did members of later generations. In the earlier study with the water jars, the older participants were not only older than the younger participants but also members of an earlier generation. There does not seem to be good reason to subscribe to the belief that most people become increasingly inflexible in their behaviors as they grow older.

Rigidity has been applied to social and political attitudes. Here, the common belief is that older adults are less likely than younger adults to change their attitudes as the social and political climate and mores change. However, evidence again indicates that older adults tend to show flexibility rather than rigidity in regard to such attitudes. An age change in rigidity seems to be one of the myths of aging. *See also* Attitudes (Political and Social).

Roles Seniors Play

All the world's a stage. And all the men and women merely players.
They have their exits and their entrances. And one man in his time
plays many parts.

> —William Shakespeare, *As You Like It*

We do play many roles in our lives: son or daughter, spouse, parent, grandparent, worker, mentor, and so on. However, is late adulthood mostly a "roleless" time of our lives? We probably no longer play the role of salaried worker. However, other roles, such as volunteer worker, replace the former role. Throughout our adulthood our roles vary in importance—late adulthood is no exception.

In several studies by Dr. Neal Krause and his associates of the University of Michigan, the same eight potentially salient roles of older adults were identified and responded to by older participants. The roles are spouse, parent, grandparent, other relative, friend, homemaker, provider, and volunteer worker.

In one study nearly one thousand participants (average age of 74.2 years) identified the three roles that best fit the way they think about themselves. They also ranked the roles in the order of their importance. The most frequent first choice was spouse, with parent and grandparent being second and third, respectively.

The participants also identified from a list of forty-nine stressful life events which ones they had experienced in the previous year. They also evaluated the current level of their life satisfaction (*see* Life Satisfaction). The negative effects of stressful events on life satisfaction were restricted largely to events associated with the three most salient roles. Stressful events associated with less salient roles had little effect on life satisfaction.

In later studies, Dr. Krause discovered that stressors in salient roles serve to lower life satisfaction because they decrease the feeling of control of life events related to those roles (*see* Control over Life's Events; Stress and Coping with Stress).

Rural Older People (Characteristics and Problems They Face)

In the 1920s nearly one-third of Americans lived on farms. Now only about 2 percent live on farms. However, nearly 20 percent of older Americans live in small towns or in farm areas. Older adults who live in rural areas tend to have less education and are poorer than those who live in cities. They have more children than city-dwelling older people, but they are less likely to live with an adult child. They are more likely to be married and living with their spouses.

Nonfarm rural seniors have less income, poorer housing, and fewer family members to assist them than farm-dwelling or city-dwelling elders. They also report more medical problems and rate their health as poorer than those seniors in the city or those still farming.

Access to health care is difficult in rural areas. There are fewer physicians, nurses, and hospital beds per person. They are likely to visit a general practitioner and less likely to see a specialist than city-dwelling seniors.

Rural elderly people tend to be suspicious of outside help, especially that offered by government programs. However, they help their neighbors and vice versa. They usually live in the same community all of their lives.

S

Salt Intake

Not all seniors with high blood pressure are sensitive to salt. However, many of them are. It probably pays for them to be on the safe side and be on a low-salt diet. By doing so, they lower the risk of a stroke by 38 percent and heart disease by 16 percent. In addition, too much salt in a diet increases the loss of calcium from the body, increasing the risk of osteoporosis (*see* Osteoporosis). Too much salt could even contribute to the risk of stomach cancer and even cataracts. *See also* Stroke.

Sarcopenia

Sarcopenia is the term given to the loss of muscle mass and strength with normal aging. It does not require a disease for its occurrence, but chronic diseases accelerate the deterioration. It is a major cause of disability, and even morbidity for elderly adults. Resistance training helps to slow it down, but the best intervention is lifelong physical activity and a nutritious diet. *See also* Strength and Stamina.

Scams

Elderly people are often the victims of scams that cost them billions of dollars a year. They should realize that con artists often target their victims by reading obituaries to find out the names of grief-stricken widows or widowers who are especially vulnerable to deceptively attractive schemes.

Elderly men should be leery of products that sound like Viagra (but are not) that are sold through scientific-sounding companies. A common scam is one involving home repairs. If you are considering having repairs made to your home, you should ask the contractor for customer references for products similar to yours. Be sure to get all guarantees, warranties, and promises in writing, and make certain that the start and completion dates are specified in the contract. Contact your Better Business Bureau to check out contractors, especially unsolicited ones.

Elderly people are at a high risk for telephone scams. They should know that legitimate prize promotions do not require payment of a fee to qualify. Do not give your credit card number over the phone. Be skeptical of calls offering to help you to recover money already spent in sweepstakes (known as "reloading," it is really a rip-off).

If someone calls and says he is an AT&T service technician who is running a test, he may ask you to help him by dialing 9, 2, #, and hanging up. This combination may enable him to place long-distance calls on your bill. Do not do what he says. Real technicians do not call to run tests. Older people are especially targets of various telemarketing scams. According to a 1996 survey, adults age fifty and older made up more than 50 percent of the victims.

Seniors need to be aware of a possible scam involving promissory notes issued by individuals rather than by corporate or institutional investors. They usually offer interest rates that are unrealistically higher than the current market.

Seniors should also be aware that money may be stolen from their bank account through their automatic teller machine (ATM). In a relatively new scam called "phishing" the victim of the scam receives an e-mail that looks like one sent by their bank or other place where he or she has deposited money. The message directs them to a Web site where they are asked to provide information about their account. That information enables the thief to gain access to your ATM and steal money from it. If you receive e-mail from what seems to be your bank, you should call the bank and verify that the message is indeed from your bank.

There are other ways a thief may get money from your ATM. One of the steps the thief may take to accomplish this is by using a tiny camera that videotapes an elder using his or her ATM. The result is a picture of the elder's personal identification number. Seniors should cover their hands when entering their numbers, and they should ask their bank to limit the amount of money they are able to withdraw.

Some elders are victims of a scam that consists of giving fortune tellers money for their so-called advice for making money. Once you are the victim of a scam you may be approached by other scammers. The word gets around that you are an easy mark.

There are consumer protection laws, such as the Fair Credit Billing Act and the Telephone Consumer Protection Act. Possible scams are investigated by the Federal Trade Commission, the Federal Bureau of Investigation, and the Attorney General's office. If you suspect a scam is going on, contact a representative of one of these offices, or call the National Consumer League's Nation Fraud Information Center at 800-876-7060.

Searching for a Quality Nursing Home

The average age of the more than 1.5 million residents of nursing homes is eighty-five. About a million new residents are added annually. Nearly half of the residents have some degree of dementia. Many have multiple chronic diseases, and many require some assistance to feed, bathe, and toilet themselves.

Given the likelihood of disability and impairment, the quality of care residents receive is of great concern to their relatives and friends, as well as society at large. Whoever is responsible for selecting a home for a loved one wants to choose one that provides a high quality of care. To do so, they need information about the conditions that contribute to high-quality care. These conditions have been reviewed and analyzed by researchers at the University of California at San Francisco.

Large facilities were found to have more deficiencies and poorer outcomes than smaller facilities. However, they also generally have better outcomes on mental-status measures than smaller facilities. Facilities with a higher percentage of Medicaid residents tend to have more deficiencies than those with smaller percentages.

There are many benefits to a higher staffing level. Included are improved physical functioning and lower mortality of residents, fewer pressure ulcers, and fewer urinary tract infections. A high turnover of staff affects the stability of care. A high rate is associated with low staff morale and poor quality of care.

A high rate of management turnover is also associated with a large number of deficiencies. The annual turnover of nursing home administrators is estimated to be between 40 percent and 50 percent. Unfortunately, the values of the administrators and those of the nursing home's advisory board may be a mismatch. Retention of administrators tends to be higher when they are involved in decision making, treated fairly, and given goals to achieve. Those searching for a nursing home should consider for each one being considered what the status of the administrator is.

For other considerations, see the review article by Charlene Harrington et al. in the journal the *Gerontologist* (April 2003).

Sedentary Lifestyle of Many Older Women

Physical inactivity is especially prevalent among middle-aged and older women. Several factors seem to contribute to the sedentary lifestyle of many older women. Researchers at Stanford University School of Medicine conducted telephone interviews with more than twenty-nine hundred women age forty and older. Only 9 percent reported being physically active. Caregiving duties and lack of energy ranked among the top-four most frequently cited personal reasons for physical inactivity. Frequently cited environmental reasons for inactivity were lack of a neighborhood sidewalk and a lack of streetlights.

Seizures

Seizures occur more often for older people than for younger people. A seizure is caused by electricity generated by brain cells. One reason for seizures in older people is scar tissue remaining from an earlier small stroke. Another is uncontrolled high blood pressure. The reason could also be the presence of a brain tumor, but in nearly 70 percent of the cases the cause is unknown. The reason for seizures could be determined by a brain scan or an EEG (electroencephalogram) to find the problem in the brain.

Selective Attention

Suppose you are a participant in a miniature-golf tournament. Throughout your play a radio in the background blares out the broadcast of a major sporting event. Would the broadcast affect your play? Research in Sweden (where miniature-golf tournaments are very popular) suggests that it would, but only if you are an older player. Older players (in their fifties) were sufficiently distracted by the irrelevant event (that is, the broadcast) that their performance on the relevant event (the golf game) deteriorated. By contrast, younger players (average age of twenty-eight years) were unaffected by the broadcast. They played as well in the presence of the broadcast as they did in its absence.

This study demonstrates that older people, under some circumstances, have greater difficulty in selectively attending to relevant information in the presence of irrelevant information than do younger people. Some information in our environment is relevant to what we are presently doing (for example, the location of the ball relative to the cup in miniature golf). By contrast, other information present at the same time is irrelevant to our objective (for example, the broadcast of the sporting event). Selective attention refers to focusing attention on the relevant information while inhibiting our attention to the irrelevant information. In the Swedish study, the irrelevant information was auditory, and the relevant information was visual. Moreover, the irrelevant information was meaningful and interesting in its content. Despite this, the younger players were able to "tune it out."

However, there are other circumstances in which irrelevant information is clearly of little interest to the persons receiving it. Under these circumstances, older individuals appear as capable as younger individuals of inhibiting attention to the irrelevant information. This is the case when research participants listen to the occurrences of tones of one pitch as the relevant information and tones of a much different pitch as the irrelevant information. Although adults of all ages are distracted slightly by the irrelevant information, the amount of distraction is no greater for older adults than for younger adults.

Most research on age differences in the proficiency of selective attention has made use of relevant and irrelevant events that are both visual. The materials usually consist of letters of the alphabet. A popular task in gerontological research is to ask participants to examine index cards to determine which of two target letters (for example, *A* or *Y*) is present on each card. Thus, the target letters make up the relevant events. The cards vary in the number of distracting letters (that is, letters other than the target letters) that serve as the irrelevant events. Most important, the position of the target letter varies from card to card. That is, sometimes it is in the center, sometimes in the upper right corner, and so on. Consequently, a search of the card's content is needed to find the target. The time to complete the task for a stack of cards increases as the number of irrelevants present on the cards (thus increasing the amount of information that must be searched) increases. However, the increase in sorting time is much greater for older adults than for younger adults.

Older adults do have greater difficulty than younger adults in inhibiting their attention to the irrelevant events. They probably pay more attention to the irrelevant letters than is needed to determine that they are indeed irrelevant to the task at hand (finding if it is an *A* or a *Y* on each card). Suppose, for example, that one of the irrelevant letters is *Q*. This letter should be quickly identified as being a nontarget letter in that it differs greatly in its physical features from either of the target letters. Older adults, however, appear to attend to it to the point where they unnecessarily identify it as the letter *Q*. By contrast, younger adults end their attention to the *Q* much earlier once they determine that its basic form eliminates it as one of the target letters.

There are other tasks involving visual relevant and irrelevant events that have been used in research on age differences in selective attention. Some of these tasks share one important feature with the card-sorting task, namely, they require searching an array of relevant and irrelevant information. Studies with these tasks have yielded results much like those obtained with the card-sorting task. That is, older adults have been found to be moderately less proficient in selective attention than younger adults.

However, there are other tasks in which a search is not needed to focus on the relevant event. Consider, for example, a task again involving two target letters, *A* and *Y*. On each of a series of trials only one of the target letters is presented on a computer screen—and always in the exact center of the screen. Participants simply identify which of the target letters is in view on any given trial. In the absence of any irrelevant letters, the decision time for older participants averages only moderately greater than the decision time for younger participants. On some trials, irrelevant letters are added to the left and right of the target letter at the center of the screen (for example, *J U A U J*). Note that a search of the letters is not needed to find the target letter—it is always in the center. Under these conditions, both young and older participants show only a slight increase in decision times. However, the increase, relative to the condition in which there are no irrelevant letters, is no greater for elderly participants than for younger participants. The evidence seems to be clear. An age difference in the ability to ignore irrelevant information is present only when a visual search is a task requirement.

Results obtained by researchers at the University of Kansas suggest that there is little age difference in tuning out irrelevant events when both relevant and irrelevant events consist of auditory events and when adjustments are made for age differences in hearing proficiency. With such events, no search of total content is needed.

A visual search is required many times in the everyday world. For example, consider your attempt to follow the actions of your favorite player during a basketball game. When that player (the relevant event) is surrounded by other players (irrelevant events), a visual search is required to focus your attention on him or her. The laboratory evidence implies that the older spectator may have greater difficulty than the younger spectator in inhibiting attention to the other players, especially those with the same kind of uniform as the favorite player.

There are also many situations in the everyday world in which a search is not required to "tune out" irrelevant events. For example, while you are watching a television program (the relevant event), someone in the same room reaches for the potato chips in front of you (the irrelevant event). Here the laboratory evidence implies that the irrelevant event should be no more distracting if you are an older adult than if you are a younger adult.

Selective Control of Memory

We need to be able to control what information from our immediate environment is important enough to be encoded and placed in our memory store if our memory system is to operate efficiently. The problem is that our environment often presents us with an overload of information, and only a portion of it can be encoded for entry into the memory store. What portion should be selected? Usually it is information of the greatest relevance to us at the moment.

Such selectivity is a memory strategy that is usually under our control, but does the efficiency of that control diminish with aging? Laboratory evidence indicates that selective control is relatively unaffected by normal aging. For example, researchers at the Georgia Institute of Technology informed their participants not to recall words that were not in the word list they studied but were related to words in the list (for example, *bed, rest,* and *awake* are in the list, but *sleep* is not [*see* False Memory]). Older participants were just as capable as younger participants in not recalling such words as *sleep* that were not in the list.

Self-Concept

Your self-concept is the collection of perceptions you have of yourself, that is, it is a self-image. It includes your knowledge of your family and social roles, your knowledge of your personality characteristics, your knowledge of your abilities and limitations, your knowledge of your body and your physical appearance, and so on. Also included is an affective or evaluative component known as self-esteem (*see* Self-Esteem). These components influence people's self-concepts at all age levels. Most people are able to give a fairly accurate assessment of what they are like. These assessments are expected to change from early to late adulthood as individuals' social roles, family roles, abilities, and physical condition and appearance change.

In general, older adults are well aware of these changes, and they modify their self-concepts accordingly. By contrast, their personality characteristics are likely to change relatively little from those of early adulthood. Such stability is usually reflected in the constancy of this part of the self-concept. Researchers at the University of Wisconsin at Madison have found that an overall positive self-concept in elderly people has a beneficial effect on their mental health.

Self-Efficacy

Self-efficacy refers to a sense of competence or mastery an individual has when confronted by various challenging situations. There is evidence indicating that normally aging adults tend to overestimate slightly their mastery over events in their lives. However, depressed older people generally feel that they have little mastery over family relationships, management of expenditures, protection of themselves and those they love, and so on.

Does participation in an exercise program improve self-efficacy regarding exercise capability for previously sedentary elderly adults? Evidence indicates that it does—at least for a while. Sedentary adults age sixty to seventy-five were given six months of aerobic walking exercise. At the end of six months, confidence in their physical capabilities (for example, strength, agility, and motor ability) increased significantly as did confidence in their exercise capability. However, self-efficacy was found to decline over six months following completion of the exercise program. Interestingly, participants in a control group performing only stretching and tonal exercise for six months also increased their exercise self-efficacy. Older adults in exercise programs should be encouraged to continue those programs at least at regular intervals beyond six months in order to maintain their confidence in their own capabilities. *See also* Control over Life's Events.

Self-Esteem

How do you evaluate what you are in relation to what you would like to be? In asking this kind of evaluation, we are asking you to refer to a part of your self-concept or self-image (*see* Self-Concept) known as self-esteem. Self-esteem may vary from positive to neutral to negative. Of interest in gerontology is whether self-esteem is lower during late adulthood, relative to earlier periods of adulthood.

Cross-sectional studies have compared groups of younger and older adults in their self-esteem ratings. Usually, the participants in these studies are asked to rate themselves on a 1-to-5 scale (1, very true of me; 5, never true of me) for such items as "I feel I have a number of good qualities" and "I feel that my life is not very useful." Men tend to score more positively than women from the early twenties through the sixties. After the sixties there is little sex difference. Self-esteem, in general, increases from the early twenties to the sixties where it peaks. There is then a progressive decline through the seventies and eighties. The decline probably results from an accumulation of negative events in late life, such as deaths of family members and friends and poor health.

The results from several studies have also suggested that the individual differences in self-esteem among older adults are related to the same basic factors that are related to individual differences among younger adults. These factors include occupational success, educational attainment, and success in relating to family members and one's peers. Being on welfare has been found by University of Michigan researchers to lower the self-esteem of elderly men but not of elderly women (average age of seventy).

Self-Evaluation and Adjustment to Stressful Transitions

Do you believe you are able to handle most of the difficult situations you encounter? If so, you have a positive self-evaluation. If not, you have a negative self-evaluation.

Unfortunately, many older adults have negative self-evaluations. This presents a serious problem. Late adulthood is a time of life when people encounter stressful transitions that may adversely affect their lives. They include the death of a spouse, the discovery of a serious health problem, the need to relocate (that is, a change in residence), and so on. How well seniors cope with the stress produced by these transitions depends largely on whether they have a positive or a negative self-evaluation.

Researchers at the University of Wisconsin at Madison provided convincing evidence to show that seniors with a positive self-evaluation cope with the stress caused by a transition more successfully than those with a negative self-evaluation. The transition was that of relocation. Successful coping was determined by the presence of fewer symptoms of depression and more indications of positive psychological well-being than unsuccessful coping. *See also* Stress and Coping with Stress.

Self-Rated Functioning

When older people are asked to rate their ability to take care of themselves (for example, for such activities of daily living as bathing; *see* Activities of Daily Living), their ratings generally are related highly to their actual proficiency in self-care. Self-ratings of functioning also have a strong relationship with mortality (that is, the lower the ratings, the greater the likelihood of death in the near future). These ratings were part of the annual assessments obtained for more than six hundred elderly nuns in what has become known as the Nun Study (*see* Nun Study). Ratings of good, fair, and poor have been found to be associated with twice the risk of mortality, relative to ratings of very good and excellent.

Semantic Memory

You possess a vast store of knowledge, even if it is not at the level of a *Jeopardy* champion. You know the names of the days of the week, the names of the months of the year, the names of the states of the United States, the names of most (if not all) European countries, the multiplication tables, the rules of long division, and so on. This is all part of information permanently stored in what memory researchers call semantic memory, a major part of your total memory system (*see* Memory [Overview]). A very important component of what is stored in semantic memory is your knowledge of words in your native language. This component is known as your lexicon or mental dictionary (*see* Lexicon). You have the ability to retrieve well-established information held in semantic memory quickly and seemingly effortlessly (that is, "automatically"). What is the largest city in England? Notice how quickly and automatically "London" occurred to you. Notice how quickly you read and identified the word *quickly* in the previous sentence.

Unlike episodic memory, semantic memory holds information that is stored without reference to the context in which it was acquired. Information about when and where you learned that London is the largest city in England, or when and where you learned the meaning of the word *quickly* is usually lost from storage. You also have the ability to make inferences and reach decisions on the basis of information stored in semantic memory. For example, if you were asked, "What was Napoleon's telephone number?" you would surely respond with "He couldn't have had a telephone!" Your semantic memory contains information informing you that Napoleon died in the early 1800s and that the telephone was not invented until years after his death. To respond, you simply had to put the two facts in relationship to each other.

In general, semantic memory is remarkably resistant to declines in its functioning with normal aging. Gaining access to its information does tend to slow down a bit in late adulthood, and temporary failures to access information in it (known as tip-of-the-tongue states) occur somewhat more frequently in late adulthood than in earlier adulthood (*see* Verbal Ability). More important, the amount of information held in semantic memory tends to increase from early to late adulthood. This is apparent, for example, in the higher vocabulary-test scores generally obtained by older adults than by younger adults. Whatever declines that occur in semantic memory functioning with normal aging are much less pronounced than declines that may take place in episodic memory functioning. Interestingly, a reasonable argument may be made that semantic memory develops earlier in childhood than does episodic memory. There is an old developmental principle that states that the functions that develop earlier in childhood are subject to later and less age-related declines than are functions that develop later in childhood.

Senile Dementia

Senile dementia is characterized by severely impaired mental functioning in late adulthood. The symptoms include poor memory functioning, poor intellectual functioning, and poor orientation in regard to time and place. Senile dementia is found mainly in patients with Alzheimer's disease and often in patients who have had strokes (*see* Multi-Infarct Dementia).

Creutzfeldt-Jakob disease is a rare form of dementia that usually has its onset earlier than Alzheimer's disease and then goes through a rapid progression of the severity of the dementia. It is suspected of being transmitted by a virus. Pick's disease is a form of dementia that is often indistinguishable from Alzheimer's disease. It is suspected of being caused by a single dominant gene. Some of the brain changes with the disease resemble those found with Alzheimer's disease. However, the high frequency of senile plaques and neurofibrillary tangles found in Alzheimer's disease are not characteristic of Pick's disease.

Senile dementia may also be found in some individuals with other diseases, such as Huntington's disease and Parkinson's disease. Huntington's disease is often called the Woody Guthrie disease. It is genetically transmitted by a dominant gene. It is characterized by involuntary jerky movements of the body. Children of persons with the disease have a 50-50 chance of inheriting the disease. Some individuals in the late stages of Parkinson's disease may show signs of dementia (*see* Parkinson's Disease).

Researchers in Germany estimated the percentage of senile dementia in people age seventy to be about 12 percent, and it increased exponentially each five years after age seventy. Researchers in California found that the decline in cognitive functioning with dementia was slower in women than in men and in patients with more education than in those with less. Presenile dementia is a mental dysfunctioning occurring earlier in life, usually middle age; it may occur in some cases of Alzheimer's disease and multi-infarct dementia.

Researchers in Italy found that awareness of one's own dementia goes through three stages. The first is a period of stability before the decline in mental functioning is noticed, the second a period of declining awareness as the severity of the dementia increases, and the third a period of no further decline in awareness as the dementia stabilizes at a very low level of mental functioning. Of importance is the time lag between the onset of symptoms of dementia and referral for neuropsychological testing (average is 13.8 months). The longer that lag, the longer the delay in initiating care and treatment.

There is a less severe form of dementia known as mild cognitive dementia (MCD). It is defined by a score on the Mini-Mental State Exam (*see* Mini-Mental State Exam) that is below average for a person's age, but not as far below as scores earned by severely demented persons. It is estimated that about 12 percent of those with MCD progress to Alzheimer's disease per year. Researchers in Sweden discovered that MCD is usually accompanied by poor physical health that may play a role in causing the mild dementia.

Senior Centers

Senior centers, as places for education, recreation, and social interactions of senior citizens, began to appear in the early 1940s. With the expansion of the elderly population has come an expansion in the number of senior centers. It is estimated that there are now ten thousand to twelve thousand senior centers in the United States and that about 20 percent of our older population participate in center activities.

Several surveys have provided information about the most likely users of services at senior centers. Women are more likely than men to attend a center, and residents in suburban areas are more likely to attend than residents of other areas. Attendance increases with age through the early eighties and then declines. People living alone are more likely to attend than people with other living arrangements. Race does not seem to be a factor in determining attendance. In addition, users tend to have higher levels of positive health and life satisfaction and lower levels of income than nonusers. Perhaps the most important determinant is an individual's need for social interaction. Individuals reporting more frequent social interactions during the preceding year are more likely to attend than individuals reporting fewer social interactions.

Despite the benefits older adults receive from senior centers, attendance at centers has been declining in recent years. The decline causes problems in funding, recruiting volunteer staff members, and recruiting new leaders.

To determine the reasons for this decline researchers at Midwestern State University in Wichita Falls, Texas, gathered information identifying factors that are related to how often seniors participate in center activities. From this information they were able to make recommendations for increasing participation in activities at a center.

Participation in faith-based organizations was the most significant predictor of frequency of participation in center activities. The more the participation in faith-based activities, the more the participation in center activities.

The second most significant predictor was preferred group size. If groups were larger than twenty-five or smaller than ten, they were less likely to attract participants. Another important predictor was the transportation available to reach the center.

Among the recommendations were that local pastors and priests include information about the local center's weekly activities in church bulletins, that center directors arrange for better public transportation, and that the directors plan more special-interest activities to appeal to various groups of seniors.

Senior centers receive their funding from the Older Americans Act and state and local governments, as well as from their own fund-raising projects and contributions from those who attend the centers. Some of the larger centers have a paid staff, but centers, in general, rely largely on volunteers to operate them. A problem being faced by some centers is the difficulty they are having in convincing newly retired people in their early sixties to become participants, thus creating problems in funding, recruiting volunteer staff, and finding new leaders.

Senior Olympics

Senior Olympics are held every two years. Participants qualify by competing in local events. Local organizations may join the national organization. To receive information about the Games, write to U.S. National Senior Sports Organization, 1307 Washington Avenue, Suite 706, St. Louis, MO, or call 314-621-5545.

Seniors in the Community:
Risk Evaluation for Eating and Nutrition Questionnaire

The Seniors in the Community: Risk Evaluation for Eating and Nutrition Questionnaire (SCREEN) is a test developed by researchers at the University of Guelph, Ontario, Canada, to identify elderly adults at risk of malnutrition. The test has fifteen items with five possible responses. Lower scores indicate a risk of malnutrition. The test has been found to have high test-retest reliability (that is, consistent results over repeated testing). It has also been found to correlate significantly with evaluations given by dietitians of the risk test takers have of malnutrition.

Sensory Functioning and Mental Functioning (Relationship)

Researchers at both the Max Planck Institute in Berlin, Germany, and the Georgia Institute of Technology have found a strong relationship in elderly adults between the proficiency of sensory functioning, both visual and auditory, and proficiency of performance on a number of mental tests, such as intelligence and memory tests. Elderly adults who are experiencing sensory impairments are more likely to have lower mental test scores than elderly adults who are functioning well with their senses.

One possible reason for this relationship is that both sensory and mental functioning are affected by the same general atrophy of the brain. Another possibility is that poor sensory functioning results in diminished encoding of information included on mental tests. However, the fact that age-related declines in smell sensitivity are also closely associated with age-related declines on mental tests suggests that the loss of brain cells is sufficiently widespread to affect both olfactory and other sensory functioning and mental functioning. Smell is unlikely to be involved in the encoding of most verbal mental tests.

Sensory Memory

A familiar experience is to listen to someone and before you respond to the content of that person's statement you find yourself saying, "Uh, what did you say?" You then find yourself responding without having the statement repeated. A probable reason for not needing repetition of the spoken words is that the words actually persisted in the form of an "echo" for several seconds after the speaker had finished saying them. This persistence enabled you to continue analyzing the words spoken until they were fully comprehended.

In other words, your hearing has its own form of memory in which sounds persist as sounds for at least several seconds after the source of the sound has ended. This is one form of *sensory memory*. The other senses have similar memory components that enable sensory information to be extended in time beyond the time the source of that information is physically present. In the case of auditory information, the memory component is called *echoic memory*. The exact duration of echoic memory is unknown, but it seems to be at least several seconds for adults of all ages. It may even persist slightly longer for older adults than for younger adults. This seems likely from evidence indicating that sensory stimuli, in general, persist longer for older than for younger individuals (*see* Stimulus Persistence).

Of further interest is the capacity of echoic memory. How many different sounds (for example, spoken words) may be held in echoic form at any one time? There is evidence to indicate that the capacity diminishes moderately with normal aging. However, in general, echoic memory seems to function quite well in late adulthood, assuming there are no major hearing impairments, and it helps to explain why speech perception under normal conversational conditions is relatively unaffected by aging (*see* Speech Perception). This is true even though older adults require slightly more time to analyze and identify individual spoken words than do younger adults. Echoic memory allows them extra time to identify those words.

Of the other senses, only visual memory has been widely studied. In this case, it is called *iconic memory* in which "icons" (images) of visual information persist after their physical sources cease. The persistence of the information prolongs the time that visually presented information can be analyzed and identified. It may also compensate for the fact that our eyes are in constant motion, and during periods of movement no image is being projected on the retina of the eye. The iconic image of the image registered on the retina just before a movement may persist long enough to enable us to see the events in our visual environment without interruption. Without iconic memory, our vision would perhaps consist of a series of flashes.

The duration of iconic memory is much briefer than the duration of echoic memory—it is probably no longer than half a second. As with echoic memory, iconic memory seems to be relatively unaffected by normal aging. The duration may be slightly longer for elderly adults than for younger adults. However, as with echoic memory, the amount of information held in iconic memory is probably less for older adults than for younger adults.

Sequential Method

The sequential method is an alternative to the traditional cross-sectional and longitudinal methods of studying adult age differences in behavior. It was introduced by Dr. K. Warner Schaie in the mid-1960s and has been applied primarily in studies of intelligence and personality. The method is intended to avoid the problems associated with the traditional cross-sectional and longitudinal methods in determining the extent to which observed age differences are actually attributable to a true age change. These problems occur through the possibility of cohort and historical time effects that cause age differences in the absence of true age changes (*see* Cross-Sectional Method; Longitudinal Method). The sequential method combines the simultaneous examination of cross-sectional and longitudinal age differences, together with time-lag comparisons (*see* Time-Lag Comparison), all on the same behavior or characteristic.

Services (Formal)

Formal services received by elderly people are to be distinguished from the informal services provided by family members and friends. How much use do elderly people make of these formal services? A survey of people aged sixty and older in Albany, New York, revealed that the most frequently used service is the multipurpose senior center (used by about 20 percent of those surveyed; *see* Senior Centers). Other services were less frequently used. For example, fewer than 5 percent of those surveyed reported using Meals on Wheels, fewer than 3 percent reported using financial or personal counseling services, and fewer than 2 percent reported using telephone check-in calls. Moreover, the survey indicated that the use of formal services showed little relationship to their availability or accessibility. Understandably, they were used more frequently by those people with a disability than by those without a disability. Nevertheless, it appears that only a minority of older people take advantage of the services that exist for them. A greater effort needs to be made to make such services known to older people and to make them realize the advantages they offer.

Sex Differences and Scientific Ability

In 2005 the president of Harvard University gave an address in which he noted that there are many more male scientists than there are female scientists. He did not stop there. He added that the reason is that women have less scientific aptitude than men. This created quite a furor, especially by women's organizations (the president eventually resigned in 2006). It is true that men tend to score higher than women on basic abilities that are seemingly relevant to scientific ability and aptitude. This is the case, for example, for spatial ability (*see* Spatial Ability). From early adulthood on, men score higher than women. This sex difference persists well into late adulthood. On the other hand, women score higher than men on tests of verbal ability from early adulthood on. This sex difference also persists into late adulthood. It is of interest to observe how many prominent female authors there have been over the years.

There are experts, however, who believe that men and women do not differ basically in their aptitude for science. The reason for the greater number of male scientists than female scientists is attributed by them to factors other than innate aptitude, such as motivation, differential treatment of the sexes during childhood and adolescence, and so on.

Sexual Behavior (Heterosexual)

One of the most prevalent myths about aging is that elderly people are basically asexual and that the domain of sexual behavior is limited to only younger people. Perhaps even more disturbing beliefs held by some people are that sexual activity in late adulthood is either silly or sinful. Statements like "He's a dirty old man" are not uncommon. The implication here is that many older men are too preoccupied with sex. It is important to distinguish between interest in sexual activity and actual participation in sexual activity. The two do not always coincide, especially in late adulthood.

Interest in continuing sexual activity during late adulthood is related to several factors. For example, in general, elderly people from the middle and upper socioeconomic classes are likely to be more interested in continuing sexual activity than people from the lower socioeconomic class. Evidence also indicates that the amount of education is related positively to the sexual interests of elderly people—the greater the amount of education, the greater interest is likely to be. However, interest in sexual behavior remains fairly constant throughout adulthood and is unlikely to show any pronounced decline until after people reach their seventies.

Interviews of adults of varying ages have revealed age-related declines in the frequency of intercourse reported by married couples. For couples in their twenties, the reported average frequency is slightly greater than three times per week. For couples in their forties, it is an average of twice per week, and for couples in their fifties, it has dropped to about once per week. Couples ranging in age from sixty-five to ninety-seven said they had sex about two and a half times a month—and complained that they wanted it twice as often. In a survey reported in *Modern Maturity* magazine, more than 25 percent of the respondents age seventy-five and older said they had sex at least once a week. Moreover, of those age seventy-five and older more than 60 percent said they found their sexual partner to be physically attractive (compared to 56 percent in the forty-five-to-seventy-four-year age range). Sexual activity seems to be a major factor in determining quality of life, even in late adulthood.

In a large-scale survey of men in the age range of sixty-six to seventy, whether or not they were married, 24 percent reported they no longer had intercourse, another 48 percent reported once a month, 26 percent once a week, and 2 percent two or three times a week (no one reported a still greater frequency, possibly because they thought they might be regarded as being "oversexed"). For women in the same age range, 73 percent reported no intercourse at all (women in this age range are often widowed and have no available sexual partner), 16 percent reported once a month, and 11 percent once a week (no one reported a frequency of two or more times a week).

If these percentages are accurate, it would appear that intercourse for men in the sixty-six-to-seventy-year age range is often occurring with women younger than age sixty-six. The frequency of intercourse by older people is likely to be greater for those who had experienced greater enjoyment from it earlier in life than for those who experienced less enjoyment.

Although sexual behavior does continue well into late adulthood (there are reports of men in their nineties having intercourse occasionally), there is undoubtedly a decline in the frequency of intercourse and in the incidence of total impotence (estimated to be about 15 percent of men age seventy compared with 5 percent of men age forty). Viagra, a pill approved by the U.S. Food and Drug Administration, has received considerable attention as a means of overcoming impotence. It is the first nonsurgical treatment of impotence that does not have to be injected or inserted into the penis. The biological aging of the sex organs accounts for only part of this decline in the frequency of intercourse. Other reasons for elderly men include feelings of monotony in intercourse with the same partner, physical fatigue, preoccupation with work, fear of impotence, depression, diabetes, heart disease, and hypertension. The monotony problem is resolvable by the realization that variety is the spice of life, and a little variety in the form of intercourse may relieve the monotony. Preoccupation with work is likely to diminish as increasing numbers of older people retire at younger ages. The fear of impotence is likely to be greatly reduced if elderly men are made fully aware of the normal changes that are occurring in them, especially the increase in the refractory duration (the time before the next erection can be attained) and knowledge that Viagra is available, if needed.

A decline in physical health is likely to become decreasingly important as the health status of future generations of older people shows substantial gains. There is the common belief that intercourse is likely to precipitate a heart attack in elderly men. However, deaths during intercourse are rare, and they account for only 1 percent of sudden deaths from coronary failures. Even adults who have had heart attacks are usually able to resume sexual activity eventually.

When intercourse ceases for elderly couples, it is usually at the wish of the male partner. In fact, there is evidence indicating that the percentage of women age sixty-five years and older engaging in sexual activity, including masturbation, is greater than for women ages eighteen to twenty-six. For elderly women, the major reason for the absence of intercourse per se is the lack of a sexual partner. This may change in the future as increasing numbers of older women are in the labor force. Job preoccupation and fatigue may become reasons as prevalent for older women as for older men.

Changes do occur in sexual behavior during intercourse for both older men and older women. For elderly men the time required to attain a penile erection increases (and the time needed for foreplay increases), the force of ejaculation and the volume of seminal fluid released decrease, the duration of orgasms decreases, and, perhaps, most important, the refractory period increases with advancing age.

These changes are not really manifestations of sexual dysfunctioning, but rather manifestations of normal aging. Sex therapists believe that one of the reasons for a reduction in the frequency of intercourse by older couples is the failure of older women to understand these changes in their male partner. For older women, the production of vaginal lubricant takes longer (with an increased need for longer foreplay), the vaginal opening decreases in size, the vaginal walls become thinner (resulting possibly in greater pain during intercourse), and the duration of orgasms becomes briefer with advancing age, even though the frequency of orgasms increases in each decade of life through the eighth decade.

These changes, like those for older men, have a negative effect on sexual interest. However, they are manifestations of normal aging, not sexual dysfunctioning. Other reasons include prostate problems in older men, declining health for both partners, and adverse effects of some medications for both partners.

Of concern is the possibility that elderly people with dementia show inappropriate sexual behavior. Anecdotes suggest that they do (for example, exposing themselves). However, evidence gathered by researchers in California indicates that inappropriate sexual behaviors are actually uncommon in institutional settings. They observed a number of demented residents over nine separate occasions. Inappropriate behaviors were defined as touching someone other than a spouse on the breasts or genitals and exposing breasts or genitals publicly. Only 18 percent of the observed residents displayed inappropriate behaviors. When such behaviors did occur, they were usually brief and relatively minor in extent.

Shingles

Shingles is a painful skin and nervous disease that affects nearly a million people in the United States annually. Most of the people affected are over age fifty, with the peak incidence occurring between ages sixty and seventy. In addition, the severity of the disease increases with age. The disease is caused by the virus varicella-zoster, and it appears first in childhood as chicken pox. The virus then remains dormant until it is reactivated as shingles later in life. The reason for the reactivation is not known.

The first symptoms of shingles are numbness, a tingling pain on or under the skin somewhere on the body, and mild flulike symptoms. Later a rash appears on the skin. A doctor may prescribe antiviral medicines and steroids such as prednisone. The Food and Drug Administration approved the drug Famvir as a possible means of relieving the pain that often follows shingles. Treatment within the first few days of the rash's breaking out may reduce aftereffects of the disease, such as chronic pain or visual and hearing problems (if the rash appears near the eyes or ears).

Anyone who has had chicken pox and has a weakened immune system is at risk of having shingles. This combination, of course, includes many elderly people. Shingles may be contagious. Fluid in the rash contains live chicken pox virus. If someone who has shingles touches someone who has had chicken pox, the disease could be passed on, but the probability of this happening is low.

Short-Term Memory

You have just looked up a telephone number in the telephone directory, and you have begun to dial it. Will you remember all of the digits you need to dial? This is an example of short-term memory, memory of information that lasts for only seconds. Without rehearsing the information in short-term memory, most, if not all, of it is likely to be lost from memory within twenty to thirty seconds. If you are distracted for several seconds before you can dial the telephone number, you will probably find that you have forgotten several of the digits. If the distraction lasts much longer, you will probably forget most of the digits. To maintain information in short-term memory, you need to repeat it to yourself constantly.

Short-term memory (also called *primary memory*) is memory for information that is presently in consciousness. Short-term memory is distinguishable from *long-term memory* (also called *secondary memory*) that is not in consciousness but has the potential for being retrieved and made part of consciousness (as in the retrieval of a frequently called telephone number that no longer requires you to look it up in a directory before you dial it—you have retrieved it from long-term memory).

There is frequent confusion for many people between the concepts of short-term memory and long-term memory. Many older people may often say that their short-term memory is poor. They probably mean that their long-term memory for recent events ("short-term" to them means recent, but well beyond the realm of seconds) that are stored in memory (but not in consciousness unless they are successfully retrieved; for example, the name of a new neighbor they met recently) is seemingly giving them problems. When most elderly people refer to their "long-term memory," they probably mean their *very long-term or remote memory* or events from years ago (*see* Very Long-Term Memory). In fact, older persons who complain about their "short-term memory" probably have a good short-term memory as the term is used in memory research.

Short-term memory is part of the functioning of a component of the memory system called *working memory* (*see* Working Memory). Working memory has a capacity for storing briefly a limited amount of information. Regardless of a person's age, the information held in working memory's store is in the form of the sounds needed to reproduce it. Thus, the number 8 as one of the digits in the aforementioned telephone number is stored briefly as the sound "ate." If necessary, however, working memory is flexible enough to store information in forms other than sound. This is obviously the case in that congenitally deaf individuals have short-term memory in which information is stored either in visual form or in the form of the motions needed to reproduce the information in sign language.

Are there age differences in the amount of information that can be stored briefly and recalled completely without error? That is, does the capacity of working memory's store decrease from early to late adulthood? The capacity of the short-term store may be measured by several different procedures. The most common procedure is to determine a person's memory span for either digits or words (see Memory Span), that is, the longest series of digits or words that can be retained immediately after hearing or seeing them without making an error. When capacity is measured in this way, there is little difference between young adults and older adults in span length. For example, it is about 7 digits, on the average, for young adults and about 6.5, on the average, for elderly adults. In general, the capacity for short-term storage is only 5 percent to 10 percent less for older adults than for young adults.

The amount of information that can be stored briefly can be expanded considerably by a process known as chunking. Suppose a telephone number contains the successive digits 1 4 9 2. If you immediately identify this sequence as the year Columbus discovered America, then the four numbers may be stored as a single "chunk" rather than as four separate "chunks" (one chunk for each number). Similarly, the word sequence *turtle, neck, sweater* may be stored as a single chunk (*turtleneck sweater*) rather than as three separate chunks (one for each word). Ordinarily, you may not be able to hold more than five unrelated words in short-term memory. However, if there are fifteen words and every three words form a chunk (for example, like *turtle, neck, sweater*), then you should be able to span all fifteen words. There is evidence to indicate that elderly adults are less likely than young adults to use chunking spontaneously to expand their short-term memory capacity.

As noted earlier, information held in the short-term store is forgotten quickly unless it is repeated or rehearsed. To demonstrate the rapid rate of forgetting, participants are given a series of trials in which they receive on each trial an item to be remembered, such as three letters of the alphabet that do not form a word (called a nonsense syllable; for example, *JVB*). After hearing or seeing the item, they have a retention interval that varies in duration over the trials. For example, it may be three seconds on some trials, and six, nine, twelve, or fifteen seconds on other trials. During the retention interval, they are prevented from rehearsing the item by being forced to perform some activity that blocks the opportunity to rehearse (for example, counting backward by three from a given number—363, 360, 357, and so on). Most of the items will be recalled when the retention interval is only three seconds, but most will be forgotten when the interval is fifteen seconds. The rate of forgetting is rapid regardless of one's age, and it occurs at about the same rate for older adults as for younger adults.

We have the ability to search or scan information in the short-term store to answer questions about it. For example, suppose you heard on the television news that today's baseball winners in the National League were Los Angeles, San Diego, Philadelphia, Chicago, and St. Louis. Shortly after hearing this, someone in the next room asks you, "Did Atlanta win today?" After a very rapid search of the contents of your short-term store, you find yourself saying "No." The search did not locate Atlanta in your store. If the question had been, "Did Chicago win today?" your rapid answer would have been "Yes." You would find Chicago to be part of the information held in your short-term store. The nature of searching short-term memory shows little change from early to late adulthood. Elderly adults are just as capable as young adults, but the speed of the search is a bit slower in late adulthood, in agreement with the slowing-down principle (*see* Slowing-Down Principle).

In summary, short-term memory is fairly robust in regard to declines in functioning with normal aging. Its capacity for storage changes only slightly, its rate of forgetting is about what it is in early adulthood, and its ability to search its own contents remains highly functional and reliable.

Sibling Relationships

A recent survey revealed that of the people older than age sixty surveyed, more than 80 percent reported being close to at least one brother or sister. The closeness usually dates back to childhood or adolescence, and it persists throughout adulthood. Siblings who were close during the pre-adulthood years are highly likely to remain close when they are both older adults.

In general, however, the closeness is greater between sisters than between either brothers or sisters and brothers. Sibling rivalry often intensifies in midlife, but it usually disappears before late adulthood is reached. However, it may resurface under some conditions, especially those involving an inheritance.

Dr. Victor C. Cicirelli of Purdue University studied a group of elderly persons who each had at least one living sibling. He discovered those individuals, both men and women, who had a close relationship with a sister had less depression than individuals who did not have such a relationship. By contrast, elderly women who experienced poorer relationships with a sister had a greater degree of depression. In general, sisters are viewed by both elderly men and women as playing a greater role as potential sources of help and comfort than are brothers.

Siblings are not often a main source of help with instrumental activities of living (for example, shopping or transportation). Nevertheless, they are likely to be there when the need is great.

In general, older people are more likely to believe that a sibling will come to their aid if they have more than one sibling than if they have only one. Moreover, there is some support for this belief: there is evidence to indicate that elderly people are more likely to receive assistance from a sibling when they have more than one sibling.

The incidence of negative relationships between siblings is lower for older than it is for younger adults. One probable reason is the fact that older adults generally have better control of their emotions than do younger adults (see Emotions).

Signs and Forms

We all read signs and fill out forms. However, given the visual problems many elderly adults have (see Vision; Visual Disorders), signs and forms need to be made more readable. Signs should be in large black letters or numbers on a white background rather than, say, blue on violet. Forms to be filled out should be black on white and not a different combination (for example, blue on green). If there is more than one color in the content of a sign or form, they should be easily discriminated (for example, red and yellow).

Sjogren's Syndrome

See Teeth, Gums, and Mouth.

Skin Cancer

Basal cell and squamous cell cancers are the two most common forms of skin cancer. They can be easily removed and treated more easily than the melanoma type of skin cancer.

Melanoma is the most serious skin cancer. It involves skin cells that produce a dark brown or black pigment called melanin. Each year more than fifty thousand people in the United States discover they have melanoma. The incidence increases with age. Non-Hispanic white women aged fifty to seventy-nine who have a history of nonmelanoma cancer are especially likely to develop melanoma.

Overexposure to ultraviolet radiation from sunlight greatly increases the risk of developing melanoma, as well as other skin cancers. Older adults should practice protection from the sun. This includes avoiding the sun between ten in the morning and four in the afternoon, when the sun's rays are the strongest. They should seek shade as often as possible, and they should use broad-spectrum sunscreen. Wear protective clothing, including a wide-brimmed hat, and sunglasses that provide 100 percent protection from ultraviolet light. A family history of melanoma should be a significant warning to take such precautions.

Treatment consists of surgical removal of the tumor and surrounding skin once a biopsy has confirmed the melanoma. Chemotherapy or radiation therapy may be needed to destroy remaining cancerous cells. There is also the possibility of having immunotherapy (or biotherapy) in which the patient's immune system is directed at recognizing and destroying cancer cells.

Seniors should have regular checkups with a dermatologist. They should see a dermatologist as soon as possible if they discover a suspicious-looking mole on their skin.

Skipping Meals

Some elderly people will skip one of their meals daily, usually either to lose weight or to save money. It is a poor weight-loss strategy. Those who skip breakfast may have more weight problems than those who eat a healthy breakfast. The same is true for skipping lunch. In either event, you may eat too much during the rest of the day, adding to your weight problem. In addition, you may be causing problems with various parts of your body. The damage done to your body is likely to cost you more than the cost of the meals you are skipping. If there is a need to save money, find a way to do it other than by skipping a meal daily.

Breakfast is an especially important meal. After a night's sleep your body has gone for hours without fuel to energize it. Your glucose store needs to be replenished.

Sleep

"To sleep, perchance to dream." If Hamlet had been an elderly man, he would have had some concern about the likelihood of dreaming. Dreaming usually occurs during a particular stage of sleep known as *REM sleep. REM* is an acronym for "rapid eye movement." This stage of sleep is characterized by the eyes darting about, as well as other characteristics such as the complete relaxation of the muscles, the insensitivity of the senses to external stimulation, and the presence of brain waves that resemble those present when one is awake and alert. (For this reason REM sleep is also often called paradoxical sleep.) If awakened during one of the several periods of REM sleep during a night's sleep cycle, the probability is very high that the person awakened will report dreaming. That probability is much lower if the person is awakened at a time other than REM sleep.

The amount of time in REM sleep decreases steadily from infancy through late adulthood. Researchers at the University of Florida found that their participants in the twenty-to-thirty-year age range averaged twenty-five to thirty minutes per REM period, whereas their participants in the fifty-to-sixty-year age range averaged ten to twenty minutes. Consequently, dreaming does occur less often in older than in younger adults (*see also* Nightmares). The decline in amount of REM sleep in late adulthood may have negative effects on the mental functioning of elderly adults. A University of Washington researcher reported a fairly substantial correlation in her elderly research participants between average REM sleep time and scores on an intelligence test.

REM sleep is one of five stages of sleep that occur in repeated or partially repeated cycles during a night's sleep. The four stages other than REM are often grouped together and referred to as *NREM* (non-REM) *sleep*. Of particular interest is the stage reached at the end of the first nightly cycle. It is called *stage 4*, or *deep sleep*. Recordings by an electroencephalogram reveal slow, high-amplitude waves (known as delta waves) during this sleep stage. In late adulthood, the amplitude of these waves diminishes, and the amount of time spent in deep sleep diminishes. A study at the University of Washington found that participants between the ages of seventy-six and ninety averaged only twenty-five minutes per night in deep sleep, compared with the average of sixty-three minutes by adult participants in their twenties.

These changes in sleep occur even though older adults tend to spend more time in bed (ten to twelve hours) than younger adults. They also spend more time in bed with their sleep commonly disrupted by difficulty in getting to sleep and frequent awakenings once they are asleep. As a result, older adults average less sleep per night than do younger adults. The diminished nightly sleep often results in drowsiness and lack of mental alertness during the daytime hours. Interestingly, researchers at the University of Florida discovered that their elderly participants who napped less than an hour during the day did not experience any added difficulty in getting to sleep in the subsequent night. Irregular bedtimes and late-night television watching may disturb normal sleep, as may physical illness and pain.

In a study of women ranging in age from fifty-six to seventy-seven it was found that they averaged forty-five minutes of out-of-bed sleep over twenty-four hours. The amount of out-of-bed sleep correlated significantly and positively with age (the older the woman, the greater the amount). No other variable was found to correlate significantly with the amount of out-of-bed sleep (for example, use of sleep aids or amount of caffeine consumed).

Sleep has been related to longevity and life expectancy. In general, people who sleep ten or more hours per day or less than five hours a day die younger than people who sleep between six and nine hours per day. The optimal life expectancy has been found among people who sleep about seven hours per day. Thus, sleep joins other characteristics (for example, years of education; *see* Educational Level) as a predictor of life expectancy, and is likely to be one of the variables included in tables that predict life expectancy at any given age.

The relationship between the amount of sleep and longevity is not fully understood. Conceivably, those people who sleep too much are doing so because they are in poor health, which, in turn, could lead to decreased longevity. In addition, prolonged sleep results in diminished activity, which, in turn, could be another contributor to a shorter longevity. Too little sleep may add to a person's tension level and lead to a decrease in physical health.

Researchers at the University of Pittsburgh School of Medicine compared three groups of elderly men (sixty-one to eighty-nine years of age). As diagnosed by various criteria of sleep quality, the groups consisted of good sleepers, relatively impaired sleepers, and poor sleepers. The poor sleepers, relative to the others, were found, in general, to have had more recent negative life events and less support from family members and friends. The poor sleepers were also largely the oldest participants in their study. Researchers at Stanford University found that poor sleepers with high levels of stress had greater difficulty falling asleep than did poor sleepers with lower levels of stress. For good sleepers, they found no relationship between amount of sleep and level of stress.

Sleep Complaints

Complaints about poor sleep are among the most frequent complaints expressed by elderly people. The complaints include difficulty in falling asleep, difficulty in remaining asleep, and not feeling rested in the morning. There are reasons for the legitimacy of these complaints (*see* Sleep). Complaints are given most often by elderly women and elderly people with less education, more cognitive impairment, poor self-rated health, psychiatric disorders, and depression. Complaints are also given more frequently by whites than by African Americans.

Caregivers of elderly patients with dementia report more sleep complaints than age-matched individuals who are not caregivers. Their most common complaint (84 percent) is having to get up at night or early morning to care for the patient. The frequency of complaints does not appear to be related to the quality of the relationship with the patient or to the patient's source of dementia.

Sleep Disorders

Surveys of community-dwelling, normally aging elderly people indicate that more than a third of them state they have problems with their sleep. Sleep problems occur among both older men and women, but the incidence may be somewhat greater for men. One of the most common forms of sleep disorders is insomnia. There are two forms of insomnia. The first is *sleep-onset insomnia*. In this situation the individual has difficulty getting to sleep. The second form, and the one more frequent in late adulthood, is *sleep-maintenance insomnia*. In this situation the individual awakens several times during the night and has difficulty going back to sleep once awakened.

Elderly adults who report insomnia have been found to report more symptoms of anxiety and depression and to have greater fear about losing control over their sleep than do elderly adults who do not report insomnia. Researchers at the Medical College of Virginia found that older insomniacs have much stronger beliefs about serious negative consequences of insomnia than elderly self-defined good sleepers. Most of these beliefs are inaccurate. Unfortunately, these beliefs may prolong periods of insomnia and lead to a vicious circle.

Older insomniacs should consult sleep therapists not only for help in improving their sleep habits (*see* Sleep Therapy) but also for information that could ease their minds about the dangers of insomnia. The incidence of medical disorders and the use of drugs other than sleeping pills appears to be about the same for those reporting frequent insomnia and those who do not.

A third of all sleeping-pill subscriptions are written for people older than age sixty. There are, of course, many nonprescription sleeping pills (for example, Sominex and Tylenol PM). If you use one of them, be certain to read about the right amount to take and the conditions you should avoid. Sleeping pills have a short-term effectiveness in treating insomnia, but, if taken regularly, they can have many side effects. For example, individuals with *sleep apnea* (see below) may experience an increase in both the frequency and the duration of its episodes. Sleeping pills may also reduce the duration of REM sleep periods and increase the incidence of cardiac dysrhythmia. Moreover, some degree of sleep loss on some nights may actually improve the quality of sleep the next night by increasing the amount of stage 4 (deep) sleep.

A natural substance, melatonin, produced in the pineal gland (located in the center of the brain) is believed to induce sleep. It was once believed its production decreased with aging. However, a report from the National Institutes of Health revealed that men aged sixty-five to eighty-one had melatonin levels similar to those of much younger men. A nutritional supplement of synthetic melatonin is used to treat insomnia, but its effectiveness is uncertain. Foods rich in the amino acid tryptophan, such as tofu, may increase the body's production of melatonin and provide relief for insomniacs. Relief from insomnia may be obtained by moderate exercise and by sleeping pills such as Ambien (it may make you groggy in the morning) and Benzodiazepine. Indiplon is a new medication that has been very effective in treating insomnia in clinical trials. It is expected to be evaluated in 2006 for approval by the U.S. Food and Drug Administration. Declines in mental functioning for elderly insomniacs who are chronic users of sleeping pills (for example, Benzodiazepine) have been found by researchers to be equal to the declines for insomniacs without such pills.

It is estimated that nearly one-third of the elderly population has sleep apnea, with men being twice as likely to have it as women. Elderly adults with high blood pressure are also more likely to have it than those with normal pressure. It consists of periods lasting ten seconds or longer in which there is a cessation of air flow in breathing. Apnea and other abnormal respiratory events during sleep are considered pathological conditions if they occur at a rate of five or more episodes per night. Some elderly people may have hundreds of episodes during a night's sleep. Apnea must be taken seriously by those adults who have the disorder. Researchers have discovered that elders with apnea are about twice as likely to have a stroke or to die as are elders without the disorder.

Apnea is usually accompanied by blood oxygen desaturation (hypoxemia), a condition that may cause mental dysfunctioning. However, researchers at the Medical College of Virginia found only negligible differences in mental functioning of older adults with mild to moderate apnea compared with those without apnea. On the other hand, pathological apnea may be associated with such health problems as obesity and hypertension.

Elderly people with apnea tend to have much slower reaction times than elderly people without apnea, a condition that makes them especially susceptible to accidents while driving an automobile. Obesity may also contribute to sleep apnea. Conceivably, body fat pushes down on the air passages, interfering with breathing. In addition, sleep apnea may cause weight gain. Victims of apnea are usually too tired to do much exercising. Weight gain and apnea tend to feed on each other.

There seems to be a relationship between snoring and apnea. Like apnea, the prevalence of snoring increases with age, and like apnea, snoring is more prevalent in men than in women. Treatments for sleep apnea include avoiding sleeping on your back, losing weight, and avoiding respiratory depressants and stimulants. Avoidance of alcohol is especially important. For more information about apnea, write to the American Sleep Apnea Association, 2025 Pennsylvania Avenue, Suite 905, Washington, DC 20006, or contact its Web site at http://www.sleepapnea.org.

Periodic leg movements also increase in late adulthood. They are characterized by the "restless leg syndrome" and the urge to move the legs repeatedly with rapid and stereotyped flexions. The cause is unknown. Its presence increases the number of awakenings after falling asleep. Afflicted individuals may jump out of bed and move about the house. A common treatment is the administration of the drugs used to treat Parkinson's disease, such as Mirapex and Requip. Some seniors have a strong presleep urge to move their legs repeatedly. The result is often sleep-onset insomnia.

The incidence of some sleep disorders in late adulthood is low. One of these disorders is *narcolepsy*. Narcolepsy is characterized by the inability to control wakefulness, with the narcoleptic individual experiencing periods during the normal waking hours in which he or she suddenly falls asleep. Another uncommon sleep disorder in late adulthood is *sleep walking*.

Dr. William C. Dement, a prominent sleep researcher, offers a number of tips for having a healthy sleep. They include avoiding caffeinated drinks in the evening, avoiding eating close to bedtime, having a regular bedtime, and having a regular ritual, such as reading a few pages of a book. You should also make certain that your bedroom is quiet, dark, and not too warm. Exercise, but not just before going to bed.

Several surveys of nursing home residents have revealed that they have greater sleep problems than community-dwelling elderly adults. They rarely spend a single hour completely in sleep. In general, both brief periods of sleep and wakefulness are observed during every hour of the twenty-four-hour day, although sleep is least likely near sunset. Their sleep pattern is greatly distorted by frequent daytime napping caused largely by lack of activity and by frequent awakening at night by loud roommates.

Some sleep researchers believe that sleep measures may provide an effective early diagnosis of Alzheimer's diseases. The sleep of patients with Alzheimer's disease is usually greatly distorted. The time in bed actually sleeping is likely to be diminished considerably, and the fragmentation by awakening periods is especially pronounced. As the dementia becomes more severe, so does the magnitude of the sleep disturbance.

Some patients with Alzheimer's disease display what is called the *sundown syndrome.* It is characterized by agitation and confusion during the awakening periods, often accompanied by straying from bed and wandering about the residence. Other symptoms include vocalizations and pacing during the evening hours. The syndrome is associated with such factors as dehydration, incontinence, sleep disturbance, and social isolation. There is also evidence indicating that patients with Alzheimer's disease have less deep sleep than normally aging adults and that it takes patients longer to reach the REM stage of sleep. *See also* Visual Disorders (Sleep Problems).

Sleep (Inefficient)

The loss of continuity and depth of sleep for many elderly people (*see* Sleep) constitutes what is called *inefficient sleep.* Many people suffer from inefficient sleep after age seventy-five, with the possible consequences being daytime sleepiness and declining mental functioning.

Researchers at the University of Pittsburgh discovered two interventions for improving sleep efficiency in normally aging seniors. One treatment consists of sleep-restriction therapy in which time in bed is restricted by thirty minutes nightly for one year. The participants did show improvement in sleep efficiency as measured by sustained sleep continuity and greater sleep depth.

The other therapy consists of sleep-hygiene education (for example, the effects of caffeine, alcohol, medications, and the benefits of moderate exercise and so on). The participants showed less improvement in sleep efficiency than those in the other treatment condition. However, they did show initial improvement in their feeling of well-being during the daytime.

Sleep Therapy

Sleep centers are now located at many universities and hospitals across the United States. They provide diagnostic tests of individuals who report sleep disorders. Most important, they also offer behavioral methods of treating sleep disorders, especially insomnia. These methods are generally preferred over the excessive use of sleeping pills.

A popular behavioral therapy is called the *stimulus control method.* Clients are trained to use their beds only for sleep, to establish a regular sleep schedule, and to get out of bed after every ten- to twenty-minute period of sleeplessness, and do something else. Researchers at Washington University in St. Louis have demonstrated that this method is as effective for insomniacs over age sixty as it is for younger insomniacs.

Another behavioral therapy is called the *countercontrol method.* Clients are trained to engage in a nonarousing activity during sleepless periods. For example, they are to read a dull book or to listen to the radio. Clients are also advised not to nap after three in the afternoon and to reduce their caffeine intake, especially in the afternoon and evening. They also should not drink alcoholic beverages at night. Above all they are trained not to panic if they do not fall asleep immediately. The researchers at Washington University have also discovered this method to be as effective for older insomniacs as for younger insomniacs.

There is another therapeutic program called *cognitive sleep therapy* that seems to be effective for elderly people who awaken during the night and have difficulty getting back to sleep (maintenance insomnia). The program calls for both education about the effects of aging on sleep, the effects of sleep deprivation on later sleeping, and the application of a modified stimulus-control procedure (for example, go to bed only when sleepy, leave the bedroom if awake for more than twenty or thirty minutes, and return when sleepy). Researchers in North Carolina tested the program for six weeks, with a follow-up at six months. They found it to yield a 54 percent reduction of wake time during the normal sleep period.

Perhaps the most interesting form of sleep therapy is that of acupuncture. Researchers in Taiwan found that it greatly reduced the sleep problems of the elderly participants in their study (*see* Acupuncture).

There is a workshop available for elderly people to help them sleep better. The materials used in the workshop include a ten-minute video about sleep and informative brochures about sleep and sleep disorders. Write to the National Council on Aging (Attn: Health Promotion/Sleep), 409 Third Street Southwest, Washington, DC 20024. *See also* Sleep (Inefficient).

Slowing-Down Principle

Many components of human behavior are slower in their execution for older adults than for younger adults. This slowing-down principle applies to reaction times and the times needed to perform various behaviors. It also applies to the speed of conducting mental operations, such as those involved in perceiving and identifying visual forms. Consider the time it takes to determine whether two letters have the same name. When the two letters are physically the same (for example, both uppercase *A*s), younger adults usually require less time to decide they have the same name than older adults. When the two letters are no longer physically identical, but still have the same name (for example, an uppercase *A* and a lowercase *a*), the time needed to make the same name decision increases for both younger and older adults, but disproportionately more for older adults.

If young participants averaged about 100 milliseconds to perform with physically identical letters, we would expect elderly adults to average about 150 milliseconds. If the average time for young adults to perform the name-identity task in the absence of physical identity is 200 milliseconds, we would expect the average time for elderly adults to be about 300 milliseconds. The mental operations time for elderly adults averages about one and a half times that of young adults.

The slower time to perform mental operations for elderly adults is a contributor to their diminished performances on some memory tasks.

Some evidence for this position comes from a study by researchers at the University of Victoria in Canada (*see* Longitudinal Studies of Aging's Effects on Health and Cognition). They evaluated age differences in the speed of comprehending reading material as an index of speed of mental operations and related them to age differences in episodic memory and working memory (*see* Episodic Memory; Working Memory). They found that the slower rate of elderly adults accounted for much of the adverse effects of age on both forms of memory.

Researchers at Washington University in St. Louis found that speed of processing is related to physical performances, such as standing up from a chair, climbing one flight of stairs, and a fifty-foot floor walk. They proposed that excessive slowing down of mental processing with aging could be a significant contributor to frailty in the elderly population. *See also* Speed of Behavior.

Smallpox

Smallpox is a highly contagious viral disease that may attack people of all ages. About 30 percent of those afflicted with the disease die. For centuries it killed many people, and scarred those it did not kill. Dr. Edward Jenner developed a vaccination in 1796 that was effective in preventing the disease. Eventually, smallpox was eliminated in most countries, including the United States.

As a result, vaccinations were no longer given in mass inoculations after

1972. Most people, especially older adults, who received vaccinations are unlikely to be protected now after so many years after vaccination. Today the threat of biological terrorism has made it essential for the vaccine to become available again.

Smell

The epithelium (tissue lining the inner surface of the nose) becomes thinner with increasing age over the adult life span. This thinning is accompanied by a loss of olfactory (smell) receptor cells that enable us to detect the presence of an odorous substance; therefore, diminished smell sensitivity occurs during late adulthood. As with all of the other senses, sensitivity refers both to the threshold sensitivity and to the suprathreshold (above the threshold) sensitivity.

Threshold sensitivity refers to the ability to detect a weak odorous substance. The minimum concentration of a given odorous substance that must be present before the odor is just barely noticed defines the threshold value for that substance. Different odorous substances have different threshold values, with greater concentrations of some substances needed for detection than for other substances. Regardless of the substance, a greater concentration is needed for detection, on average, by elderly adults than by young adults. For some odorous substances, the threshold value may be nine times greater for older adults than for young adults. Overall, the age-related decline in threshold sensitivity is much greater for smell than for taste. The decline in smell sensitivity, on average, is greater for men than for women.

Suprathreshold sensitivity refers to the ability to discriminate among varying intensities of an odorous substance, all of which are well above threshold value. As the concentration of the substance doubles or triples, do we also perceive the intensity of the odor as doubling or tripling? There is evidence that elderly adults have less suprathreshold sensitivity than do younger adults and that this is especially the case for sweet-smelling substances.

A related problem for older people is their diminished ability to identify odorous substances (for example, banana or lemon) by name. Odor identification peaks around the early to midthirties and then declines steadily with increasing age. Some indication of the extent of this decline is evident from the results obtained by researchers at the John B. Pierce Foundation Laboratory. Both young and elderly adults were given a number of familiar odorous substances to identify. The young adults correctly identified about 50 percent of the substances; the elderly adults correctly identified about 30 percent. Older women tend to be slightly better than older men in identification. There are exceptions, however—some odorous substances are more readily identified by elderly than by young adults. This is especially true for odors that were more prevalent when current elderly people were younger than they are now (for example, lye soap). Some cognitive abilities tend to correlate with the ability to identify the names of odorous substances (for example, the speed of processing information).

People do have memories of different odors in their environment. Researchers in Sweden discovered that memory for odors is, in general, poorer for elderly people than for younger people. That is, memory of an odor seems to be forgotten faster in late adulthood than in earlier adulthood.

The age-related decline in smell sensitivity and discriminability is a major factor in affecting elderly adults' ability to identify food substances. Smell plays a greater role in discriminating among foods than does taste (*see* Taste).

Smoking

In the year 2005 for people of all ages about 20.9 percent were still smokers. The incidence is a decline from the 24.7 percent of smokers in 1997— it is hoped the decline will continue until the percentage reaches zero. Unfortunately, some seniors represent a segment of the total smoking population. The American Lung Association estimated that in 2005 about 10 percent of seniors age sixty-five or over remained as smokers. A third of those who were still smokers said their physicians never advised them to quit. Given both the health and financial reasons associated with smoking, the percentage may soon become zero.

The incidence of smoking among older adults is greater for African Americans than for whites, Hispanics, and Asian Americans. Smokers enter nursing homes earlier than nonsmokers, and at a younger age than nonsmokers. Researchers at Duke University found that religiously active older people are less likely to smoke cigarettes than less religiously active people.

The lower rate of smoking for older people than for younger people is related to the fact that many former smokers have been forced to quit smoking in late adulthood because of their poor health status. Emphysema, heart disease, and cancer are only worsened by continuing to smoke. The mortality rate for elderly smokers is about twice that for elderly people of the same age who never smoked.

The major health problems related to smoking for older people are cancer and heart diseases. For seniors, smoking is responsible for 87 percent of deaths from lung cancer, 21 percent of deaths from heart disease, and 18 percent of deaths from stroke. Women over age sixty who smoke are more than twice as likely to develop lung cancer as men of the same ages who smoke. Women may be more vulnerable to the carcinogens in tobacco, or they may inhale more of the carcinogens with each puff. Alternatively, they may not be examined as thoroughly for lung cancer as are men. Added to the health problems of smokers is evidence indicating that they have many times the risk of needing root canals for their teeth than do nonsmokers.

Smoking cessation is advantageous to the health of people of any age, including those in late adulthood. The mortality rate for elderly people who quit smoking is between that of those older people who never smoked and those who continue to smoke.

Researchers at the National Center for Health Statistics reported that smokers average a gain of about ten pounds in weight after they quit smoking. Why? Nicotine in cigarettes suppresses weight gain. Once it is withdrawn, the body makes up the difference. The weight gain, however, is a small price to pay for reducing the risk of cancer and heart disease.

Does smoking increase the likelihood of developing Alzheimer's disease? A study in the Netherlands of nearly seven thousand men and women age fifty-five and older reported that smokers were 2.2 times more likely to develop dementia and 2.3 times more likely to develop specifically Alzheimer's disease.

Behavior modification programs (see Psychotherapy) have become popular in the United States as a means of helping people to stop smoking. These programs are offered at many medical centers and psychological clinics across the United States. The use of nicotine patches, as prescribed by a physician, has also been a popular aid for people to stop smoking. However, a survey by the U.S. Surgeon General's Office indicated that as many as 90 percent to 95 percent of the smokers who do quit do so without external help (that is, by going "cold turkey").

Older smokers who are still smoking after years of doing so are probably smokers who have not been able to stop smoking on their own. They represent difficult cases for behavior-modification programs to produce a cure (that is, stopping smoking). Nevertheless, it is well worth the effort for elderly smokers to try these programs to break the cigarette (or cigar) habit. Smokers age fifty and older who face the health consequences of smoking realistically and view smoking as being addictive are the most likely candidates for quitting.

For more information about aging smokers, contact the American Lung Association at http://www.lungusa.org.

Socially Inappropriate Behavior

A common belief about older adults is that they are more likely than younger adults to express themselves with socially inappropriate language and behaviors when they are irritated or frustrated. In general, it has been found to be true for a number of older adults. They seem to have experienced a decline in their ability to inhibit inappropriate language and behavior.

Those suffering from Alzheimer's disease may have a similar failure of inhibiting behaviors that could be embarrassing to their caregivers when they are together in a restaurant or other public place. Caregivers could inform workers that their companion suffers from the disease and that is the reason for the inappropriate behavior. Cards provided by the Alzheimer's Association that explain the problem could be handed out in advance.

Social Networks

Researchers in Michigan conducted a survey of more than one thousand people in the Detroit area who were age sixty and older. Older age was found to involve smaller, less frequently seen, and less proximal networks, with a higher proportion of relatives and a lower proportion of friends as members of the networks. African Americans had smaller networks, more contact with members of the network, and more relatives in the network than did whites. African Americans and whites were similar in regard to the proximity of their networks.

Source Memory

"I heard that Senator Jones is retiring from the U.S. Senate." "Oh, where did you hear that?" "On the radio." This exchange illustrates what memory researchers call source memory. Note that it is not the content of memory (Jones is retiring) that is pertinent, but rather the source from which the content was acquired (the radio). Source memory, like that of some other forms of memory (for example, temporal memory; *see* Temporal Memory) is for a noncontent attribute of an event (that is, information that supplements content in terms of such features as when or where the event in question occurred).

Note further that in the everyday world, our source memory is likely to be incidental in form. We surely do not intend to remember where we heard about Jones's retirement, nor are we likely to rehearse the source in an attempt to ensure its memorability. Yet we often do remember sources of information we have acquired, but not always ("Was it on the radio or TV?"). Source memory may have a number of different kinds of information associated with it. For example, was the news reporter on the radio a man or a woman?

Age differences in the proficiency of source memory are studied by giving participants a series of items from different sources and later testing their memories for the source of each item. For example, researchers at the University of Toronto used trivial factual statements as items, with half of the statements delivered by means of an overhead projector and the other half delivered verbally by the investigator. When tested later for the source of each statement (projector or investigator), the proportion of correct identifications was moderately greater for young adult participants than for older participants.

A similar outcome has been found in other laboratory studies with somewhat different content items and somewhat different sources for those items. In fact, Swedish researchers found the age-related deficit in memory for the source of items to be greater than the age-related deficit in memory for the content of the items. The implication is that elderly adults generally are somewhat less proficient than young adults in their everyday applications of source memory. However, in most cases, the accuracy of identifying sources of information is of little consequence, and it is a form of memory that should be of little concern to older people unless it functions very poorly.

There is some evidence to indicate that source memory involves the brain's frontal lobes, and extremely poor source memory could be a sign of frontal lobe dysfunctioning (*see* Brain and Aging). Researchers at the University of Arizona found with the use of magnetic resonance imaging that seniors with pronounced deficits in source memory show declining frontal lobe functioning. Seniors who perform well on source memory tasks show little decline in frontal lobe functioning.

Even benign problems with source memory could result in some mild disagreements between spouses or friends, as is evident by such exchanges as "We saw that on the television news" and "We did not—we read it in the newspaper."

There is a special case of source memory in which accuracy is seemingly very high for adults of all ages. From what source did you hear that President Kennedy had been shot? The majority of people who were adults in 1963 will tell you whether they heard the news on the radio, the television, or from a friend, spouse, or another source—and with great confidence in the accuracy of their source identification. Memories of dramatic and highly emotional events are often remarkably preserved in their details (memory of the news about the bombing of Pearl Harbor and memory of the news about the plane crash of John F. Kennedy Jr. are other examples). For this reason, they are called *flashbulb memories*. Flashbulb memories commonly include the location of where you were when you heard about the dramatic event as well as the source of the news. That is, flashbulb memories consist of both spatial memory (*see* Spatial Memory) and source memory. Flashbulb memories are usually independent of the age of the adult who experienced the news about the dramatic event. However, recent evidence has revealed that distortions of some of the details of a flashbulb memory are not unusual.

Span of Apprehension

How much information can you "see" in a brief glance? If several letters of the alphabet were flashed on a screen for fifty milliseconds, how many letters could you recall seeing? The amount of information that can be seen in a glance is called the span of apprehension, a characteristic of our iconic memory, a form of sensory memory (*see* Sensory Memory). For young adults, the span of apprehension averages four or five letters. There is limited evidence indicating that older adults may have a slightly lower span of apprehension.

Some indication of your own span of apprehension may be given by a simple procedure. Have someone throw several beans on a table and then quickly cover them. If asked how many beans there were, you will probably be correct if the number is no more than four or five. If the number is much greater than this, you would need more time than allowed by a glance—enough time to allow you to count the beans before they are removed from view.

Spatial Ability

What would the resulting figure look like if you were to place this segment < side by side with this segment > ? The answer, of course, is a diamond-shaped figure. This is a simple example of your spatial ability. Spatial ability refers to your ability to visualize mentally how objects will appear if they are physically manipulated. This example involves the ability to integrate separated segments to form a whole. Spatial ability also includes the ability to visualize the third dimension of objects from their two-dimensional drawings, and to reproduce three-dimensional designs from two-dimensional drawings.

Spatial ability is measured by several components of intelligence tests, including the space test of the Primary Mental Abilities test (*see* Primary Mental Abilities Test [PMA]) and the block-design subtest of the Wechsler Adult Intelligence Scale (*see* Wechsler Intelligence Tests). Both cross-sectional and longitudinal studies have revealed substantial age-related declines in spatial ability as measured by these tests. For example, scores on the block-design test show about an 8 percent decline per decade (relative to scores in early adulthood) in cross-sectional studies.

Aging's effects on spatial ability parallel those for the use of imagery in other mental performances (*see* Imagery), and they suggest the possible faster rate of decline with normal aging in the brain's right hemisphere than in the left hemisphere (but *see* Brain and Aging).

The decline in spatial ability with normal aging is unlikely to affect the daily lives of most older people. Men tend to score higher than women beginning in early adulthood and continuing through late adulthood. There are professions, such as engineering and architecture, in which proficient spatial ability is very important, and even the decline by middle age may affect job performance and require greater assistance from younger colleagues. Age-related declines in scores on spatial-ability tests have been found for engineers with years of experience. However, older engineers and architects score well above nonengineers and nonarchitects on such tests, suggesting that they had unusually high spatial abilities when they were young adults (if they did not, they probably would not have become successful engineers or architects). Architecture and engineering do tend to be predominantly male professions (*see* Sex Differences and Scientific Ability).

One minor problem elderly people may encounter is with "you are here" maps found in shopping malls and other large facilities. Canadian researchers have found that older people have much greater difficulty than younger people in navigating through the facility when the map is not upright and is not coordinated with the viewer's position while viewing the map. *See also* Gender and Sex Differences in Aging; Sex Differences and Scientific Ability.

Spatial Learning

Do you know where the canned vegetables are in your favorite supermarket? If you start to shop in a new supermarket, how many visits to the store would be required before you knew where they were? Do you know where the Amtrak station is located in your city? Where the bathroom is located in your neighbor's house? You undoubtedly could describe the location in each case. In so doing, you are using mental or cognitive maps of your supermarket, your city, and your neighbor's house. These mental maps are the products of spatial learning that are acquired through frequent exposures to each of these areas.

Are there age differences in the rate at which spatial learning takes place? This is an important question. Adults of all ages do move to different cities, to different neighborhoods within the same city, and to different residences. The acquisition of new mental maps is essential for the adjustment of anyone who has moved from a familiar environment.

To simulate spatial learning in the laboratory, researchers have introduced tasks that are more closely related to everyday spatial learning than the older task of maze learning (*see* Maze Learning). In effect, participants "take a walk" through a novel environment. Movement through the environment is simulated by having the participants view a series of slides that show various scenes and locations in a strange (to the participants) neighborhood or building. After such a "walk," older participants have consistently been found to have acquired less information about components of the novel environment than younger participants.

This does not mean that normally aging people are incapable of mastering a novel environment. It simply means that it usually will take them longer and require more exposures to the environment before their spatial learning is complete. It also suggests that it would benefit elderly people to take notes for future reference when they begin their exploration of a new environment.

Spatial learning is especially a problem for residents of a nursing home, even those residents who are mentally alert and ambulatory. Researchers at Oklahoma State University provided a dramatic demonstration of this problem. They showed nursing home residents slides from various areas of both the exterior and the interior of their nursing home. The residents were asked to locate on a map of the home where each area in a slide would be found. Even highly distinctive areas, such as the dining room and nursing station, were correctly located by relatively small percentages of the residents. These researchers also found that the older the resident, the lower the accuracy of locations. Surprisingly, they also found that duration of stay in the nursing home was unrelated to accuracy. Spatial learning for residents of nursing homes would surely be greater if the managers of those homes made areas within them more distinctive. Currently, most hallways look alike, as do most rooms.

Spatial Memory

"Now where did I leave my keys?" "I don't remember where I parked my car in the mall's lot!" These are examples of the importance of spatial memory in our everyday lives. Unless we always leave our keys in the same place and always park our car in the same location every time we go to the mall, we are likely to discover frequently the imperfections of spatial memory. Spatial memory is memory for where objects are located in geometric space.

At one time, memory theorists believed that spatial memory was an automatic form of memory in the sense that spatial information is recorded in memory with little effort on our part and without any effort to rehearse that information. As a form of automatic memory, spatial memory was thought to show little decline in proficiency with normal aging. Laboratory studies, however, have demonstrated that the memory for spatial locations is better when we know our memory will be tested later (intentional memory) than when we are unaware of any future memory test (incidental memory). Some rehearsal that occurs when we are trying to remember spatial locations does seem to help us remember those locations better. In addition, laboratory research has revealed a moderate decline in spatial memory proficiency from early to late adulthood.

A variety of laboratory tasks have been used in spatial memory research. One of the most frequently used tasks is one in which the participants examine a box containing a number of compartments. A different object is placed in each compartment (for example, a comb in one, a key in another, and so on). After examining the filled box for a period of time, the participants are given the same box now emptied and asked where the comb had been, where the key had been, and so on. Another popular task is one in which participants study a map with different kinds of buildings located at various places on the map. They are then asked the location of the gas station on the map, where the church was, and so on. For both of these tasks older adults remember moderately fewer locations than young adults.

In a variation of these tasks, researchers at Lincoln University had participants view four small rooms for fifteen seconds each. Each room contained five common objects. After three minutes of performing a distracting task, the participants identified the room in which each object was located. The age difference in correct identifications was slight, but it increased in magnitude when recall was delayed until thirty minutes after viewing the rooms. Laboratory evidence confirms the frequent complaint of elderly people that they have difficulty in remembering where things are located.

Many of the problems of older people with regard to spatial memory could be reduced if individuals recognized their decline in proficiency and tried to bypass spatial memory as much as possible. For example, individuals should try to place their keys in the same place every time they set them down, and they should try to park in the same general section of the parking lot every time they visit the mall. However, such consistency is not always possible. There are certainly occasions when your favorite section of the parking lot is full and you have to park your car in a different location.

Memory training experts believe your memory for where you parked will be improved if you do other things besides simply looking where you are and trust that your location will be automatically recorded in your memory. These other things really amount to rehearsing where you are located. One memory aid is forming a mental image of the mall's overall structure and adding to that image a further image of your car in relation to that structure. It is hoped that you will later be able to retrieve the total image and easily find your car. However, older people are not as proficient in imaging as are younger people, and they are unlikely to find this memory trick to be of great value. Another approach may be more helpful. Translate the spatial location to a verbal code. Observe where you are and say it to yourself. For example, "I am parked on the west side of the mall, about three-fourths of the distance from the front of the lot." Even the later retrieval of only part of the code should help you find your car. Yet another approach is not to rely on memory at all. Instead, carry a notebook with you. Sketch a map of the parking lot in it and include a picture of your car where it is located in the lot.

Speech Perception

"What did you say? Would you mind repeating it?" Such requests are more likely to be made by elderly people than by younger people. There is a moderate decline with normal aging in speech perception. When asked to listen to a series of individual words and name each one after hearing it, older adults are likely to misidentify more words than younger adults, with errors being more pronounced among the old-old (people in the eighties and older) than for the young-old (people in their sixties). The misidentification of words occurs for words that have low-pitched sounds as well as for words with higher-pitched sounds. Only high-pitched sounds are likely to be affected by the changes in the ear that accompany normal aging (*see* Hearing). The difficulty encountered with words of a lower pitch suggests that some of the speech perception impairment in late adulthood is caused by some neural loss in the language centers of the brain that are located in the temporal lobe (usually the temporal lobe of the left cerebral hemisphere).

Most everyday conversations require the comprehension of spoken sentences as a meaningful whole, and not necessarily the complete comprehension of every word in that sentence. Consider, for example, the spoken sentence "Yesterday I saw several ducks swimming in the lake in the park." Even if you did not fully comprehend the word *swimming*, your mind would probably fill it in. There are few words other than *swimming* that would make sense with the rest of the sentence. Thus, the loss in spoken-sentence comprehension with normal aging is not as great as might be expected, thanks to our ability to fill in unheard words when listening to meaningful sentences and also thanks to the existence of a lingering sensory memory for the last word or two of a sentence that enables analysis of those words to occur even though the physical sound has ended (*see* Sensory Memory).

When sentences are spoken at a normal conversational rate (about 140 words per minute) and at a loudness well above the listener's threshold value, there is little loss in comprehension until older adults are in their eighties, and even then the loss is only about 10 percent, in relation to young adults. Nevertheless, it is probably wise to speak a little louder to an older audience than to a younger audience, given the greater thresholds for elderly people. It may also be wise to try to lower the pitch of your voice when you speak to an elderly audience. The extent of hearing impairment for elderly people is much greater for high-pitched sounds than for low-pitched sounds. You should also try not to talk in "baby talk" for most elderly people (*see* Baby Talk [Elderspeak]).

Speech is not always delivered under ideal conditions. For example, there may be a noisy background that must be overcome to hear the spoken sentences. Here, an elderly listener is likely to experience a much greater loss of comprehension than a younger listener. This is also likely to be true when the speech is delivered at an excessively fast rate or when there is reverberation in the speech (as may be heard over the loudspeaker at a stadium or an airport). Fortunately, researchers at the University of Calgary found that much of the difficulty experienced by older listeners with reverberated speech may be eliminated when the speaker pauses before saying important words in the sentences. The lesson should be clear for those who use loudspeakers.

Sometimes seniors have difficulty understanding all that has been said to them, even under seemingly ideal conditions. This is a condition known as *phonemic regression*. Speakers should be aware of this possibility and take steps to try to improve understanding by their older listener. This includes speaking somewhat slowly and using few words that contain high-frequency consonants that are difficult to discriminate between (for example, "fit" and "sit"). They should also make sure they are facing the listener to provide clues from mouth movements.

Speed of Behavior

The movements of older adults are slower than those of younger adults. The slowing down of behavior with aging (*see* Slowing-Down Principle) has been noted for movements requiring a wide range of tasks, including the writing of words or sentences and digits, the movement of a lever from side to side, sorting cards, and dialing a telephone number. In general, age-related slowing becomes disproportionately greater as the complexity of the behavior increases.

For example, the age difference in speed favoring young adults is much greater for writing unfamiliar sentences than it is for writing familiar sentences. For many tasks, the slower behavior of older adults is of little consequence (after all, the tortoise did win the race). It should matter little how rapidly the cards are shuffled in a card game or how fast they are dealt to the players; the job is completed anyway. Of course, the slower dialing of a telephone number does allow greater time for the number to be forgotten as it is being dialed; however, the number can always be looked up again in the telephone book, or the person dialing the number can keep repeating it to himself or herself while dialing (*see* Short-Term Memory).

A potential serious consequence of the slowing down of behavior with aging occurs when an older adult is required to take some evasive action to avoid being struck by a moving vehicle or a flying object.

Spelling

Does spelling ability decline in proficiency from early to late adulthood? The evidence is somewhat ambiguous. Researchers in England did find a decline from the fifties to the sixties, but only for low-frequency words (that is, words not in common use). Researchers at the University of California at Los Angeles also found that misspellings increase with age, but more so for high-frequency words (words used often but difficult to spell) than for low-frequency words. The older participants in their study were aware of their declining ability to spell correctly. The age difference was not associated with educational background, hours per week spent reading, or time spent solving crossword puzzles.

The difficulty elderly people encounter in spelling stems from the greater difficulty they have in getting orthographic information (that is, the visual appearance of words) out of the lexicon. *See also* Lexicon; Verbal Learning.

Spinal Stenosis

Spinal stenosis is a condition affecting some older people. It results in pain (called sciatica) experienced while walking or standing that results from pressure on the spinal cord from the narrowing of the tunnel containing the cord. Sitting usually relieves the compression and the resulting pain. Anti-inflammatory medicines, such as ibuprofen, may also relieve the pain.

Stimulus Persistence

Suppose you see the pattern ⅃⊓I, followed a second or so later by the pattern ⁻⊦⁻. You will undoubtedly see them as two different nonsense figures. Suppose, however, the second pattern follows much less than a second after the first. Now you are likely to see the word 5AT instead of the two distinctive patterns. It takes time for the stimulation within the nervous system produced by an external event (or stimulus) to be "cleared" (that is, to disappear). In other words, the stimulation persists for a time after the event itself has terminated. If the second event occurs after the first event has "cleared" the nervous system, then the two events will be perceived separately and independently of one another.

This is the case when a second separates our two patterns. However, if the time separation is much shorter, the two events will fuse, and you will see the product of that fusion (in this case, the word). Elderly adults experience the fused event after longer separations of the two patterns than will younger adults. Stimulation in the nervous system seems to persist longer in late adulthood than in earlier adulthood. Evidence supporting the existence of an age difference in the *duration of persistence* is derived from numerous studies employing patterns, such as the ones encountered above as well as other kinds of external events. The likely age difference in stimulus persistence seemingly explains the age differences in a number of sensory phenomena, such as visual aftereffects (*see* Aftereffects [Visual]).

Stomach Cancer

In the United States, more than twenty thousand people are diagnosed with stomach cancer each year. Actually, the incidence of stomach cancer has decreased by half in the United States over the past twenty-five years, probably because of better nutrition. Stomach cancer is more common in men than in women, and it usually occurs between the ages of fifty and seventy.

Fewer than 25 percent of the cases of stomach cancer are for people under age fifty.

In the United States, the disease is more common in poor people, in African Americans, and in the northern states. There is no evidence to date on the best way to use diet to prevent stomach cancer.

The disease may occur without apparent symptoms. The symptoms that may occur are loss of appetite, weight loss, abdominal pain, and vomiting blood. Unfortunately, the disease may not be detected until it is in an advanced stage and has spread to other organs.

A blood test for anemia (low red blood cell count) is the usual means of diagnosis, but a computed axial tomography may be used to examine the inside of the stomach (*see* Brain and Aging).

Strength and Stamina

The typical 170-pound man has about 70 pounds of his weight in muscle at age thirty. By late adulthood, only about 60 pounds of that muscle is likely to be retained. The lost muscle is gradually replaced by fat, and the remaining muscle slowly declines with aging in strength, flexibility, and tone. Strength declines with aging are generally greater for leg and trunk muscles than for arm muscles. Men, on average, have greater strength (about 30 percent) than women at every adult age level. Strength of a man's handgrip at midlife has been found to be related to physical limitations twenty-five years later. Researchers found that men with the lowest handgrip strength at midlife had twice the risk of physical limitations twenty-five years later than those men with the highest strength.

Physical performances that are dependent on muscular status usually show progressive decline from early to late adulthood. An exceptionally thorough study of age differences in physical performances was conducted in 1981 (the Canada Fitness Survey). Almost seven thousand adults ranging in age from the early twenties to the late sixties were evaluated on such abilities as grip strength, situps, and pushups. Relative to the scores for men in the twenty-one-to-twenty-nine-year age range, men in the sixty-one-to-sixty-nine-year age range showed a loss of about 18 percent in grip strength, about 60 percent in situps, and about 72 percent in pushups. Comparable losses for women in the sixty-one-to-sixty-nine-year age range (relative to women in the twenty-one-to-twenty-nine-year age range) were about 12 percent, 75 percent, and 62 percent.

Age-related declines are also seen for events such as running a sprint, hurdle racing, and marathon racing, but the degree of decline varies greatly among such events. In general, the age-related decline is greatest for those events that require a massive power output. Running short sprints shows much less decline from the forties to the sixties than does running a steeplechase or a marathon, even for regular participants in those events.

How much of these declines is related to lack of physical fitness and regular exercise, rather than the inevitability of physical declines with normal aging? Muscle atrophy (that is, loss of some muscle) that occurs with aging probably cannot be reversed. However, muscle strength can be increased despite such loss of muscle, given the maintenance of physical fitness with regular lifelong exercise. *See also* Sarcopenia.

Stress and Coping with Stress

The alarm clock did not go off this morning, so you overslept and were late for work. You spilled your first cup of coffee on the brand-new blouse you were wearing. These are example of daily stressors experienced by adults of all ages. Usually, the stress created by them is mild, and it disappears quickly, regardless of age. Another kind of stress is that created by major negative life events. In such cases, one needs to find a way to cope with the stress caused by these events.

Coping means the use of thoughts and actions to eliminate, or at least diminish, the distress and negative emotions produced by a stressful event. Researchers at Wayne State University found that older adults have greater control over their impulses and greater ability to reinterpret what would otherwise be stress-provoking situations than do younger adults.

A popular belief is that late adulthood is an especially stressful period of life, given the negative events likely to be encountered. They include death of a spouse, deaths of friends, retirement (to some elderly people), and similar negative events less likely to occur earlier in life. However, other periods of life have their own stressful events that are less likely to occur later in life. They include a faltering marriage, divorce, a new job, loss of job, and so on.

Negative life events may be less stressful for many elderly people than younger people believe they would be. Events may be less stressful in that they are not unexpected and therefore are somewhat anticipated. Especially stressful are those unexpected life events, such as the death of a grown child or the loss of one's savings by bad investments. For this reason, divorce in late adulthood is likely to be more stressful for an elderly person than in earlier adulthood. In fact, divorce has been found to be more stressful for an elderly person than is the death of a spouse (*see* Divorce). When the latter occurs at older ages, the incidence of subsequent illness and death is lower than it is when widowhood or widowerhood occurs at earlier ages (*see* Widowhood and Widowerhood)

However, the number of negative life events experienced by older people during a six-month period is a reasonably good predictor of their physical health status when their initial (before the negative events) health status is considered. Elderly people who are psychologically healthy and well adjusted experience less stress from negative events than do elderly people who are not as well adjusted. However, for some older people, an accumulation of negative events has been found to be predictive of a decline in mental functioning and the occurrence of depression. In general, the existence of a good social network of friends helps to prevent such mental deterioration.

People play various roles during their lives, those of spouse, parent, grandparent, friend, church member, and so on. For older adults, stressors that occur in roles that are highly important to them have more negative effects on their life satisfaction than do stressors that occur in roles that are less important to them (*see* Roles Seniors Play). Researchers at the University of Michigan surveyed adults age sixty-five and older to determine which roles are highly important to them and which are less important. The most important role was found to be that of spouse, with parent and grandparent being second and third, respectively. Less important roles included those of friend, church member, and volunteer worker.

Of interest to researchers of stress is the source to which people attribute their problems and who (or what) is responsible for finding a solution to their problems. Researchers have identified several models that may be followed.

The first is the *moral model*, in which people see themselves as creating their own problems and accept responsibility for solving the problems themselves. The second is the *compensatory model*, in which people believe they are not responsible for their problems, but they accept the responsibility for solving them. They see themselves as being handicapped in some way by their environments or by forces beyond their own control. The third model is the *enlightenment model*, in which people accept the responsibility for causing their own problem, but not the responsibility for solving them. For example, they may see their own weakness as being responsible for their excessive drinking, but they turn to Alcoholics Anonymous to solve the problem. The final model is the *medical model*, in which people accept neither the responsibility for their problems nor responsibility for solving them. They need expert help to identify their problems and to find solutions to them. Unfortunately, studies in this area have found a greater tendency among older people than among younger people to accept the medical model.

Psychologists have discovered that there are several broad types of coping behaviors when people are confronted by negative life events. One type is called *problem-focused coping*. Here, the individual directly tackles the problem causing stress. Thus, if one is experiencing symptoms of illness, problem-focused coping with the stress would be to seek medical diagnosis and advice. A second type is called *emotion-focused coping*. Here, the person would take an optimistic view and believe that the symptoms are temporary and will soon be gone. A third type of coping is *resignation*, in which the individual experiencing a negative event, such as symptoms of illness, simply accepts the stressful event and is prepared to take its consequences (for example, resigned to die after experiencing the physical symptoms) and makes no effort to cope with it. Elderly people are more likely to use problem-focused coping than either emotion-focused coping or resignation. In general, if one's resources (health, financial, and social) decline in late adulthood, then one's ability to cope effectively with stress diminishes. However, if these resources remain intact, the older person should be able to cope with stress as well as a younger person.

The decisions we are often required to make may be stressful. Having to decide when to retire may be such a stressful event for many older people, as may also be having to decide where to live after retirement. Of interest is how elderly people, compared with younger people, cope with difficult decisions.

A recent study in Los Angeles compared the coping strategies of middle-aged and elderly men to the conflict created by a difficult decision. Each participant described a major decisional conflict they had recently encountered and how they coped with the problem it created. The researchers identified three different strategies of coping with the conflict: *problem solving* (direct action to find the best solution), *avoidance* (trying to escape the problem without making a firm decision), and *resignation* (accepting the stress without doing anything about it). Both the middle-aged and elderly participants favored the problem-solving strategy for most decisions. The elderly participants made less use of avoidance than did the middle-aged participants, and there was no age difference in the relatively infrequent use of resignation.

An especially harmful way of coping with stress is to engage in excessive drinking of alcoholic beverages. The number of older people with drinking problems is probably fairly low. Those who do have a drinking problem, however, are more likely to be experiencing a chronic source of stress than those who do not have a drinking problem.

Adults who are especially confronted by stressful conditions are those who are caregivers of family members with Alzheimer's disease or some other form of dementia. Experts recommend a number of steps that may be taken to cope more effectively with caregiving stress: recognize the stress and realize you must take care of yourself before you can take care of a loved one; admit to yourself that you need support gained by talking to someone about your feelings, perhaps of guilt; keep updating information about your loved one's condition; join a support group and make use of respite centers (*see* Respite Care); rely as much as possible on home services; and seek counseling as a means of learning coping strategies.

We need to note finally that stress is not necessarily harmful. Challenges that create stress, such as public speaking and meeting a deadline, may serve to release a protein that strengthens the immune system of the body. *See also* Disability (Adaptation).

Stroke

A stroke occurs when there is a disruption in cerebral blood flow, most often from a blood clot in the brain. A stroke may also be caused (about 30 percent of strokes) by fat deposits in the carotid artery that block the flow of blood from the heart to the brain. Blockage may be detected by echocardiography (an ultrasound procedure much like that of sonar). Researchers at the Washington University School of Medicine have discovered that measuring oxygen use by the brain may serve as a predictor of a stroke from a blocked carotid artery. A patient diagnosed as a high-risk case could then receive a bypass surgery in which the carotid artery is repositioned to route blood flow around the blockage. If the blockage is severe, surgery may be required in which cuts are made in the carotid artery and fatty deposits are removed. If less severe, medical treatment may be sufficient (for example, a baby aspirin daily).

It is estimated that more than half a million Americans have strokes each year, and this could be an underestimation. Stroke is a leading cause of death in the United States, with about 160,000 deaths resulting from a stroke annually. The risk of a stroke nearly doubles every decade after age fifty-five, and two-thirds of strokes occur in people over age sixty-five. More than 60 percent of the deaths from stroke occur for women (strokes kill twice as many women as breast cancer). The risk of death from a stroke is nearly twice as high among African American men as it is among white men. The racial difference may be genetic in nature. The risk is also higher for women than for men and for diabetics than for nondiabetics. The highest risk, however, appears to be for patients who have had an earlier stroke before they had heart surgery.

Early treatment of a stroke is essential to avoid either death or severe impairment. Among the warning signs of an impending stroke are sudden numbness in the face, arm, or leg, usually on only one side of the body; mental confusion; trouble speaking; inability to walk; dizziness; and a severe headache.

Most victims of a stroke arrive at a hospital too late to use the medication (TPA; tissue plasminogen activator) needed to dissolve the clot that causes most strokes. The medication must be used within three hours after the onset of symptoms (for example, slurred speech), but most victims delay getting treatment. Fewer than 4 percent get to the emergency room within three hours.

Recent evidence indicates that the risk of stroke for elderly people who have thickening of the walls of the heart is three times greater than the average risk for other elderly people. The reason for the connection between such thickening and the risk of stroke is unknown. The thickening of the wall may be detected by echocardiography. The procedure is expensive, but is beneficial for those known to be at high risk who may benefit from preventive measures (for example, smoking cessation and avoidance of alcoholic beverages).

High blood pressure and a high level of cholesterol are known to be factors that place elderly people at an especially high risk of stroke. Treating high blood pressure in middle age can significantly lower the risk of small so-called silent strokes (transient ischemic attacks) in later life. People who had strokes late in life have consistently been found to have had high blood pressure when they were in their forties.

Drugs that lower bad cholesterol (LDL) levels seem to help to reduce the likelihood of a stroke for people considered at high risk for a stroke. A baby aspirin a day, or less often, is frequently prescribed by physicians as a means of preventing thrombolytic stroke (a blood clot in the brain). However, two or more aspirin a day may double the risk of hemorrhagic stroke (a break in the walls of a blood vessel in the brain). Coumadin, a blood thinner, may also help to prevent blood clots that result in a stroke. However, its use should be frequently monitored by blood tests to determine if you are receiving too much Coumadin that could cause serious bleeding. Women who participated in the Women's Health Initiative Study (see Women's Health Initiative) and were taking estrogen and progestin therapy (see Estrogen Replacement Therapy [Hormone Replacement Therapy]) were found to have a 41 percent increase in strokes compared to women who were not on the therapy. A more moderate increase in the incidence of strokes was found for women who had estrogen-only therapy.

Five or six daily servings of fruits and vegetables may lower the risk of a stroke caused by a blockage of a blood vessel. Especially beneficial are cruciferous vegetables (the cabbage family, such as broccoli, brussels sprouts, and cauliflower), green leafy vegetables, and citrus fruits. A low-salt diet is often recommended as well (see Salt Intake).

The parts of the brain that are affected by the loss of blood supply during a stroke are no longer capable of normal functioning. The consequences, contingent on the location of the area of the brain in which the stroke occurs, may result in declines in physical, mental, and emotional functioning (see Multi-Infarct Dementia). The symptoms of a stroke may include paralysis in one side of the body, difficulty in speaking (aphasia) or understanding speech (apraxia), memory impairment, depression, and uncontrollable crying or anger.

A medicine has been discovered that may reduce the extent of brain damage caused by a stroke if it is given within a few hours of the onset of a stroke. The medicine is tissue plasminogen activator (TPA), a genetically engineered protein. There are, however, risks associated with TPA. A new drug seems to function as well as TPA, even when given between three to six hours after symptoms begin. Perhaps an even more effective drug for reducing brain damage will be available in the future. Electrical stimulation in the motor area of the brain may serve to activate new motor behavior for strokes involving that area of the brain.

Therapists attempt to shift some brain functions from damaged parts of the brain to undamaged parts. The standard procedure is for therapists to support the limbs on the side of the body affected by the stroke and strengthen the unaffected side. Researchers at Washington University in St. Louis have discovered a technique called constrain-induced movement that prevents stroke rehabilitation patients from using their good side and forces them to focus on moving the muscles weakened by the stroke.

Care of a patient who has had a stroke usually begins with hospitalization during the acute phase of the stroke. The acute phase may last for days and even weeks. Rehabilitation training with one or more therapists (for example, physical and speech therapists; see above) follows the acute phase. The objectives of rehabilitation are to allow the patient to recover as much of the impaired functions as possible and to teach ways of compensating for those functions that cannot be recovered. The length of the rehabilitation period varies greatly with the severity of the stroke and may last several months to a year or longer.

The welfare of older patients affected by strokes is influenced by the degree to which they are able to find continuity with their lifestyles before the stroke. In a survey of a number of stroke patients, Dr. Gay Becker of the University of California at San Francisco found that many patients do find ways to accomplish this continuity. Those who demonstrated the greatest success in finding some form of continuity were the ones most likely to persevere in their efforts to recover from the stroke.

Other researchers have found that the size of the patient's social network is related to the degree of physical limitations after the stroke. Frequent contacts and interactions with friends and family members and participation in group activities are associated with improved physical functioning after the stroke. Perhaps most important, motor impairment of the limbs following a stroke may show recovery in some patients through unaffected areas of the brain's motor system developing new neural networks. This is part of the plasticity of the brain (*see also* Brain and Aging; Plasticity Theory).

Our discussion thus far has been about full-fledged strokes. In addition to these strokes, many Americans, especially older ones, suffer ministrokes (technically called transient ischemic attacks). They are caused by temporary blocking of blood flow to the brain. Symptoms last from a few seconds to twenty-four hours. Although they rarely cause permanent brain impairment, they are often predictors of a full-fledged stroke. Most people who suffer a ministroke are unaware they have had one. Possible symptoms that could lead to a diagnosis of a ministroke are numbness in the face or arm, usually on one side of the body; difficulty seeing; difficulty walking; and a severe headache. People over age sixty who have experienced these symptoms for more than ten minutes, feel weak, and have had a history of diabetes are especially vulnerable to a later full-fledged stroke. *See also* Aspirin; Attention and Stroke Recovery; Cardiovascular Diseases: Flaxseed.

Subjective Age

How old do you feel? Younger or older than your actual (chronological) age? Our reference is to your subjective age in contrast to your true age. There is some evidence that subjective age in late adulthood may be more closely related to performances on various tasks than is chronological age. However, this is an area of research that has not received the attention it deserves.

Psychologists measure subjective age by asking participants four questions: What age most clearly corresponds to the way you feel, the way you look, the age of the person who has interests and activities most like yours, and the age you would like to be if you could choose your age right now? Your subjective age is then found by averaging the answers to these four questions.

Researchers at Brandeis University determined the average subjective age for groups of men and women ranging in age from their teens through their early eighties. What they discovered is that adults of all ages tend to have subjective ages that are lower than their actual ages. Moreover, this discrepancy between subjective age and true age increases progressively from early to late adulthood, and the discrepancy is greater for women than for men. For example, for the true age of thirty-five, men and women averaged subjective ages of about thirty-four and twenty-eight, respectively. For the true age of sixty-five, the average subjective ages were about fifty-five (men) and forty-seven (women), and for the true age of seventy-five, they were about sixty-five and fifty.

Why do older adults maintain younger subjective age identities? A popular theory has been that it is a way of denying their age and thereby avoid the stigma they believe is associated with old age. Moreover, the denial of aging has been regarded by some gerontologists as being important in promoting successful aging and higher life satisfaction. That is, older people with lower subjective ages should have greater life satisfaction than older people with higher subjective ages.

In the Brandeis University study, participants were evaluated in terms of their fear of aging and their current life satisfaction. Contrary to the denial theory, the researchers found that fears of aging for their older participants were not strongly related to their subjective ages. The researchers also found no relationship for older men between their subjective age and life satisfaction. They did find a relationship between subjective age and life satisfaction for the older women in their study. However, the relationship was the opposite of that predicted by theory—the older women with the least discrepancy between their subjective age and their true age were found to be the most satisfied with their current lives.

Successful Aging

A popular concept in gerontology these days is that of "successful aging." Which of our seniors are aging successfully, and what is it that distinguishes them from other seniors? The MacArthur Foundation Study of Successful Aging that began in 1987 with a team of medical, biological, psychological, and sociological researchers provided information that resulted in a now widely accepted view of what constitutes successful aging. The emphasis in the study was to compare seniors who appeared to be aging successfully with seniors who were not in order to determine the factors underlying the distinction between the two.

The results of the MacArthur Foundation Study of Successful Aging are published in the book *Successful Aging* (Pantheon Books, 1998) written by John W. Rowe, M.D., and Robert L. Kahn, Ph.D., the head investigators of the study. From the results of this study, Drs. Rowe and Kahn concluded that successful aging has three main components. They are avoiding disease, maintaining high cognitive and physical functioning, and actively engaging in life. Moreover, it is the combination of all three components in interaction with one another that is essential for successful aging.

Achievement of these three components requires lifestyle choices that include diet and regular exercise, as well as pursuing mental challenges. Also, social bonds or connections with both family members and friends are important for successful aging. Close social relationships were found to increase longevity, seemingly because they involve support that affects health positively.

Successful Aging: An Alternative Perspective

Are the three components identified by Drs. Rowe and Kahn as needed for successful aging (*see* Successful Aging) too stringent? Some health experts believe they are. Are Americans aging unsuccessfully if they do not meet the three criteria or components? Only about 20 percent to 33 percent of Americans would be considered to be aging successfully. Should older adults who have diabetes, but no other disease, and who maintain high levels of mental and physical functioning and actively engage in life be considered aging unsuccessfully?

How do seniors perceive themselves as aging successfully? Researchers at the Human Population Laboratory in Berkeley, California, had nearly nine hundred women and men ranging in age from sixty-five to ninety-nine rate themselves. Slightly more than half of the participants believed they were aging successfully, a percentage well above the 18 percent who qualified as aging successfully by the criteria of Drs. Rowe and Kahn. Perhaps gerontologists need to find an alternative way of identifying what should define aging successfully.

Suicide

Older adults have the highest risk of suicide of all adult age ranges. Those at greatest risk of suicide are white widowed men over age seventy-five who are depressed or alcoholic or both. Overall, the highest risk of suicide is much greater for the oldest old (age eighty and older) than the younger old (age sixty-five to seventy-nine).

In terms of actually committing suicide, adults age sixty-five and older have the highest rate. They account for nearly 20 percent of all suicides. The incidence for all age groups combined is about eleven suicides per one hundred thousand. For the sixty-five and older age group it is about fifteen suicides per one hundred thousand.

Researchers at the Max Planck Institute for Demographic Research in Rostock, Germany, analyzed the suicide rates for age groups fifty to sixty-four, sixty-five to seventy-nine, and eighty and older. For both men and women in the fifty-to-sixty-four and sixty-five-to-seventy-nine age ranges there was a decline from 1972 to 1999. By contrast, the rate stayed nearly constant for both men and women age eighty and older. The suicide rate in 1998 for the oldest old was much higher than that for either middle-aged or younger adults.

Other factors leading to a high risk of suicide are loss of health, work, and friends or family members and a poor financial status. Warning signs of a potential suicide include loss of appetite, insomnia, sadness, unexplained tiredness, increased use of alcohol, buying a gun, a sudden interest or lack of interest in religion, and talking about suicide. No specific illness is associated with suicide for elders, but poor self-perceived health is a factor. However, researchers in San Diego County investigated suicides for young adults and elderly adults (sixty to eighty-eight years of age) and found that the two groups did not differ in frequency of being friendless or lacking outside interests.

The elderly adults were less likely than the young adults to have made previous unsuccessful suicide attempts, and the elderly adults were actually less likely than the young adults to have financial problems. Others have found that the ratio of attempted suicides to actual suicides differs between young and older adults. For young adults the ratio is about seven unsuccessful attempts to one successful attempt. By contrast, the ratio for older adults is about eight successful attempts to one unsuccessful attempt.

The suicide rate for elderly adults is lower among white women and nonwhite men and women than among white men. The high incidence of suicide among older white men is seemingly related to the perceived loss of economic, business, and social power experienced by a number of white men after retirement. The large difference in suicide rates between elderly men and women overall is somewhat misleading in that more elderly women than men attempt suicide. The probable reason for the difference is a sex difference in the choice of method used to attempt suicide. Women are more likely to choose less lethal methods (for example, sleeping pills) than men (for example, a gun). Of nearly fifteen thousand cases of suicide by elderly white men from 1989 through 1991, 77 percent were committed with firearms.

Surgery Survival

Are you ever too old to have surgery? A study of centenarians who had various surgeries implies that you are not. The rate of their survival, forty-eight hours, one month, and one year after surgery, was the same as that of centenarians who did not have surgery of any kind.

Both age and prior physical condition are predictors of the duration of hospital stay after surgery. That is, the older the patient and the poorer his or her physical condition, the longer the stay. For many kinds of surgery, age is not a critical risk factor. Physical health and functional status (mobility and the ability to perform the activities of daily living) are much more important. Since these conditions correlate with age, postsurgical complications do tend to increase with age. The oldest patients have more than one complication three to four more times than younger patients.

Survival after Death of a Spouse or Significant Other

In a five-year study of more than one million people, researchers in Finland found that after the death of a spouse or a significant other person, the surviving partner had a greater risk of dying from an accident, from violence, or from alcohol-related causes than age-matched people who did not lose a spouse. Moreover, those who lost a spouse or significant other had a 20 percent to 30 percent greater risk of dying from heart disease or lung cancer than the others. Men had a higher risk of dying soon after the deaths of their spouses than did women after the deaths of their spouses (*see also* Widowhood and Widowerhood).

Swallowing

Older adults make up a large proportion of the more than fifteen million Americans who suffer from a condition known as *dysphagia* that may severely hinder the pleasure of eating and drinking. The condition is quite dangerous in that it may severely restrict air from reaching the lungs.

Dysphagia is a medical term meaning difficulty in swallowing. Although many of the sufferers of dysphagia are older adults, it may occur at any age for people who have cerebral palsy, muscular dystrophy, cancer of the mouth or throat, as well as several other disorders. It may also bear a causal relationship to pneumonia, dehydration, malnutrition, and perhaps even death.

Dr. Jo Anne Robbins of the University of Wisconsin Medical School is an authority on the problems of swallowing. She offers a number of important suggestions for safe swallowing for older people or anyone else as well. Even if you do not presently have a swallowing problem, there are steps you should take to avoid a critical incidence of blocking your airways from improper swallowing.

When eating, you should sit upright in a chair that gives you good support. Eat in a quiet, comfortable environment that is free of disruptions, such as the blasting of a television. If you wear dentures, make sure they fit securely in your mouth. Do not talk with food in your mouth. Finish swallowing before taking the next bite or sip of liquid. Wash down food with fluids. Take small bites of food, and do not eat too fast. If we eat too fast, our swallowing system cannot keep up with the food input. Talking opens the airways.

Dr. Robbins has been joined by two other experts in dysphagia in writing a book that should be of interest to anyone with a swallowing problem or who has a loved one with a swallowing problem. The book's title is *Easy to Swallow, Easy to Chew.*

Switching Tasks

Suppose you perform a series of additions. Or you perform a series of subtractions. Now consider a situation where you have to alternate between the two arithmetic tasks. That is, your mind-set has to change quickly from addition to subtraction and then back to addition again.

In general, older adults are slowed more by switching than are younger adults (*see* Trail Making Test). Such switching does take place in some everyday situations. For example, you may add several new deposits to your checking account, and then you need to subtract the amount of a recent check you wrote. Laboratory evidence implies that older adults will take longer to make the switch than will younger adults.

Syncope

Syncope is a dizziness or fainting produced by cerebral anemia (that is, diminished blood supply to the brain) that is often caused by unknown body conditions. It presents a dangerous problem for elderly people in that falls resulting in fractures may be the consequence. In addition, one-fourth of elderly people with syncope are dead within two years after the initial diagnosis (compared to 8 percent in younger patients). Syncope may be a critical indicator of a serious cardiovascular disease (*see* Dizziness; Falls).

Syntax

Stored in our permanent memory is our knowledge of the rules of grammar, that is, the *syntax* of our spoken and written language. These rules are automatically and effortlessly employed whenever we speak or write a sentence. You surely realize that people do not become "ungrammatical" as they age. There is no evidence to suggest that normal aging is accompanied by any major changes in the ability to use syntax effectively. However, some more subtle changes in the use of syntax occur as people age. Older adults tend to have greater difficulty than younger adults in comprehending complex sentences (those containing embedded clauses). Interestingly, Dr. Susan Kemper at the University of Kansas has examined diary entries of people who kept a diary for many years. She discovered a tendency for sentences entered in the diaries to be syntactically less complex when the diary writers were old than when they were younger.

T

Taste

If you believe everything you hear from elderly people, you are likely to believe that many of them are "tasteless." Familiar statements by older people are "Everything tastes alike to me now" and "Food just doesn't taste the way it used to taste." Although such statements are probably exaggerated (unless there is a specific biological disease affecting the taste and smell systems), there is some degree of truth behind them.

In classic studies by Dr. Susan Schiffman, young adults and adults in their seventies were tested for their ability to identify, while blindfolded, a number of blended foods (blending was necessary to prevent identifications by means of the substance's texture). For most of the blended foods, the young adults were considerably more accurate in their identifications than were the elderly adults. For example, the percentages of those identifying apple, strawberry, and fish were 81 percent, 78 percent, and 78 percent, respectively, for the young adults and 55 percent, 33 percent, and 59 percent, respectively for the elderly adults. However, it is important to note that there were some reversals, specifically for tomato (69 percent for elderly adults, 52 percent for the young adults) and potato (38 percent for the elderly adults, 19 percent for the young adults).

The problem in assigning the responsibility for the greater difficulty of older people in food identification to age-related declines in taste sensitivity is the fact that taste plays only a relatively minor role in these identifications. The texture of food in your mouth provides useful information, and the smell of the food is especially important information. The importance of smell is clearly indicated when young adults are deprived of smell and texture by having them hold their nostrils while attempting to identify blended food substances. When this is done, their accuracy in food identification is no greater than that of older adults. It is apparent that not only is smell important in discriminating among foods regardless of age, but also it is the diminished sense of smell with aging (see Smell) that is largely responsible for the difficulty experienced by many older people in making these discriminations.

Recent evidence, however, indicates that the sense of taste may not be completely blameless for the reason foods seem to lose much of their taste as we grow older. Age affects sensitivity to the intensity of taste. Older adults have difficulty telling the difference in the concentrations of a sour substance and a salty substance. Especially important is sensitivity to the concentration of salt. This may explain why some older adults shake excessive amounts of salt on their food in order to detect the presence of salt. They have to use a lot of salt to add to the flavor.

If everything does seem to taste alike to an elderly person whose appetite is suffering as a result, perhaps he or she should follow the advice of some experts and flavor his or her foods with one of several healthful supplements. If foods seem to have lost their zest, concerned individuals should consult with the nutritionist at one of their local hospitals about these additives. Researchers in the Netherlands were concerned about nursing home residents not eating sufficiently. They compared a group over sixteen weeks that was given flavor enhancers on their food with a control group without the enhancers. Those with the enhancers ate more, increased more weight, and had hungry feelings more often than those without the enhancers. The enhancers were chicken flavor, beef bouillon flavor, turkey flavor, and fish flavor. In addition, foods that taste bland could be seasoned with bacon bits, cheese chunks, croutons for salads, and so on.

What happens to taste itself with aging? We must recognize first that there are only four basic tastes: bitterness, saltiness, sourness, and sweetness. Common foods have varying combinations of these basic tastes, thus accounting in part for their varying tastes (along with their variations in odor and texture). Of interest in aging research is the extent to which sensitivity to each of the four basic tastes decreases with normal aging. As with all of the other senses, sensitivity refers both to threshold sensitivity and suprathreshold (above the threshold) sensitivity.

Threshold sensitivity refers to the ability to detect weak amounts of a taste substance. For example, how much salt must be added to water before you are able to detect the presence of the salt on half of the trials in which it is present? That amount defines your saltiness threshold value. Similarly, how much of a bitter substance, a sour substance, and a sweet substance must be present before you are able to detect bitterness, sourness, and sweetness on half of the trials in which they are present? These amounts define your bitterness, sourness, and sweetness thresholds.

Studies comparing individuals of various ages indicate that there is only a modest decline in sensitivity for saltiness from early to late adulthood. That is, there is only a modest increase in the absolute threshold for older adults, on average, relative to young adults. Moreover, the decline in sensitivity may be even less for detecting bitterness, sourness, and sweetness. For all of the four basic tastes, the threshold value for older adults, in general, may be no more than two to two and one-half times that of young adults.

The magnitude of the increase in threshold (or decrease in sensitivity) is much less than that found for the other senses. This is especially true for the sense of smell (*see* Smell). Part of the moderate decline in taste sensitivity in elderly adults may result from the taking of certain medicines that dull taste sensitivity. These medicines are more likely to be taken by older adults than by younger adults.

Suprathreshold sensitivity refers to the ability to discriminate among varying intensities of a taste substance, all of which are well above threshold intensity. Does a concentration of salt that is twice as high taste twice as salty, less than twice as salty, or even more than twice as salty? In general, the evidence indicates that elderly adults have less suprathreshold sensitivity than do young adults, but, as with absolute sensitivity, the age difference is relatively modest.

Older participants do need a greater increase in the concentration of a taste substance than do younger participants before they are able to perceive the fact that the concentration has indeed increased. This seems to be the reason older adults generally prefer stronger tastes (for example, more tart) than do younger adults and why older adults may put too much salt on their food. That is, the greater concentration of the taste substance is actually perceived as being weaker than it really is by most elderly adults. The exception, however, is for sweetness. There is evidence to indicate that the preference for less sweet tastes increases from early to late adulthood.

Tea

Elderly people should be aware of the possible health benefits gained from drinking black or green tea. Drinking one cup or more of black tea daily has been found in some studies to reduce by half the risk of a heart attack, relative to nondrinkers. However, the tea must be brewed from leaves, and it should not be instant tea. Both green tea and black tea may reduce the risk of cancer, although the evidence is a bit conflicting. Green tea appears to be more effective than black because it contains a greater concentration of the antioxidant that helps to inhibit the growth of cancer cells.

Researchers in Taiwan studied a group of men and women who were age thirty and older at the beginning of their study. They found that those who drank an average of nearly two cups of tea (any one of the three main kinds of tea—black, green, or oolong) daily for ten years or more had a 6.2 percent greater hip bone density than occasional tea drinkers. Some of the chemicals in tea of all of the three main kinds seem to help preserve bone-mineral density.

Tear Secretion

Tears are drops of a saline solution that are secreted by the lacrimal glands.

The drops are spread between the eye and the eyelid to moisten their parts and aid their motion. One of the problems confronting older people is a reduction in the amount of tear secretion (it may be as much as a 40 percent reduction). This reduction may produce visual problems for some elderly people. An examination of tear flow should be part of regular eye examinations for elderly people. There are medications to reduce the symptoms of dryness in the eyes.

Teeth, Gums, and Mouth

It is estimated that about 60 percent of people age sixty-five and over have some or all of their teeth. However, many of these elderly people make insufficient use of dental services, primarily because most health insurance plans provide no dental coverage and Medicare pays only for the removal of tumors from the mouth. Consequently, many elderly people have considerable discomfort from their teeth and gums. Teeth are likely to be less sensitive to hot or cold substances in late adulthood than in earlier adulthood because nerve and blood supplies to the teeth decrease with age.

In a survey of nearly one thousand elderly people, only 44 percent reported the use of some dental service within the previous year. Only 13 percent had a private dental insurance policy, with nearly 70 percent of the dental expenditures being paid by the patients themselves. The users of dental services were better educated and had better financial resources than nonusers. Other researchers have found that poor physical functioning is negatively associated with the use of dental services by people age seventy-five and older (that is, the poorer the functioning, the less the use of dental services).

About 50 percent of adults between the ages of sixty-five and seventy-four years have some form of periodontal (gum) disease, and more than 95 percent have lost some gum tissue, exposing tooth roots and making them susceptible to decay. Gum disease develops when plaque accumulates between the teeth and the gums and causes the gums to recede from the teeth. Infection then forms in the resulting open spaces, producing swollen or tender gums, unpleasant breath, and a bad taste in the mouth. Elderly adults with diabetes are at particular risk of infections that result in periodontal problems. Dentists should check their senior patients regularly for signs of diabetes. Gum infection may contribute to heart disease (*see* Cardiovascular Diseases). Researchers at the University of Michigan found that adults age sixty and older with advanced periodontal disease were four and a half times more likely to have heart disease than those without periodontal disease.

Being edentulous (toothless) even with dentures increases the risk of a significant weight loss. Elderly men consistently have more periodontal disease (and also more cavities) than elderly women. A drug called Periostal is used to treat gum disease. It suppresses the enzyme causing a breakdown of the gums and eventually the teeth.

Elderly people who wear dentures also need to visit their dentists at regular intervals. The mouth tends to change its shape somewhat with aging. Consequently, dentures do not fit properly, and they need to be adjusted. Dentists should check regularly for the possible presence of oral problems other than those of the teeth themselves.

Xerostoma (dry mouth) occurs for some older people because their salivary glands do not function as they should. This is a side effect of many of the medications taken by elderly people. Persons affected by xerostoma feel thirsty frequently and have difficulty in speaking. Dry mouth may contribute to tooth decay and periodontal disease. Dentists often recommend that those with dry mouth use sugar-free mints, home air humidifiers, fluoride rinses, and artificial saliva solutions. Also, they should carry a squeeze bottle filled with water.

There is a form of dry mouth called Sjogren's Syndrome that is caused by white blood cells entering the salivary glands and disrupting the production of saliva. It may accompany other diseases such as rheumatoid arthritis and lupus. The prescription medicine Salagen may stimulate the salivary glands to begin producing saliva again. In addition, there are artificial salivas that may be found at a pharmacy.

Oral cancer (abnormal, malignant tissue growth in the mouth) often goes undetected in older people because they visit their dentists infrequently and because there is little pain early in the disease. The disease affects more elderly men than elderly women, especially men who are older than forty. The cancer most commonly involves the lips or the tongue, but it may affect other areas of the mouth as well. Early symptoms consist of skin lesions, lumps, or ulcers. In its early stage treatment usually consists of surgery. In later stages radiation therapy and chemotherapy are likely to be applied. Elderly people who have the greatest risk of oral cancer are those elders who smoked or chewed tobacco for years and were heavy consumers of alcohol for a number of years.

Telephone

Elderly adults who are unable to use a standard telephone because of hearing or visual impairment or difficulty in handling the equipment should have adaptive telephone equipment with a large-number dialing structure and hearing-aid adaptability. *See also* Visual Disorders (Coping with Macular Degeneration).

Television Viewing

The most frequent reason people give for watching television is its entertainment value. This is true for both young and elderly adults and for both men and women. Elderly people also report that they watch television to get most of the news they receive daily. Elderly adults like to watch family-oriented shows and shows that feature older people in highly positive roles. This undoubtedly is a major reason for the long-standing popularity of reruns of such shows as *The Andy Griffith Show, Matlock,* and *Murder She Wrote.*

Temperature Sensitivity

What room temperature do you prefer to feel comfortable? There is a modest age difference in this "comfort-point" temperature, with middle-aged and elderly adults averaging only about half a degree higher than young adults. This evidence implies that there is little change with aging in *temperature sensitivity.* In agreement with this position is the limited evidence indicating the slight age difference in the threshold value for detecting the presence of either cold or heat on the skin. *Threshold* here refers to the minimal intensity of the source of cold or heat needed to report the experience of cold or heat.

Conflicting with this evidence, however, are studies suggesting that older people are less capable than younger people of estimating the temperature of their environments and less capable of detecting a temperature change in their environments.

The diminished capability is probably a contributing factor to the higher incidence of hypothermia (a below-normal body temperature—95 degrees Fahrenheit or lower), heat stroke, and frostbite among older adults than among younger adults (*see also* Heat Stroke). A survey by researchers at Southwest Texas State University conducted from 1979 to 1985 revealed that there were more than five thousand deaths of people age sixty and older related to excessive heat or cold. Moreover, the risk of death from hypothermia is more than three times greater for people age eighty-five and older than for people in the sixty-five-to-seventy-four-year age range.

To avoid hypothermia, keep the thermostat set at 68 to 70 degrees Fahrenheit. If living alone, have a neighbor or family member check on you at least once a day. Avoid drinking alcoholic beverages, and eat and drink more hot foods and beverages.

The incidence of deaths per year in which excessive temperatures played a role is probably underestimated. The researchers in Texas found deaths related to cold were responsible for more than three-fourths of the temperature-related deaths. Indicators of low body temperature include irregular heartbeat, very slow breathing, weak pulse, low blood pressure, and mental confusion. The presence of these indicators calls for immediate emergency treatment.

What should you do if you are stuck in snow and extreme cold while driving? The American Red Cross has a number of tips for survival. You should not walk unless you know for certain there is a place nearby. Tie a brightly colored (preferably red) cloth to the antenna of your car. Dig the exhaust pipe of your car clear of snow and run your car's engine and heater for ten minutes every hour. Move your arms and legs to keep the blood flowing and to stay warm. Open a window away from the wind, just a crack, to get fresh air and to avoid carbon monoxide poisoning (*see also* Winter Storms).

The researchers in Texas also found that the overall incidence of deaths was about the same for older men and older women. However, older women were found to die more frequently from excessive heat than from excessive cold, whereas the opposite was true for older men. More than 70 percent of the deaths occurred among elderly adults living in metropolitan areas. By mid-July 1999 more than one hundred people, mostly elderly adults, died from the excessive heat gripping the East and Midwest of the United States.

Most deaths of elderly people attributable to excessive temperatures could be avoided. Older people forced to live on a meager income often save money for food and rent by reducing their heating and cooling bills. Those who are in danger of death by so doing could readily be discovered by daily visitations to their homes from community volunteers, visiting nurses, or Meals on Wheels personnel. Financial aid for adjusting the temperature in their rooms could then be provided by various agencies and services. In addition, to avoid hypothermia during cold weather elderly people should be encouraged to wear layers of warm clothing both indoors and outdoors, to wear a hat outdoors, to use extra blankets in bed, and to keep active physically.

Temporal Memory

"Did I go grocery shopping last week on Wednesday or Thursday?" "When did we last play bridge together?" Events are remembered not only for their contents, but also to some degree for the time of their occurrence. Temporal memory is memory for the timing of events in one's life. The usual procedure for studying temporal memory in the laboratory is to have participants receive a series of events and then make temporal judgments about those events. Usually, the events are familiar words (for example, *apple* and *pencil*) presented in a lengthy series. After the series is presented, participants may be asked such questions as which word appeared more recently in the series, *apple* or *pencil*?

Alternatively, the participants may be asked to reconstruct the order in which the words appeared, and their reconstructed order is compared in accuracy with the actual order. Regardless of the task, older adults have been found to be considerably less proficient in temporal memory than are young adults.

The diminished proficiency of temporal memory with normal aging is further demonstrated when words in a series are replaced by actions performed in the laboratory (for example, touching your nose, shaking your head; *see* Action Memory). After the last action is performed, subjects are asked to reconstruct the order in which they were performed. Elderly adults are generally far less accurate than young adults in reconstructing the temporal order of the actions they had just performed. Temporal memory for events does seem to be much more adversely affected by normal aging than is memory for the frequency with which events occur (*see* Frequency-of-Occurrence Memory). The adverse effect of aging on temporal memory is also probably greater than the adverse effect on spatial memory (*see* Spatial Memory).

Terminal-Drop Phenomenon

In the early 1960s psychologist Dr. Robert Kleemeier discovered a peculiar phenomenon known as the terminal-drop phenomenon. He discovered that older people who showed a pronounced decline in intelligence test scores from one time of testing to a later time of testing had an unusually high probability of death within a relatively short period of time after the second testing.

Later investigators have generally supported the existence of the terminal-drop phenomenon. Declines in scores for several of the subtests of the Wechsler intelligence tests (especially the vocabulary subtest; *see* Wechsler Intelligence Tests) appear to be particularly associated with impending death. In the Seattle Longitudinal Study (*see* Longitudinal Studies of Aging's Effects on Health and Cognition), significant predictors of mortality for older participants over a seven-year period were declines in verbal meaning, spatial ability, reasoning, and psychomotor speed.

Some researchers have found that the best predictor may be a battery of cognitive tests that includes tests of learning and memory as well as various components of intelligence tests (especially vocabulary). A general decline in cognitive functioning signals impending death. The decline is most likely the result of an extensive neurological or brain degeneration.

Terminal Illness

Many seriously ill elderly hospital patients who ask their physicians to issue orders for them not to be resuscitated do not get their request fulfilled. Patients should name some person they trust to represent them if they are incapacitated. They should also write out their wishes about application of life-sustaining treatments when they are well and before they are seriously ill (these are called advance directives; *see* Advance Directives). They should also inform family members of their wishes not to be resuscitated when there is no chance of recovery and considerable ravishing of their bodies has taken place. There is a growing sentiment in the United States that death with dignity is a more humane choice than life with great suffering. Physicians can write orders not to resuscitate only with consent of the patient or the patient's family. The use of such orders has increased from 3 percent of terminally ill patients to nearly 13 percent in the past ten years.

Testicular Cancer

Testicular cancer is a relatively rare form of cancer in men (about eighty-five hundred new cases annually in the United States). The most common form is a seminom (cancer in the cells that produce semen). It is usually diagnosed in men between the ages of thirty and thirty-five. However, there is a second peak in occurrence for men age sixty-five and older. It occurs more often in white men than in African American men. Risk factors include late descending testicles, a family history of the disease, and an HIV infection.

If caught early, testicular cancer is curable for the vast majority of cases. One of the first signs of the cancer is a painless lump that may be felt by gently rolling your fingers upward over the testicles. The usual treatment is surgical removal of the cancerous testicle. The relapse-free rate after three years is 95.9 percent for those receiving radiation and 94.8 percent for those receiving chemotherapy (a nonsignificant difference).

Men with testicular cancer in one testicle have a higher than average chance of developing cancer in the other testicle. However, the risk is low, and the survival rate is high. Most testicular cancer patients who try to have children after their treatment are successful in doing so.

Tetanus

You should have a booster shot to prevent tetanus at least at age sixty-five if you have not had a shot since childhood. In fact, some experts recommend having a booster shot every ten years. Tetanus is a rare severe disease that occurs mostly in elderly people and may be prevented by immunization. Unfortunately, researchers at the National Center for Health Statistics found that fewer than one-third of people age seventy and older have protective levels of tetanus antibodies.

Time Estimation

As people grow older, they often say that the years go by faster than they did when they were younger. William James, the great psychologist of the nineteenth century, wrote in his classic book *The Principles of Psychology* (1890) that "the same space of time seems to grow shorter as we grow older."

Does the estimation of time's durations actually change as we grow older? We obviously cannot lock up people of different ages in cells that prohibit looking outside and maintaining contact with the outside world—and wait to have them tell us when they believe a year has passed by. If we could do that, would we really find that older people perceive time passing more quickly than do younger people? That is, would they say a year has ended after only ten months, compared to younger people adults saying it is over after twelve months?

What we can do, however, is to have younger and older adults estimate briefer periods of time (for example, thirty seconds or sixty seconds). For example, they may be asked to push a button when they think sixty seconds have transpired (while preventing them from counting or from seeing a clock or watch). On such tasks older people tend to give longer estimates than younger people. Thus, older people may average pushing the button after seventy-five seconds, younger people after sixty-one seconds. What this age difference suggests is that time seems to pass more slowly for older than for younger people. This is the opposite of what would be expected if the years really go by faster as you grow older. However, it is in agreement with the slowing-down principle (*see* Slowing-Down Principle).

Time-Lag Comparison

Time-lag comparisons are possible when the same task is given at widely separated times to groups of adults who are of the same age at each time the task is administered. Thus, the task may have been given to a group of elderly adults in 1930 and again in 1990. The comparison between the average score on the task in 1930 and the average score in 1990 is a time-lag comparison.

If the two averages are approximately equal, then it suggests that performance on the task in question is unaffected either by generational membership or by the time period in which the task was administered. Older adults tested in 1930 obviously came from a much earlier generation than older adults tested in 1990. Similarly, the two tests occurred in very different time periods. This is the case, for example, with the digit-span task in which it is determined for each participant the longest series of digits that can be remembered in order without an error (*see* Memory Span). The average digit span for older adults was about 6.5 in 1930, and it was also about 6.5 for older adults tested in 1990.

However, if a time-lag comparison indicates that the average score earned at one time differs greatly from the average score earned at another time, then it is likely that either the variation in generational membership or the variation in time period has affected performance on the task in question.

Time of Day and Memory Performance

The time of day when adults of different ages are tested for age differences in memory performance greatly influences the magnitude of age related deficits in performance scores. Pronounced age deficits are found when all participants are tested in the late afternoon or evening. Deficits are much less pronounced when they are tested in the morning. This is especially true when older adults are tested in the morning. Elderly adults seem to be more alert in the morning. For younger adults, variation in the time of day when they are tested has less effect on their memory performances.

The time of day effect probably accounts for at least part of the age-related deficit found for episodic memory performances. Most memory studies are conducted either in the late afternoon or in the evening—times unfavorable to older participants. The reason is that the tester is usually a graduate assistant who has classes during the morning hours and is unavailable as the tester during that time.

Interestingly, when elderly adults are given memory tests in the evening, they come much closer to matching the scores of younger participants if they are allowed to consume twelve ounces or so of caffeine coffee thirty minutes or so before they are tested. The caffeine seems to increase their mental alertness.

Tinnitus

Tinnitus is a condition in which the affected individuals "hear" noises, such as a ringing or a buzzing sound, either intermittently or constantly. Occasionally, a person standing near someone with tinnitus may hear a clicking sound, probably due to rapid contractions of the ear muscles of the person with tinnitus. Tinnitus may result from various diseases, or it may be the consequence of an allergy, an obstruction in the ear canal, or the buildup of wax in the ear canal.

Whatever the direct cause, it seems to involve spontaneous nerve activity in a part of the brain that leads to the noise. The condition may be accompanied by some hearing loss, and it tends to worsen as hearing sensitivity decreases with normal aging. Many drugs, including aspirin, may exaggerate tinnitus.

Although the percentage of older people with tinnitus is small, those who have it find it to be especially stressful. Treatment of the condition in terms of permanent relief is often unsuccessful. If treatment is unsuccessful, elderly people with tinnitus should consult their physician about the use of tranquilizers to reduce the stress they experience or about the acquisition of a "masker" (a device producing noise at frequencies that could cancel the inner ear noise).

In some cases, a hearing aid may also lessen the annoyance produced by inner ear noise. For some people, uttering a specific sound gives relief; for others, relief comes from certain breathing exercises; and for still others, relief may come from an herbal ear drop. For more information about tinnitus, call the American Tinnitus Association at 800-634-8978.

Toilet Seats

Rising from a toilet seat is difficult for many elderly people. Most of the toilet seats in the United States are 14.5 inches from the floor, whereas other seats, such as one in a wheelchair, are about 19 inches from the ground. Toilets with higher seats are available, but they are expensive. The most common solution is a raised toilet seat that sits on or is clamped to the top of the toilet. They do make it easier to stand up. However, there is the risk of the added-on seat slipping and causing a fall.

Tomatoes

Tomatoes are considered to be one of the healthiest foods because of the lycopene (an antioxidant) they contain. They may serve to reduce the risk of prostate cancer (*see* Nutrition and Diet; Prostate Cancer) and other diseases as well. Researchers in Scotland have found that there seems to be another health benefit from tomatoes. The yellow jelly surrounding tomato seeds contains a substance that prevents blood clots. It seems to interfere with the clumping of platelets in blood that could cause circulatory problems.

Touch

The degree to which *touch sensitivity* declines with aging varies with different parts of the body. The decline is particularly pronounced for the fingers. This decline is largely the result of the loss of many touch receptors in the skin of the fingers during late adulthood. Some related decline in the ability to locate and identify objects by touch is to be expected as a consequence of normal aging.

The fact that the sense of touch declines in sensitivity with aging does not prevent seniors from having both physical health and mental health benefits when they receive caring touch from someone. For example, widows and widowers in their seventies and eighties who became deprived of caring touch from their late spouse were found to have less depression and anxiety when they either gave massages to others or received massages from others (*see AARP the Magazine,* January–February 2006, for additional information).

Trail Making Test

The Trail Making Test has been part of a battery for evaluating degree of dementia for many years. The test consists of two parts, Part A and Part B. For Part A a client connects, with a pencil, 25 circles numbered 1 to 25 as quickly as possible. For Part B a client connects 13 circles numbered 1 to 13 and 12 circles labeled *A* to *L,* alternating between the two series. The score is the time to complete the two parts. As dementia increases in severity, time scores increase drastically. Time scores also increase with normal aging, but not nearly to the degree they do with dementia.

Transfer of Learning/Training

After finally learning the names of all of the president's cabinet members, a new president is elected, and the process of learning cabinet members' names has to start all over. Now instead of Secretary of State Sanders it is Secretary of State Simpson. This is a situation in which previous learning is likely to have a negative effect on the new learning. The previous name of Sanders keeps intruding while you are trying to learn to relate Simpson to the position of secretary of state, and by so doing interferes with and slows your rate of new learning. This is an example of what learning psychologists call *transfer of training*—the effect of previous learning (or training) on new learning. In this case, it is an example of *specific negative transfer,* meaning that the specific content of previous learning interferes to some degree with new learning.

To bring specific transfer into the laboratory, participants are asked to learn successive lists of paired words (paired-associate learning; *see* Verbal Learning) in which the first word of each pair from the first list is also the first word of each pair in the second list. However, the second word of each pair in the first list is replaced by a new and unrelated word in the second list. For example, *apple* and *king* may be words of a pair in the first list, and *apple* and *pencil* the corresponding words in the second list. Note that *apple* plays the same role as *secretary of state* and *king* and *pencil* the same roles as *Sanders* and *Simpson* in our previous example. Adults of all ages tend to show specific negative transfer in learning the second list. Their rate of learning is slower than if the pairs in the first list had been completely unrelated to the pairs in the second list. The interference from *king* slows the learning of *pencil* as the new response to be given to *apple,* just as the interference from *Sanders* slows the learning of *Simpson* as the new response to be given to *secretary of state.* Most important, the amount of negative transfer (or slowing down in rate of learning) has generally been found to be no greater for older participants than for younger participants, despite the common belief that elderly people are more susceptible to interference from prior learning (*see* Forgetting).

Specific transfer is not unusual in learning motor skills. Consider having learned to drive a car with an automatic transmission. Then, for some reason, you must learn to drive a car with a stick shift. Your previous learning with the automatic shift may make learning the use of the stick shift somewhat more difficult than if you did not have the previous experience with the automatic shift.

Specific transfer may also be *positive* in its effects. Prior learning may facilitate subsequent learning. Consider a basketball fan in Milwaukee in the 1970s. The city already had a men's professional basketball team known as the Milwaukee Bucks. A professional women's basketball league was then formed, and Milwaukee was one of the cities involved. The name of the new team? The Milwaukee Does! Having already learned to associate Bucks with Milwaukee should make it easier to learn now to associate Does with Milwaukee. Positive transfer is the expected outcome. It probably is no coincidence that cities with both professional baseball and professional football teams often have team names that lead to positive transfer (for example, Chicago Cubs and Chicago Bears).

To bring specific positive transfer into the laboratory, participants receive successive lists in which the pairs of words are, for example, *apple* and *king* in the first list and *apple* and *queen* in the second list. Here the task is like learning *Milwaukee* paired with *Bucks* in the first list and *Milwaukee* paired with *Does* in the second list. Evidence indicates that elderly participants show less positive transfer (facilitation) on the second list than do younger participants, presumably because they are less likely to take advantage of the relatedness of content.

There is another form of transfer known as *learning-how-to-learn* or *nonspecific transfer*. The reference is to mastering the skills needed to learn a particular kind of task or needed to perform more proficiently on a task, and then applying these skills to a new version of that task even when the specific content changes with successive tasks. This is the case when participants are given successive lists of paired words in which there is no commonality of the words across the lists (for example, *apple-pencil* as a pair in the first list is replaced by *table-lion* in the second list). Rate of learning tends to improve from the first to the second list and perhaps even from the second list to a third list as participants learn skills that make learning faster. Nonspecific transfer is always positive (that is, it facilitates new learning), and it is likely to be as facilitative for older participants as it is for younger participants.

Nonspecific transfer also occurs, again in about equal amounts, for both younger and older participants when they are given extensive practice on some reasoning tasks. In such cases participants are acquiring, with practice, more effective skills for solving the kinds of reasoning problems they receive. Older people are not only capable of learning new content but also quite competent in learning skills that benefit a wide range of mental performances.

Traveling

Today's senior citizens look for more adventure and education in their travels than in the past. Today many travel agencies have specialists in senior travel. Current elderly people are more interested in spending money on themselves than were past generations of elderly people. They spend about 30 percent more on vacations than do younger people. Many senior citizens are looking for travel experiences that lead to personal growth (for example, *see* Elderhostel) rather than emphasize old age (for example, senior cruises).

A problem facing elderly travelers to foreign countries is the risk of contracting an illness while away from the United States. Elderly people planning such a trip should consider visiting a travel clinic that specializes in travel medications, immunizations, and vaccinations. Personnel at such a clinic include physicians and nurses who are qualified to inform you about the health risks you may face in the country you are to visit. The staff will make certain that elderly travelers know where to go if they do encounter illness while away and will be able to give advice about health insurance for foreign trips.

When away from the United States, it is safe for seniors to eat peeled fruit. Local water is safe to drink if it has been boiled. Tea and coffee are safe to drink, and so are beer, wine, carbonated drinks, and canned drinks. Ice could be made from unsafe water. To be safe, avoid its use. Avoid all raw food, unpasteurized milk, and cheese made from such milk. All meat and fish should be cooked thoroughly. If you get diarrhea, make sure you have Immodium on hand. If it is a severe case, get medical help.

In a motel do not accept an isolated room in the rear of the motel or at the end of a long corridor. Never leave your door open, and always lock it when you leave it. If staying in a hotel and you have difficulty descending many flights of stairs, do not accept a room that is on a high floor. In case of a fire or other emergency, the elevators will not be in use. *See also* Vaccinations and Shots for Traveling.

Tremor (Essential)

Four to five million Americans have a condition known as *essential tremor.* The condition is characterized by the head bobbing in a "yes-yes" and "no-no" manner. The hands may often shake as well, but not in all cases. The disease may strike both young adults and older adults. In about 25 percent of the cases, the disease develops after the age of fifty.

The disease has a strong genetic connection. A child whose parent has the disease has a 50 percent chance of inheriting the gene. However, not everyone who has the gene shows signs of tremor. Essential tremor may be confused with the tremor shown by patients with Parkinson's disease (*see*

Parkinson's Disease). However, in Parkinson's disease the tremor appears when the hands and legs are at rest, and it slows down when the limbs are being used. With essential tremor, the tremor occurs when the hands are in motion, and not when they are at rest.

Beta-blocking drugs, such as Inderal, may control the tremor. Training to relax muscles may help to reduce the tremors. Not treating the tremors usually does not impair physical health. However, people with essential tremor may be impaired in their social and leisure activities, in the performance of the activities of daily living (*see* Activities of Daily Living), and in their psychological adjustment.

Tuberculosis

Tuberculosis is a chronic bacterial lung disease that for years has been a serious health threat. In 1992, 33.4 percent of the cases of tuberculosis were of people age fifty-five and older. The incidence is higher in men than in women and higher in African Americans than in whites. The disease is usually transmitted from person to person by inhaling airborne droplets containing the bacteria. Symptoms often develop gradually and are likely to be vague. They include a cough, fatigue, weight loss, sweating or chills at night, and chest tightness. Diagnosis for older people is often delayed, or the symptoms are misdiagnosed as those of pneumonia or congestive heart failure with pleural effusion. In one study, it was found that 60 percent of the deaths from the disease were for people age sixty-five and older.

Twins

Identical twins have long played an important part in psychological research. They have identical heredities, making them a critical research asset for determining the relative contributions of inheritance and the environment to individual differences in many kinds of behaviors. Especially important are comparisons between identical twins who were reared together during childhood and identical twins who were separated soon after birth and reared in different environments.

If pairs of adult twins are found to be highly similar in a given behavior, regardless of their childhood environments, then there is good reason to believe that heredity is a major determinant of proficiency in that behavior. That is, with the same heredity, variation in the environment seems to have little effect on the behavior. Scores on intelligence tests earned by identical twins, even during late adulthood, tend to be highly similar whether or not they had been reared together. Moreover, psychologists at Pennsylvania State University have discovered remarkable similarities in several personality traits between older identical twins (average age fifty-nine years, with many of the twins being much older than fifty-nine), again regardless of their togetherness or separation while growing up. The traits are those of emotionality, activity level, and sociability. Twins in Denmark were found to be very similar in the difficulties they had in performing the normal physical activities of daily living (for instance, dressing or combing hair), again whether or not they grew up together. This too implies a large role played by heredity in determining our proficiency in performing such acts.

Identical twins may be expected to be similar in many ways throughout their adult life spans. Their identical heredities ensure their similarities. Of particular interest in gerontology is the similarity identical twins may have in longevity, given their identical heredities. There is evidence indicating that identical twins die several years closer to each other in age than do fraternal twins (*see* Longevity). However, the role of environmental factors in determining longevity cannot be denied. Swedish researchers studied the records of more than thirty-six hundred identical twins and nearly seven thousand fraternal twins. They discovered that only one-third of the variability in age at death was attributable to heredity and the rest to environmental factors.

Type A versus Type B Behavior

See Retirement (Involuntary).

U

Underdiagnosis of Illnesses

Elderly patients are much more likely to be underdiagnosed by physicians than are younger patients. Among the many reasons for this are symptom denial by older patients, patient noncommunication with their physician, and physicians attributing symptoms simply to "old age." Underdiagnosis is less likely to occur when diagnosis is made by a geriatric physician rather than by a nongeriatric physician. Especially likely to be missed in diagnosis by a nongeriatric physician are metabolic problems, early cancers, untreated infections, reversible causes of incontinence, and even dementia. *See also* Barriers to Health in Older Men; Physicians (Communication with); Problems Physicians Have with Older Patients.

Unsolicited Support and Advice

If an individual offers, without being asked to do so, an elderly person support of some kind or advice on some matter, does it mean that the individual believes the elderly person is incompetent? Do elderly people believe that it does matter more than young adults and middle-age adults believe it does, and, if so, do they feel it more intensely?

To answer these questions, researchers in Germany created a number of situations involving unsolicited support and advice in seven different areas. For example, one of the areas was health (someone suggests you should be eating more vegetables) and another was finance ("Let me help you organize your finances"). Contrary to what many may believe, fewer elderly participants (45 percent) reported bad feelings or displeasure about support or advice than either young participants (60 percent) or middle-age participants (55 percent). In addition, the intensity of displeasure was about the same at each age level.

Untreated Hearing Impairment (Effects on Spouses)

Husbands with untreated hearing impairment create not only a negative effect on the quality of their lives but also a negative effect on the quality of the lives of their wives. Especially a problem for wives is that the poor communication they may already have with their husbands is exacerbated by their husband's hearing impairment. The consequence is likely to be a decline in wive's psychological well-being (*see* Well-Being [Psychological]). Husbands need help for their impairment! The communication needs of older women are greater than those of older men. Consequently, the well-being of husbands is unlikely to be affected by their wives' untreated hearing impairment.

Urinary Incontinence

A common health problem in late adulthood is urinary incontinence (involuntary urination). It is estimated to be present in about 38 percent of community-dwelling elderly women (more often in white women than in African American women), about 19 percent of community-dwelling elderly men, and in more than half of elderly nursing home residents.

A substantial percentage of incontinent men and a somewhat smaller percentage of incontinent women report spontaneous remission to continence over a period of months. The sex difference in remission rates is seemingly related to the different types of incontinence present in elderly people. Men are more likely than women to have *urge incontinence* (uncontrollable urination with no warning) brought about by physical conditions (for instance, urinary infection or bowel dysfunctions). Women are more likely to have *stress incontinence* in which there is a loss of urine at times of exertion (such as when laughing, sneezing, or bending). Stress incontinence is related to anatomical problems that usually require treatment of some kind.

When older people begin to experience incontinence of either type, it is usually mild and may eventually become moderate. Reversals from moderate to mild incontinence are not uncommon. Men whose incontinence progresses from mild to moderate usually experience a change from urge incontinence alone in the mild form to a combination of urge and stress incontinence in the moderate form. Similarly, women whose incontinence progresses from mild to moderate usually have a change from stress incontinence alone in the mild form to a combination of stress and urge incontinence in the moderate form.

In a study in Italy of more than twenty-three hundred men and women age sixty-five and older, evidence was gathered of any association between incontinence and various physical impairments. For women, three different diseases or ailments were associated with increases in incidence of incontinence. They were chronic respiratory disease, Parkinson's disease, and hip fracture. For men, only chronic diarrhea was associated with incontinence. In addition, disability increased the incidence twofold, and incidence increased by 50 percent for women with sleep disturbances.

A common belief about older people is that incontinence results in social embarrassment and withdrawal from social contacts and that it is likely to lead to loss of self-esteem, depression, and anxiety. However, the results obtained by researchers at the University of Michigan indicated that incontinence, even in a severe form, is only weakly related to increases in depression and negative emotions and to a lowering of life satisfaction.

Experts recommend a number of steps to manage incontinence. The crucial first step is to avoid denial. The problem cannot be managed without being aware of its presence and the willingness to do something about it. Other steps include avoiding the intake of bladder irritants, such as caffeine and spices, and eating foods high in fiber and carbohydrates. Seniors with incontinence should live a lifestyle that includes exercise to strengthen the pelvic muscles that support the bladder, urinate whenever it is convenient even when the urge is not very great, and avoid wearing tight clothing that could weaken the pelvic muscles. They could avoid embarrassment by taking such preventive measures as alerting the flight attendant on an airplane to the fact that they may have to get up even when the "Fasten seat belt" sign is on and asking for directions to the nearest restroom when scheduling an appointment in an unfamiliar building.

Dr. Kathryn L. Burgio of the University of Alabama at Birmingham uses biofeedback (*see* Psychotherapy) to help women learn to control incontinence by contracting and relaxing their bladders. In her study she found that women in her biofeedback group reduced their incontinence by 81 percent. Women in a medication group reduced it by 69 percent, and women in a placebo group by only 39 percent. There is a diagnostic test of incontinence called Urodynamics that evaluates the bladder's ability to store and empty urine. A computer identifies the probable cause of incontinence. The test takes about an hour, and it does not require medication. Behavior modification (*see* Psychotherapy) may be used to treat incontinence. The patient keeps track of the amount and type of beverages consumed and the time since the last urination. Also likely to be included is pelvic muscle exercise and bladder retraining with the use of biofeedback. Younger patients and those with more severe cases of incontinence are the most likely to benefit from behavioral therapy. Surgery may be used in some cases. It now has better long-term results than in the past, and it is less painful than it once was.

Older women with urge incontinence have been found to have significantly more symptoms of depression than women without incontinence. Older men with and without urge incontinence have been found not to differ in the number of symptoms they have of depression. Urge incontinence and depression are both reliable predictors of institutionalization for men but not for women.

Incontinence is especially a problem for nursing home residents who have Alzheimer's disease or some other form of dementia. Much of the problem stems from their difficulty in remembering where a facility for urination is located. There is evidence to indicate that some help in solving this problem may be obtained by painting signs on the walls in areas where patients congregate. The intent of the signs is to aid them in finding the facility in each particular area of the nursing home. The most effective signs are those with the word *toilet* printed in large black letters, with arrows pointing in the direction of the facility. The frequency of incontinence for nursing home residents has been reduced significantly by a prompted void program in which they are checked to see if they are dry, and, if they are, they are prompted or encouraged to use the toilet.

There are organizations dedicated to improving the lifestyle of people with incontinence. One is called Help for Incontinent People (HIP). It publishes a newsletter and other educational materials with useful information about incontinence. HIP may be contacted by writing to HIP, P.O. Box 544, Union, SC 29379 (telephone 800-BLADDER). A similar organization is the Simon Foundation for Continence, P.O. Box 835, Wilmette, IL 60091 (telephone 800-23-SIMON). *See also* Urination.

Urination

Why do many seniors get up during the night to urinate? During the day, being vertical most of the time draws fluid from circulation. At night the fluid seeps back into circulation. This seepage becomes greater as people age. Seniors should wear compression stockings during the day to reduce daytime fluid seepage. Bladder muscles that contract at night are another reason for frequent urination at night, as is decreased production at night of the antidiuretic hormone. Seniors should not drink caffeine beverages or alcohol after five o'clock, as they stimulate urine production. There are medications that may reduce the amount of bladder contraction. Seniors should consult with their physician regarding taking such medications.

Blood in the urine is usually a symptom of a urinary infection. A common home remedy for urinary infections is cranberries or cranberry juice. However, given blood in your urine, you should not be content with just a home remedy. You should see your physician for diagnosis and treatment as soon as possible.

Uterine Cancer

Uterine cancer occurs most often in women older than age fifty. Especially at risk of uterine cancer are women who have never given birth, who are obese or diabetic, and who have high blood pressure. In addition, women who have been taking the hormone estrogen may be at a higher risk than women who have not been taking it (*see* Estrogen-Replacement Therapy [Hormone Replacement Therapy]).

There are other benign conditions of the uterus, such as fibroids. Fibroids grow in the muscle of the uterus. They occur mainly in women who are in their forties. They often require no treatment. Endometrial hyperplasia is most common after age forty. It is an increase in the number of cells in the lining of the uterus. It sometimes develops into cancer. Physicians may recommend surgical removal of the uterus.

Some women with uterine cancer who had their uterus surgically removed also have their ovaries removed as well. This is done to avoid presumably the risk of late ovarian cancer. However, there is evidence to indicate that the removal may actually increase the risk of breast cancer. The ovaries produce hormones that need to be replaced once the ovaries are removed.

V

Vaccinations and Shots for Traveling

Elderly people who plan to visit countries where cholera, typhoid fever, and yellow fever are potential risks should have shots for them. They should also be vaccinated against hepatitis B, if they are at risk of contracting it, and they should have a vaccination for hepatitis A, if they plan to visit third world countries where the water and food are subpar and the hygiene is poor (this vaccination protects the individual for about ten years). If likely to be exposed to ticks, they should consider the Lyme disease vaccination (especially if they will be in high risk states, such as Minnesota, Wisconsin, and states in the Northeast). *See also* Influenza (Vaccines); Pneumonia; Tetanus; Traveling.

Variability of Behavior

Variability on a given task usually refers to the spread or dispersion of scores around the average score earned by individuals. Consider a given task to be playing golf and scores on the task to be the number of strokes needed to play eighteen holes. One group of golfers in a charity tournament has an average score of 100 strokes. However, within the group, scores vary from 70 to 130, with many scores falling between the two extremes. A second group of golfers in a different tournament also has an average score of 100 strokes, but the scores vary only between 90 and 110. Variability of performance within the group is surely greater for the first group than for the second group. Such within-group variability is quantified by a statistic known as a *standard deviation* (*see also* Norms). For our golf example, the standard deviation would be considerably greater for the first group than for the second group.

In terms of performances on many mental tasks, groups of older participants tend to be more like the first group of golfers and younger participants more like the second group of golfers. That is, within-group variability around an average is likely to be greater (a larger standard deviation) for older than for younger participants. Greater variability in performance scores for elderly adults than for younger adults has been found for intelligence tests, memory tasks, and reaction-time tasks, among others. In addition, Australian researchers recently found that variability in the amount of decline over a period of several years in scores on memory and reaction-time tasks (but not for scores on a test of crystallized intelligence; *see* Intelligence) increases with age for people age seventy and older.

Why is there greater variability among elderly groups of people than among groups of younger people? Probably because the effects of aging on performance on a particular mental task vary greatly among elderly people. Some elderly people show little effect of aging. They may be individuals who have been regular physical exercisers for many years or have maintained very active mental lives or both. By contrast, other individuals, for various reasons, may have shown fairly pronounced declines in the mental ability in question, and many others fall somewhere between the two extremes.

Variability of behavior is also used to refer to variability in performance on the same task on different occasions for the same individual. Consider golf again as an example. One golfer may score 80 on some days, 90 on other days, and 100 on still other days, while another golfer always scores between 90 and 100. The first golfer is obviously more variable in his or her performance than is the second golfer. A popular belief is that elderly people are more variable in their performances on the same mental task than are younger people. However, there is evidence to indicate that this is usually not true. Variability in this case is determined by finding the reliability of scores. Participants in a group perform a given mental task on at least two different occasions. The correlation between scores earned on that task on the different occasions defines reliability or the consistency of the performances for the members of the group over separate occasions. This correlation has been found to be as high for elderly groups of participants on a number of mental tasks as for groups of younger participants. There is no reason to believe that normally aging older people are any less consistent in their performances on many tasks than are younger adults.

Nevertheless, seniors' inconsistency (intraindividual variability) scores for speed of responding correlate negatively with scores on several memory tasks (for example, word recall or recalling the content of a story). That is, older adults with a high degree of inconsistency in speed of responding tend to perform more poorly on memory tasks than do other older adults with a low degree of inconsistency (that is, their speed of responding shows little variation from one test session to another). Greater consistency seems to indicate greater stability in cognitive functioning.

Verbal Ability

Verbal ability refers to someone's command of his or her native language.

One index of verbal ability is vocabulary level. In general, the extent of vocabulary, as measured by vocabulary tests, grows from early to late adulthood (*see* Intelligence; Wechsler Intelligence Tests), strongly suggesting that at least one important component of verbal ability increases with normal aging.

On a vocabulary test a participant is given words and asked to define each (for example, "What does the word *psychology* mean?"). There is another component of verbal ability, however, that seems to show a slight decline from early to late adulthood. It is the ability to find the right word to label a specific idea or thought. Age differences in this ability are tested by giving participants what, in effect, is the opposite of a vocabulary test. For example, you may be asked, "What is the name of the mythical animal that is very large and breathes fire?" The use of this kind of test reveals that older participants generally have more difficulty than younger participants in providing the right word.

There is also evidence to indicate that elderly adults experience more tip-of-the-tongue states than do younger adults. A tip-of-the-tongue state occurs when you know a particular word, but you just cannot seem to say it. Often you have an idea of what the missing word sounds like (for example, *secant* when you are trying to use the word *sextant*). You usually find a way to circumvent the problem by using a synonym of the missing word (for example, "an instrument used in navigation"), and you often discover that the missing word suddenly occurs to you at a later time (when you no longer need it).

Age differences in tip-of-the-tongue states are determined by having people of various ages keep a diary for some weeks in which they record each occurrence of such a state. Elderly people, on average, tend to report about twice as many tip-of-the-tongue experiences per week as young adults. However, there is also evidence to indicate that older adults are about as effective as younger adults in gaining access to the missing word when they exert effort to do so.

Is it age per se that causes differences in the frequency of these experiences? Elderly people, in general, possess more general knowledge, including vocabulary, than younger people. Researchers in Indiana found that when the age difference in level of knowledge is taken into account, the age difference in frequency of tip-of-the-tongue experiences disappears. The implication is that the greater store of knowledge older people have, and therefore the greater the amount of information to be searched in looking for a specific item, may be the reason for the greater number of tip-of-the-tongue experiences of older people. In addition, increased tip-of-the-tongue experiences that are induced in the laboratory are mainly found for old-old participants (for example, eighty years and older) and not for young-old participants (aged sixty to seventy-four years), relative to young adults.

Verbal Fluency

Fluency in the use of language does not seem to be greatly affected adversely by normal aging. The standard laboratory task for measuring age differences in verbal fluency is to give participants individual letters of the alphabet (for example, *S*) and ask them to give as many words beginning with each letter as they can in a designated period of time (for example, one minute). Alternatively, participants may be given names of categories (for example, animals) and asked to name as many as possible in the designated time.

In some studies, younger participants have been found to average moderately more words per letter or exemplars per category name than older participants. In other studies, older participants have been found to average moderately more words per letter or exemplars per category name than younger participants.

If there is an age-related decline in the production of words, it is probably the result of an age-related decline in the speed of mental operations needed to produce words (*see* Slowing-Down Principle). However, verbal fluency involves the frontal lobes of the brain, and a serious decline in fluency could be a sign of a possible stroke.

Verbal Learning

Elements of language are always involved in verbal learning. They may be words, names, or numbers. In your lifetime, you have had many verbal learning experiences. For example, you learned that the name of Chicago's professional football team is the Bears, that the capital of Illinois is Springfield, and that the name belonging with a specific face is Johnson. What you learned in each case is a paired associate that, in turn, is the product of *paired-associate learning*. Paired-associate learning is one of the two most widely studied forms of verbal learning.

In paired-associate learning, you learn to associate two originally unrelated events with each other. Often more than one pair of unrelated events must be learned at essentially the same time. Thus, you probably learned the capitals of Illinois, Ohio, and other midwestern states at the same time. The need for paired-associate learning continues through late adulthood. Regardless of age, we try to learn the names of new cabinet members each time there is a vacancy (the new secretary of defense is Jones, the new secretary of labor is Smith, and so on). We also try to learn the names of new football teams each time the league expands (for example, Carolina Panthers), and the names to associate with the faces of our new neighbors. Of interest is what happens to paired-associate learning proficiency during late adulthood.

To study paired-associate learning in the laboratory, participants receive a list of initially unrelated elements (usually ten or twelve pairs). The pairs are composed of either words as both elements or faces as one element and surnames as the other. For example, the words *apple* and *table* may make up one pair, the words *pencil* and *king* another pair, and so on. The pairs are studied together until participants are able to say "table" when *apple* is presented alone, "king" when *pencil* is presented alone, and so on for each of the pairs in the list. Numerous studies have revealed that, with such materials (and with face-name pairs as well), elderly participants do learn paired-associate lists. However, these studies have also revealed a rather substantial age difference in the rate of learning. Learning progresses more slowly for elderly participants than for younger participants.

The main reason for this age difference seems to be in the kind of rehearsal favored by older and younger adults. Older adults tend to rehearse the paired elements rotely by simply repeating the elements to themselves (for example, *apple table, apple table*). Rote rehearsal of this kind is not very efficient in promoting rapid learning. By contrast, younger people often short-circuit rote rehearsal by finding some way of relating the seemingly unrelated elements of each pair. This is often through the use of imagery. For example, *apple-table* could be visualized as a large and highly polished red apple located squarely in the middle of a kitchen table. If the image is firmly established, then the word *apple* when presented alone should serve to recover the entire image that, of course, contains the correct word. Older people generally have less capacity for imaginal activity than do younger people (*see* Imagery). Consequently, they are less likely to use this form of imaginal rehearsal, and they must therefore rely heavily on rote learning.

The other widely studied form of verbal learning is *serial learning*. In serial learning, you must not only learn a number of verbal elements but also learn the order in which they occur. Examples of past serial learning in your life are learning the names of the months of the year in the correct order, the names of the U.S. presidents in the correct order, your Social Security number, and many telephone numbers. You still need to learn new telephone numbers, new ZIP codes, spellings of new words in your vocabulary, unique names (for example, many adults of all ages at one time learned to spell Ayatollah Khomeini), and perhaps even lines of poetry.

To study serial learning in the laboratory, participants receive a list of eight to twelve words, and they practice the list until it can be recited in the order given. As with paired-associate learning, there have been numerous studies of age differences in serial learning. Older participants clearly learn serial lists, but, as with paired-associate learning, the rate of learning is much slower than it is for younger participants. It is learning the order of the words that is especially difficult for older participants. Retaining order information is an example of temporal memory, a form of memory known to decline substantially in proficiency from early to late adulthood (*see* Temporal Memory).

Two other aspects of serial learning are of interest. The first is that older participants make many more errors of omission while practicing a serial learning list than do younger participants. An error of omission refers to saying nothing when asked what word comes after another word. By contrast, younger participants make many more errors of commission than do older participants. An error of commission refers to saying a word but at the wrong place in the serial order. The high omission rate of elderly participants is often cited as evidence for the greater cautiousness of elderly people than for younger people (*see* Cautiousness).

The other aspect of interest is the pronounced difference found for rate of learning of words at different positions in a serial list. The words in the middle of the list are much more difficult to learn in their correct order than are the words near the beginning and the end of the list. These differences in learning among positions are known as *serial-position effects*. They are as ubiquitous for elderly participants as they are for younger participants. A familiar everyday example of serial-position effects is the fact that spelling errors occur much more frequently for letters in the middle of a word than for letters at either end.

Verbosity

Elderly adults are commonly believed to be excessively talkative, or verbose, in the sense that their conversations seems to wander aimlessly away from the topic at hand and therefore prolong their conversations unnecessarily. Are elderly adults truly verbose? Probably more so than younger adults, but only for a minority of older adults.

Researchers at Concordia University in Canada conducted interviews with a number of adults of all ages. They analyzed the contents of the answers of the participants to the questions they were asked in terms of the information given that was irrelevant to those questions (for example, information about themselves, comments about the interviewer, and so on). They discovered that the percentage of elderly adults who were verbose was relatively small, but it was, nevertheless, higher than the percentage of younger adults. Those older adults identified as being verbose were generally socially outgoing people who were having some difficulty in functioning well in their daily lives. The more verbose elderly participants were also found to be more socially active, more extroverted, and experiencing greater stress than the less verbose elderly participants. Researchers in Montreal found that people age sixty-five and older who experienced more frequent and less desirable life changes were more verbose than those who experienced fewer changes. In another study by researchers in California it was found that off-topic speech by elderly adults occurs for autobiographical topics but not for simply describing pictures.

Verbosity if present seems to occur usually when older people are talking about themselves. The researchers at Concordia University also found no difference in memory functioning between their verbose and nonverbose older participants, but they did find that their verbose participants scored lower on a test of nonverbal intelligence than the nonverbose participants and also showed more signs of difficulty in inhibiting irrelevant thoughts.

Very Long-Term Memory

Try to remember—what was your third grade teacher's name? How many names of your grade school teachers can you recall? High school teachers? How is your memory for the foreign-language words you acquired in your high school language class? The names of television shows from ten years ago? These are all examples of *very long-term memory* (also called *remote* or *tertiary memory* by memory researchers) for impersonal events experienced years ago that you shared with other people. You certainly were not the only person who had Miss Johnson for a third grade teacher, the only one in the language class, or the only one watching television ten years ago. Very long-term memory refers to the retention of such past information, in contrast to long-term or secondary memory, which refers to the retention of newly acquired information (*see* Episodic Memory). Very long-term memory also consists of memory for your own personally experienced events, that is, autobiographical memory (*see* Autobiographical Memory). Our present interest is only for those remote events of a more impersonal nature, such as teachers' names.

There is convincing evidence that many of these events are rapidly forgotten, with most of the forgetting taking place within six or so years after the events were encountered. Usually, only 20 percent to 40 percent of the information seems to be retained and held in what is called a "permastore" state (that is, permanently available and highly resistant to forgetting from interference created by similar events occurring both before and after the events to be remembered—for example, names of other people, including names of your children's teachers, or names of other television programs before and after those of ten years ago).

Those events that remain in permastore are likely to be those that were especially well learned or overlearned. Thus, memory for those events is likely, on average, about what it was some years ago, and probably as good for elderly adults as the memory for comparable events for people aged thirty, forty, or fifty who are beyond the "six-year barrier." Elderly people frequently remark that their memories for remote events (tertiary memory) are very good; it is their memories for recent events that are not as good (secondary memory). Many of them are probably correct in their assessment of their own memories.

Vigilance

Vigilance refers to one's ability to maintain alertness to detect a change in otherwise constant conditions. For example, the parent of a sleeping infant stays vigilant until the infant begins to stir and cry. Here the constant condition is silence from the infant's crib. And the change is the occurrence of sounds from that crib. Similarly, a quality-control inspector observes a steady stream of objects. The inspector maintains a state of vigilance while looking for an occasional object that fails to meet some standard established by the industry and must therefore be withdrawn.

The possibility of a decline with aging in the ability to detect occasional "odd" events in a series of otherwise like events has been investigated in a number of studies. Research has been directed at two kinds of vigilance. The first kind is *simple vigilance*. In tests of simple vigilance the demand placed on the observer is slight in that the "odd" event is clearly distinguishable from the like events. Laboratory research has concentrated on age differences in the accuracy of detecting the occurrences of the odd events.

This research has made use of a clocklike device with a single moving hand and a large number of markers that resemble those indicating seconds on a true clock. Participants in research with this device watch the hand move from marker to marker for an hour. During that time the hand moves thirty-six hundred times, of which only twenty-three are odd events. An odd event consists of a double jump of the hand. Participants are asked to signal when each double jump occurs. These double jumps occur at random times during the hour.

As might be expected, accuracy in detecting a double jump decreases during the course of the hour. Fatigue does set in, and it makes its presence felt by failures to detect the double jumps that occur late in the series of jumps. However, there is convincing evidence to indicate that the decline in accuracy over time is no greater for older adults than for younger adults. In fact, accuracy throughout the tedious hourlong session is as high for elderly adults as for young adults.

The second kind of vigilance is *complex vigilance*. Here, conditions are such that it is more difficult for the observer to detect the difference between the odd event and the like events. Consider, for example, the greater difficulty of a parent in detecting an infant's crying when the parent is busy vacuuming a rug rather than sitting in silence.

Researchers at Catholic University created a laboratory situation in which complex vigilance had to be maintained. Their participants watched a series of numbers displayed on a screen. They were to signal whenever a zero appeared. Complexity was varied by the amount of visual degrading (blurring) of the numbers projected on the screen. Regardless of a participant's age, accuracy in detecting the zeros decreased as the degree of blurring increased. In addition, they found their older participants to be less accurate than their young participants, even when the degree of blurring was relatively low.

Other researchers have investigated age differences with various other ways of increasing the complexity of maintaining vigilance. They also found older adults to be less accurate than younger adults. Unlike simple vigilance, complex vigilance seems to decline moderately in proficiency with normal aging. The exception seems to be evidence in a study by researchers at the National Institute on Aging. They found that the performance decrement at the highest level of degradation was equivalent for young, middle-aged, and older participants.

Vision

Visual impairment is one of the most prevalent physical impairments confronting elderly people. It is estimated that 13 percent of the overall elderly population of the United States has some form of visual impairment. For those age eighty-five and older it is estimated that 27 percent are visually impaired. Visual impairment with normal aging brings with it a number of problems in daily living. Older people with considerable visual decline report greater difficulty in performing the normal functions of daily living (for example, preparing meals) and in maintaining social interactions than elderly people who have relatively little visual decline.

Visual decline is usually thought of initially in terms of *static acuity* (the ability to discriminate the fine details of a spatial pattern). Static acuity is measured by the familiar Snellen chart (rows of letter of different sizes that are read during an eye examination) and expressed by such scores as 20/20. Static acuity begins to decline at about age forty. By age seventy it has decreased by about 30 percent relative to the static acuity of people in their twenties. However, even with this decline it is estimated that only 1 percent of the elderly population meets the criterion for legal blindness (20/200 or worse vision in the better eye or a field vision constricted to 20 degrees or less). The decline in static acuity is by no means the only form of visual impairment with normal aging.

An even more dramatic decline occurs for *dynamic acuity*. Dynamic acuity is basically defined in terms of the smallest movement of an object that can be detected as movement by the observer. The decline in dynamic acuity begins at an earlier age than the decline in static acuity, and it progresses to the point where the loss is, on average, nearly 60 percent for people in their seventies relative to people in their twenties. However, evidence indicates that the impairment in dynamic acuity experienced by many older people may be greatly reduced when the moving target is exposed at a high level of illumination. The implication is that at least part of the decline in dynamic acuity is the result of the reduction of illumination that reaches the retina through the lens.

A number of other visual impairments accompany normal aging. One of the visual changes with aging is called *presbyopia*. It is a progressive decline in the eye's ability to focus on near objects. By middle age many people may need reading glasses (or hold objects farther from their eyes if they do not have glasses). By late adulthood people with nearsightedness may need to remove their glasses to read by holding print close to their eyes. Presbyopia is not corrected by laser surgery.

Other problems include the fact that elderly people are more susceptible to the disrupting effects of *glare* than are younger people. Also, the ability to locate the past position of objects in the visual field is less accurate among elderly people than younger people. This may be demonstrated by projecting on a computer screen a visual object at a certain position and then terminating the exposure. Participants are then asked to locate by a cursor where the target had been located on the screen. Research with this procedure has indicated that elderly participants are about 40 percent less accurate than young adult participants in correctly identifying the locations. On the other hand, researchers at Washington University in St. Louis found only minor age differences in the pattern of eye movements (*saccadic movements*). The implication is that the brain mechanism controlling eye movements is relatively unaffected by normal aging.

Older adults are less sensitive in detecting weak-intensity lights than are younger adults. That is, elderly adults have a much higher absolute threshold for brightness than young adults. The absolute threshold is measured by presenting initially very dim lights and then increasing the brightness of the light until an intensity is reached where the light is detected half of the time it occurs. This intensity is the absolute threshold. The age difference in brightness sensitivity is also apparent for brightnesses that are well above the absolute brightness threshold. For example, if a light doubles in its physical intensity, older adults will perceive it as increasing less than will younger adults. *See also* Color Perception; Constancies of Perception; Dark Adaptation; Depth Perception; Form Perception; Visual Disorders.

Visual Disorders

The visual impairment that occurs with normal aging (*see* Vision) is compounded by abnormalities of the eye that are more common in late adulthood than in earlier adulthood. Foremost among these abnormalities are *cataracts* and *glaucoma*. A cataract is a clouding of the lens that lessens the sharpness of the image transmitted to the retina, resulting in blurred vision and an increased susceptibility to glare. The chance of having a cataract is 50 percent greater in women than in men. Cataracts may be removed surgically by a procedure that is performed thousands of times annually in the United States. Microsurgery may be used to remove lenses clouded by cataracts. The lenses are then replaced by plastic lenses. In about 95 percent of the cases the surgery improves vision, but a follow-up laser treatment may be needed later.

It is estimated that more than 3 million Americans have glaucoma, and 120,000 have suffered blindness from the disease. Those who are at a high risk of having glaucoma are people with a family history of glaucoma, people with dark eyes, and African Americans over age fifty. Glaucoma, a disorder that rarely occurs before age forty, consists of an elevated pressure within the eyeball that may, if not treated, damage visual receptors in the retina. Pressure has been tested for many years by a device called a Goldmann tonometer in which a flat tip touches the eye's cornea briefly. This test does give a moderate rate of false readings. A recent digital tonometer with greater accuracy is beginning to replace the earlier device.

Often the symptoms of glaucoma are not noticed by individuals until the disease has progressed considerably. Consequently, regular eye examinations are important for early detection, especially for individuals age forty and older.

Treatment of glaucoma requires normalizing pressure within the eye. It may be done by drops such as Cosopt, Xalatan, and Brimonidine Tartrate or by laser surgery. Medicare helps to pay for eye examinations for people who are considered to have a high risk for glaucoma.

Other visual disorders that are less prevalent in late adulthood than cataracts or glaucoma, but more prevalent than in earlier adulthood, are *macular degeneration* and *diabetic retinopathy*. Macular degeneration consists of degeneration of visual receptor cells (cones) in the macular section of the retina (at its center is the fovea, the area most densely packed with cones and the most sensitive part of the retina), where most of our perception of finer details takes place. The disease affects about 25 percent of people older than seventy-five (90 percent have the dry form rather than the wet form; see below).

Elderly whites are more susceptible to degeneration than are elderly African Americans. Smoking may double the risk of having macular degeneration. It depletes the body of the nutrients that protect the eyes from the disease. Macular degeneration is the leading cause of legal blindness among Americans over age sixty. Loss of receptors in the macular area results in the inability to resolve finer visual details. Consequently, reading and driving become very difficult tasks to perform. The receptors in the periphery of the retina are rarely involved; thus, affected individuals are usually able to see sufficiently to move about and to take care of themselves.

There are two kinds of macular degeneration, dry and wet. In dry degeneration (the more prevalent form with about 90 percent of those with degeneration), there is no leaking of fluid into or below the retina. In wet degeneration, a pool of fluid and blood accumulates beneath the retina. Wet degeneration is sometimes (5 percent or less) reduced by means of laser coagulation. Laser surgery may sometimes halt further macular degeneration, but it works in only about 15 percent of the cases where retinal damage is visible. It seals leaking blood vessels and inhibits their growth. However, new blood vessels may grow in nearby areas. They may need additional laser treatment. Radiation therapy seems to have beneficial effects. In one study, it was found that those treated with radiation lost only half of the vision within one year that others without radiation lost.

There is a medical treatment that benefits only 25 percent to 50 percent of those with the severest forms of macular degeneration. The treatment consists of injecting a drug called visudyne into a vein in the arm. It eventually begins destroying new blood vessels in the retina when activated by light from a non-heat-generating laser. A new drug called Lucentis was approved in 2006 by the U.S. Food and Drug Administration for treatment of the wet form of macular degeneration. It shows considerable promise of slowing down the progression of macular degeneration. In clinical trials nearly 95 percent of the participants maintained their vision after one year of monthly injections in the eyes, compared to about 50 percent of the participants receiving a standard treatment. The injections presently cost nearly two thousand dollars each. In addition, high doses of vitamins A, E, and C along with zinc and copper have been found to slow down the progression of dry macular degeneration.

As little as one glass of red or white wine daily may reduce by half the risk of macular degeneration. Obtaining a combination of vitamins C and E, zinc, and beta-carotene from foods may serve to prevent progression of the degeneration after it has begun. Vitamin C is contained in citrus fruit and juices, green peppers, broccoli, and potatoes; vitamin E in whole grains, eggs, nuts, and vegetable oils; zinc from meat, poultry, whole grains, and dairy products; and beta-carotene from carrots and spinach.

Diabetic retinopathy, or damage to the retina from vascular hemorrhages, may occur after years of diabetes. In some cases it may be treated by laser therapy or by surgery. Lasers may be used to seal leaking blood vessels associated with diabetic retinopathy.

Still other visual disorders more common in late adulthood than in early adulthood include *floaters in the eye* and *arcus senilis*. Floaters are specks of debris floating in the back two-thirds of the eye. They move across the field of vision when the eyes move. For normal floaters it may be best to ignore them (but seek the advice of your ophthalmologist). More serious cases could indicate that the retina is degenerating. Arcus senilis consists of a ring of degeneration around the periphery of the cornea that may be seen in some elderly people. Its extent increases with age, and at a somewhat faster rate for men than for women. About 25 percent of men and 15 percent of women age fifty and older have either half or complete arcus senilis.

Visual disorders are much more likely to be present in nursing home residents than in others of the same ages living in the community. A survey of about five hundred nursing home residents in Baltimore found them to be more than ten times more likely to be blind than were community dwellers. Many of the visual problems nursing home residents have could be corrected simply by having them obtain new glasses. The need for new, updated glasses is often overlooked by caregivers in nursing homes. Their attention is likely to be concentrated on more life-threatening illnesses of their patients. Relatives of residents in nursing homes should make sure that they receive eye examinations at regular intervals. Improving the vision of residents should greatly increase the quality of their lives.

Some elderly people adapt better to visual impairment than do other elderly people. Researchers at the Lighthouse Research Institute found that attitude is closely related to successful adaptation. Those who adapted best found ways either to bypass their impairment or to alter their lifestyles somewhat. Elderly people who adapt best are those who find new goals to keep their minds off their impairment and who have a good social support system. Elderly people with visual impairment should be aware of the fact that there are large-print publications available (and even large-number playing cards) as well as various magnifying devices. In addition, they may be taught to read more slowly, to practice new methods of grooming and cooking, and to change their environments to fit their needs. For those seniors who are totally or partially blind, a new handheld device was introduced in 2006 (the Kurzwell National Federation of the Blind Reader). The device converts printed material to spoken audio material. *See also* Adapting to Fading Eyesight; Visual Disorders (Coping with Macular Degeneration); Visual Disorders (Sleep Problems).

Visual Disorders (Coping with Macular Degeneration)

A critical attribute for those suffering from macular degeneration is the degree of control they believe they have over the events in their lives. Stronger control beliefs have been found to be associated with greater functional ability (performing the activities of daily living), more favorable adaptation to vision loss, and more frequent feelings of positive emotions. Seniors suffering from macular degeneration should be offered help in strengthening their belief in their ability to control everyday events. *See also* Control over Life's Events; Visual Disorders.

Visual Disorders (Sleep Problems)

Blind adults report more sleep problems than sighted adults. One reason is that no light reaches the sleep-wake centers in the brain. Light deprivation seems to lead to dysfunctioning of these centers and therefore poorer sleep.

Elders who are not blind but suffer from visual impairments that reduce the amount of light reaching the brain's sleep centers may similarly experience poor sleep. Researchers have found that this is indeed the case.

For example, in one study 35 percent of the participants with visual impairments reported difficulty falling asleep compared to 17 percent of the participants without visual impairment.

Elders with visual impairment should be encouraged to spend more time outdoors when there is sunlight. It could cause more light to reach the sleep centers of the brain, resulting in better sleeping at night.

Vitamin D Supplements

Vitamin D deficiency is common for older people. It is estimated that 50 percent of nursing home residents have a vitamin D deficiency. The deficiency in healthy community-dwelling elders is associated with low bone mass, decreased physical performance, and a high risk of osteoporosis that may result in hip fractures. Researchers at the Beth Israel Deaconess Medical Center in Boston found that the deficiency in community-dwelling elderly women can be corrected in the majority of cases by three months of vitamin D supplements of 400-800 IU/d. However, the degree to which the supplements reduces the risk of hip fracture is debatable (*see* Fractures [Hip]).

Voice

In late adulthood the voices of many people tend to increase slightly in pitch as the vocal cords stiffen and vibrate at a higher frequency than earlier in life. For some elderly people, the volume of their voices may decrease somewhat, and there may also be a quaver in the voice through some loss of control over the vocal cords. However, it remains uncertain whether these voice changes are a normal consequence of aging for many people or whether they are the consequences of poor health and the presence of a disease.

Voice changes, such as deepening and frequent throat clearing, should be checked with a physician if they have lasted for more than two weeks. Viral infection of the larynx could be the reason, but they usually last less than two weeks. The problem could be the result of small noncancerous growths called vocal polyps. An uncommon possibility is cancer of the larynx. While experiencing the voice changes, avoid whispering because it strains the vocal cords and larynx and also avoid clearing the throat.

There is also a group of speech impairments known as dysarthria caused by neurological disorders that are fairly common among elderly adults. The impairments range from mild to severe. With mild impairment speech is likely to be intelligible even though it sounds as if it is being spoken by a drunken individual. With severe impairment speech is likely to be unintelligible. Speech therapists recommend that affected individuals be encouraged to speak slowly and to use short sentences.

Voters

The percentage of eligible voters who actually vote in national elections is depressingly small. However, this bleak picture does not apply to elderly voters. For example, in the 1996 congressional elections 20.3 percent of the voters were age sixty-five and older (in 1980 it was 16.8 percent). This is nearly twice the percentage of people age sixty-five and older in the total population of the United States. In the 2004 presidential election exit polls indicated that 25 percent of those who voted were sixty and older. In the year 2040 the percentage of voters age sixty-five and older is expected to be 41.4 percent.

A Nobel Prize–winning economist has a theory that people base their choices between alternatives on what is best in their own interest. This applies to voting. If true, it is no wonder that candidates focus on Social Security, Medicare, and maintaining benefits for seniors. They know that seniors get out to vote. However, this ignores the evidence regarding generativity (see Generativity). Seniors, in general, are very concerned about younger generations. For the most part they base their choices in voting on what benefits our entire country—and not just on what benefits seniors.

Seniors who vote in most elections are generally married, attend church regularly, and live in nonsouthern states.

W

Walkers

A number of elderly people need to use a walker to enhance their mobility and comfort while walking. Most walkers fall into three categories: walking frames, two-wheeled walkers, and four-wheeled walkers (also known as rollators). Walking frames have no wheels. They are designed to assist with balance and are used primarily to help someone rise from a sitting position. Movement requires lifting the frame and placing it ahead of the person walking. It provides slow movement but greater security when shifting from walking to sitting.

Two-wheeled walkers allow a person to slide forward easily. However, when weight is applied, rubber at the back of the walker resists motion. They are well suited for people with Parkinson's disease in that they do not roll too far ahead of the walker. Four-wheeled walkers have become very popular with elderly people. They usually have adjustable handle height. Some elderly users do complain that the brake is difficult to operate, largely because they do not have the grip strength to apply it. Elderly people with arthritis in the hands are especially likely to have a problem operating the brake.

Walking

More than one hundred community-dwelling older adults in Singapore estimated the duration and frequency of performing various habitual activities, such as low-intensity or habitual walking and gardening, each day for several weeks. They averaged eighteen minutes per day for walking, the most frequently performed activity. Walking was the only activity that correlated positively with peak oxygen consumption scores and physical performance scores (for example, faster gait speed the more minutes of walking). Researchers at Duke University found that walking eleven miles a week helps to prevent excessive fat from accumulating around your stomach and abdomen, fat that may lead to various serious health problems (*see* Body Build and Body Characteristics).

Older adults with greater involvement in habitual or low-intensity walking appear to have better physical fitness and better physical performances than older adults with less involvement in such walking.

Unfortunately, many older American adults decline many opportunities they have for engaging in low-intensity walking. For example, they park their automobiles in the parking lot of a store as close as possible to the doors of that store to avoid as much walking as possible. They should be parking some distance from the doors to ensure some extra walking that day. They should also be out walking their dog more often and for longer distances.

Seniors who give up on a walking program because the walking "wears them out" should consider walking with the use of two trekking poles. This would give them two additional points of contact with the ground besides their two feet. This should enhance their balance and lower the impact walking has on their knees and lower back.

Wandering

Mentally impaired elderly people who wander present a danger to themselves as well as to others. Researchers at the University of Washington observed a number of patients with Alzheimer's disease, 75 percent of whom lived with a spouse. They found that the greater the cognitive impairment of the patients, and the greater the impairment in performing the activities of daily living (see Activities of Daily Living), the more frequent the wandering behavior. Distress for the caregivers increased significantly with increase in the frequency of a patient's wandering.

Researchers at the University of Florida discovered that 37 percent of wanderers with dementia were found less than one mile away from their home, 49 percent between one and five miles away from home, and 14 percent farther than five miles away. Wanderers who die while wandering usually die from exposure after going into woods or fields. Caregivers should make certain their patients have a bracelet with their name on it and a telephone number to call for assistance. The patients should be registered with the Safe Return Program of the Alzheimer's Association (see Alzheimer's Association). Law enforcement officers should be taught how to spot wanderers and how to communicate with them.

Warnings

"Warning: Don't take this medicine if you are experiencing shortness of breath." Warnings are a familiar sight on various products, materials, appliances, and properties. Elderly adults were found by researchers at the Georgia Institute of Technology to be less likely to notice such warnings than are younger adults, and elderly adults are less likely than younger adults to comprehend and comply with them. Warnings must be in print large enough to be noticed readily by seniors, and they should be written in language that is easy to follow and comprehend.

Weather (Tornado)

Elderly adults with mild memory problems may have difficulty remembering the distinction between a tornado watch and a tornado warning. A watch means that conditions are favorable for developing a tornado. They should be prepared by listening to a radio or television station for the latest information. They should know where they should go if the conditions get worse. A warning means that a tornado has been sighted or detected by radar nearby. They should take immediate action by going to a safe place. If in a public place, go to an interior hall on the lowest level and stay away from windows and from areas with large free-span roofs. If in an automobile, do not try to outrun the tornado. Instead, get out of the automobile, and hide in a nearby ditch or large depression while covering your head.

If you are at home in a house with a basement, go to it. Avoid windows and chimneys. If there is no basement, hide under a stairwell or furniture and cover your head. Go to the lowest level in the northeast section of your house. Stay preferably in a small room, hallway closet, or under a stairway. Stay away from external walls and windows and cover your head. If in a mobile home, get out of it and seek shelter in a nearby building. If none is around, find a ditch or ravine and cover your head.

Web Sites (Use for Medical Information)

More than 30 percent of seniors questioned in a large survey reported using Web sites to find medical information of use to them. Web sites can provide valuable information to supplement the diagnosis and treatment provided by a physician. However, there is the danger that some older patients may use information on a Web site as a substitute for a physician's diagnosis.

Misdiagnosis from information in a Web site is not the only problem. If the site has a ".com" address at the end, it could mean that the creators of the site are trying to sell you some product mentioned favorably in the given information. The product may actually be harmful for many seniors with different disorders. Check the date when the site was last updated. If that date was some time ago, the information contained in it may no longer be valid.

There are sites that are viewed as being highly reliable by health professionals. Several are provided by the federal government and may be identified by the ".gov" at the end of the address. They include Health Index (Department of Health and Human Services, http://www.healthfinder.gov) and the National Cancer Institute (www.cancer.gov).

Wechsler Intelligence Tests

For a number of years the Stanford-Binet test was the only individually administered intelligence test. This test was developed by Lewis Terman to measure the mental ages and intelligence quotients (IQs) of children and adolescents, and its use with adults was generally viewed as being inappropriate. The void in individually administered intelligence tests was finally filled in 1939 by the appearance of the Wechsler-Bellevue Intelligence Test. The test was developed and standardized by Dr. David Wechsler, a psychologist at New York City's Bellevue Hospital.

Several revisions of the test have appeared over the years, including the Wechsler Adult Intelligence Scale (WAIS), the Wechsler Adult Intelligence Scale-Revised (WAIS-R); and the WAIS-III (the version currently in use). The Wechsler tests have had wide use in both academic and clinical settings as a reliable measure of adult intelligence.

From the beginning, the Wechsler tests have had several distinguishing features. First, the tests yield not only a global or overall IQ score but also separate IQ scores for two major components of intelligence that Wechsler called *verbal intelligence* and *performance intelligence*. Second, an individual's scores (overall, verbal, and performance) on the tests are evaluated relative to people of the same age who were included in the standardization sample. That is, there are age norms for different age ranges from early to late adulthood (*see* Norms). Thus, older adults' scores on any of the test versions are interpreted relative to people their own age rather than to scores obtained by younger adults. An adult in his or her early sixties who has an IQ of 100 on any of the versions is therefore considered to be average with respect to people of that age even though the scores earned on the test are below those earned by average younger adults.

Third, each version of the Wechsler tests consists of eleven subtests, each considered to be a component of either verbal intelligence or performance intelligence. Scores on these subtests do correlate moderately highly with each other. These correlations (that is, people who score high on one subtest have a greater than chance probability of scoring high on the other subtests as well) suggest that each subtest is measuring an ability determined in part by some general factor of intelligence (commonly called *g*) that influences to some degree each specific ability. There are six verbal subtests and five performance subtests. The six verbal subtests are information, comprehension, vocabulary, memory span, similarities, and arithmetic. The five performance subtests are picture arrangement, picture completion, block design, object assembly, and digit symbol.

Various subtests of the Wechsler tests have been widely used apart from their contributions to overall IQ scores and separate verbal and performance IQ scores. For example, the vocabulary subtest is a popular test for measuring verbal ability and for comparing adults of different ages in verbal ability (*see* Verbal Ability). Similarly, the block-design subtest is often used to compare adults of different ages in their spatial abilities (*see* Spatial Ability), and the digit-symbol subtest to compare adults of different ages in their response speed (*see* Speed of Behavior).

Adult age differences in test scores (points earned on the test before they are converted into IQ scores) have been frequently found for total scores, verbal component–only scores, and performance component–only scores. Regardless of whether age differences are determined cross-sectionally or longitudinally, the scores tend to peak for people in their early twenties and then show a progressive decline from then on. The rate of decline, however, is far more pronounced for performance scores than for verbal scores. In fact, when age groups are equated for educational level (there is a moderately high correlation between years of formal education and test scores; *see* Educational Level), scores on the verbal component have often been found to show an increase from early to late adulthood. The rate of decline in scores on the performance component has also been found to be reduced considerably when age groups are matched for educational level.

The various subtests show greatly different age effects. Some subtests are considered to be "hold" tests that show little decline in scores with advancing age (for example, vocabulary and information; but *see* Longitudinal Studies of Aging's Effects on Health and Cognition), whereas other subtests are considered to be "don't hold" tests that show pronounced decline with advancing age (for instance, digit symbol and block design). Still other subtests, such as object assembly and picture completion, fall between the "hold" and "don't hold" subtests. That is, they show age-related declines in scores, but to a lesser degree than found for the "don't hold" subtests.

Most current researchers on intelligence make a distinction between *crystallized intelligence* and *fluid intelligence* as the two basic forms of intelligence in preference to Wechsler's distinction between verbal and performance intelligence (*see* Intelligence). However, the verbal component of the Wechsler tests may be considered to approximate a measure of crystallized intelligence, and the performance component to approximate a measure of fluid intelligence. It is only an approximation, however. To many experts in intelligence testing, several subtests of the verbal component (for example, memory span) are considered to be tests of fluid intelligence rather than crystallized intelligence.

The Wechsler tests share with the Stanford-Binet test the fact that they are considered to be traditional intelligence tests that measure academic aptitude, rather than the kind of practical intelligence that older people long away from an academic setting need for living successful and productive lives (*see* Practical Intelligence). Consequently, so the argument goes, declining scores on the Wechsler tests with normal aging do not necessarily mean declining competence in everyday mental functioning.

Wechsler Memory Scale

The Wechsler Memory Scale is a widely used clinical test for diagnosing memory impairment, including moderate impairment shown with normal aging and more severe impairment with organic amnesia, Alzheimer's disease, and other forms of dementia. Included in the scale are subtests that evaluate proficiency in paired-associate learning (*see* Verbal Learning) and story memory (*see* Discourse Memory). The popularity of the scale is based largely on the availability of age norms that provide some indication of the deviation of a client from the average score for people of the client's age. However, the adequacy of these norms in determining whether an older client is experiencing a benign age-related decline in memory proficiency or is experiencing a more serious pathological decline is questionable.

Well-Being (Psychological)

Well-being is a broad concept that refers to an individual's current level of happiness or distress and his or her current satisfaction with life. Much of the research on age differences in well-being has been on the life-satisfaction component of well-being (*see* Life Satisfaction). However, other research has centered on the negative and positive affective (emotional) states of people of various ages. One of the tests used for this purpose is the General Well-Being Schedule. Participants taking this test are asked such questions as "Have you been anxious, worried, or upset during the past month?" to measure negative affect and such questions as "How happy, satisfied, or pleased have you been with your personal life during the past month?" to measure positive affect.

Research with this test and similar tests has revealed that psychological well-being as defined by emotional states is remarkably stable from early adulthood through late adulthood. That is, the subjective experience of well-being of elderly adults seems to differ little from that of younger adults. Research on life satisfaction has generally yielded the same outcome. Satisfaction with one's present life does not seem to differ greatly among adults of different ages.

Much of the research on well-being has focused on what psychologists and sociologists believe to be the major determinants of the degree of well-being in late adulthood. Of particular interest is what older people themselves believe to be the important determinants.

This information was provided by Dr. Carol D. Ryff of the University of Wisconsin at Madison. She interviewed a number of middle-aged and elderly adults. Positive well-being was found to be associated with being an individual who is "others oriented," that is, being caring and having sound relationships with other people. In addition, middle-aged individuals generally viewed a positive attitude toward one's self as being an important determinant of positive well-being. This was deemed less important by older adults. They instead viewed the ability to accept change as an important determinant of positive well-being; change was defined both in the sense of the respondents' own biological aging and in the world in which they live.

They also believed personal growth to be a contributor to positive well-being. Personal growth refers to having a sense of continued development and self-realization. Dr. Ryff's evidence indicated that personal growth declines from young adulthood to middle age and declines even more to late adulthood. She also found that women of all ages report higher levels of personal growth than do men of all ages. For the very old (age eighty-five and older), positive well-being has been found to be associated with people's independence in performing the activities of daily living (for example, doing their own shopping and managing their own finances) and with their ability to control the events of their lives.

Other researchers have found positive well-being and life satisfaction to be greater for older adults who have a number of roles in their lives (for example, employee, volunteer worker, spouse, parent, grandparent, and so on) than it is for older adults who have fewer roles to play. The positive effect of multiple roles tends to be greater for men than for women and greater for African American men than for African American women, white men, or white women. Frequent participation in such leisure activities as going to movies, plays, or concerts has also been found to affect well-being positively. Interestingly, the degree of well-being (positive or negative) of a married elderly person is a fairly good predictor of the well-being (positive or negative) of that person's spouse. The quality of social contacts is also positively related to well-being (*see also* Friendships).

Well-being is likely to be challenged when elderly people are confronted by health and financial stresses. Of interest is how control strategies affect well-being under these conditions. A control strategy refers to how people attempt to change the external world to make it fit their needs and desires. One such strategy is defined by persistence in goal striving and use of time and effort when obstacles occur. Another is positive reappraisals (for example, finding a different way of looking at things or finding something positive when the situation is bad). The third is lowering aspirations ("I don't set my goals too high—I remind myself that I can't do everything"). Older adults rely on control strategies more than younger adults do. Persistence shows a stronger positive relation to well-being for younger adults than for older adults. Positive reappraisal has a stronger positive relation to well-being in middle age and late adulthood than in young adulthood. Lowering aspirations is negatively related to well-being at all ages. *See also* Widowhood and Widowerhood.

Wheelchairs

About 1.4 million Americans use a wheelchair, many of them elderly people. Because of its ease of storage and ease of transporting in an automobile, the X-braced folding wheelchair is popular with elderly people. It is difficult to make wheelchairs that are both stiff and light. Also popular with elderly users of a wheelchair are those wheelchairs with a rigid, nonfolding frame in which the wheels can be removed by moving a release catch.

Elderly people who have little use of both arms and legs have to use a powered wheelchair. Such chairs usually have four individually powered wheels and front idling castor wheels. An option for tilting the seat is often available to aid being lifted in and out of the chair. A reclining backrest is also an option when a user has to remain in the chair for long periods of time.

The future may bring with it a strikingly different wheelchair designed by Dean Kamen. The chair will climb stairs, go over curbs, lift its occupant to eye level when talking to someone, and drive over sand beaches. The highly innovative new concept for wheelchairs was shown on a segment of television's *Dateline* show several years ago. Also soon to be marketed is a wheelchair that finds its way automatically through a moving crowd of people. The chair is programmed to move in a given direction, and it detects the movements of people in the crowd, enabling it to avoid them and move at a normal walking speed.

White House Conferences on Aging

There is a White House Conference on Aging in each decade. For each conference several thousand delegates from each state and from professional organizations gather to discuss issues relevant to the welfare of elderly people and to conclude with recommendations directed at improving that welfare. The first conference was held in 1961. Recommendations from that conference eventually led to the creation of the Medicare and Medicaid programs. The second conference, held in 1971, resulted in strengthening the Older Americans Act of 1965, including the creation of the Meals on Wheels program. The conference in 1971 is also noted for its attention to ethnic minority elders and the ethnic-related research, policies, and agencies that followed in later years.

The conference held in 1995 in Washington, D.C., was the first to address issues relevant to younger adults as well as elderly adults. Rather than proposing new legislation and new programs, the theme of this conference was to "hold the line"—that is, to maintain Social Security, Medicare, and other programs relevant to elderly people at their present levels, and to avoid forced reductions in benefits. This conference was attended by

2,217 delegates who were largely selected by governors and members of Congress. The fifty resolutions that were adopted covered topics such as housing, crime, and the independence of older people in their own homes through such services as homemaker assistance and in-home care. However, no new legislation or programs were enacted from the conference.

In the next conference, in 2005, delegates were asked to seek solutions facing seniors in the areas of the workplace of the future, health and long-term living, and social engagement, and to increase seniors' awareness that the federal government is not the panacea for solving the needs of seniors.

Why Aging? (Biological Theories of Aging)

Biological aging is as inevitable as death and taxes, yet why the human organism ages is not fully understood. Many theories have been proposed, but no single theory has become universally accepted as *the* most valid. Conceivably, aging is the result of a number of changes in the human body as we grow older, and each theory may have some element of truth.

Some biological theories of aging are based on the principle of a *biological clock* that is genetically present in all of us. Generally, the "clock" is assumed to be in some area of the brain, and a signal of some kind from the brain triggers a number of the biological changes associated with aging. One theory based on the principle of a biological clock has the pacemaker for regulating the clock located in the neurons of higher brain centers. Stimulation from these neurons causes changes in the body's endocrine system or changes in the metabolic activity of various organs or both.

Alternatively, only prematurity stages of development are programmed genetically, and genetic regulation of development ends at maturity. From this point on, the body is susceptible to the ravages of "wear and tear," in which the parts of the body accumulate defects from use and misuse and from intruders to the body from disease, pollution, and so on. The analogy here is that of a machine whose parts eventually wear out at different rates from constant use. The analogy is not a perfect one, however. Biological systems, unlike machines, have the capability of self-repair. For some systems (for example, the skin), new cells form to replace old ones; for other systems (for example, muscles), new cells are not formed, but other self-repair mechanisms occur.

Biological theories of aging also differ in the particular location where the changes responsible for aging take place. One class of theories places the location at the level of the body's cells. Theories in this class may then be further divided into genetic and nongenetic theories. Genetic theories typically view damage by radiation or mutation to cellular deoxyribonucleic acid (DNA) as the cause of aging. DNA controls the formation of the proteins that are needed by cells to sustain life. However, there is little support for this theory. Another possibility is an increase in errors of transferring information from DNA cellular molecules to ribonucleic acid (RNA) cellular molecules. Such errors are believed to produce one or more proteins that are not exact copies of the original protein in the cell. The inexact copy cannot execute its mission of maintaining cellular life, and cells age and die as a result. This theory is a promising one, but one that has been difficult to prove. Another genetic theory is that cells are programmed to reproduce themselves only so many times, and without reproduction they die.

Nongenetic theories stress that the aging and death of cells is the result of their accumulation of metabolic wastes and harmful substances (such as lipofuscin, a fibrous protein known to increase in cellular amount with aging) that interfere with cellular functioning. This theory has not received much support.

Yet another cellular theory is the *free radical theory.* Unstable chemical compounds are believed to accumulate in the cells and interact with other normal molecules to alter proteins essential for life. The evidence in support of this theory has not been great, but it has become currently popular as witnessed by the frequency with which physicians recommend that their elderly patients take antioxidants (*see* Antioxidants) to help rid the body of free radicals.

Researchers at the Massachusetts Institute of Technology believe that aging may result from a mistake in cell division that causes redundant bits of DNA to accumulate within the nuclei of cells. The "junk" may build up to the point of interfering with the normal functioning of cells. The only evidence to date in support of this theory comes from studies with yeast cells.

Evidence to support a rather optimistic cellular theory of aging may have been found by researchers at Texas Southwestern Medical Center in Dallas. They found that inserting a gene that prevents a chromosome's protective end (called a telomere) from shortening resulted in sustaining the division of cells beyond seventy or so times. They believe the procedure could eventually increase the health span of people, but it is unlikely to increase human life span (*see* Life Span).

The other major class of theories places the location at the level of a particular organ or systems of organs. One such theory, and probably the most viable one, is the *immunological theory of aging.* The body's immune system protects the body against invading microorganisms and atypical cell mutants (for example, cancer). Through the immune system the body generates antibodies that react with the proteins of foreign organisms and form defensive cells that digest the foreign bodies. Aging is known to affect the immune system. The production of antibodies declines with aging, as does the ability of antibodies that are formed to recognize mutated cells (thus accounting for the increased incidence of cancer in late adulthood). The net effect is to produce those biological decrements associated with aging.

Why Aging? (Psychological Theories of Aging)

Most psychological theories of aging stress that both decline and growth occur for mental functioning and behaviors throughout adult development. Decline is brought about by biological changes that alter the brain and other parts of the body (*see* Why Aging? [Biological Theories of Aging]) and result in slower mental processes, diminished working memory capacity (*see* Working Memory), slower reaction times, and so on.

At the same time, growth occurs through increases in knowledge and experience over the entire course of adult development. Growth is manifested in the ability to alter our behaviors in response to changes in the physical and social context (or environment) in which people live as they grow older. This position is known as *contextualism*.

Dr. Paul Baltes, a prominent gerontologist at the Max Planck Institute for Human Development and Education in Berlin, argues effectively that people play an active role in changing themselves through accumulated wisdom and experience to meet new challenges and new life crises brought about by their changing context. Further growth in the form of reversing declines that often appear in late adulthood may take place through interventions of various kinds (*see* Plasticity Theory).

Another strong advocate of positive growth in late adulthood is Dr. Gisele Labouvie-Vief of Wayne State University. She has observed that many of the age differences seen in mental performances are the result of qualitative rather than quantitative changes in late adulthood (*see* Continuity versus Discontinuity in Adult Development). Consider, for example, a likely age difference in response to information given that a wife has threatened to leave her husband if he comes home drunk one more time—and eventually he does. Young adults typically respond with the seemingly logical conclusion that she will certainly leave her husband. Many elderly adults, however, will go beyond the information given and consider situational factors, that is, the context, that may be involved. For example, the husband may have heard that day of the death of a close friend, and he had a few drinks to help relieve his sorrow.

A theoretical approach that has been followed by a number of gerontologists is the *dialecticism* introduced by the late Dr. Klaus Riegel. From a dialectical perspective, internal factors, such as physiological states and personality traits, are viewed as interacting with external factors in the physical, social, occupational, and familial environments. Crises in a person's life occur when internal and external factors are out of synchrony. The types of asynchrony and resulting crises people encounter differ at different stages of their lives. However, the ability to resolve crises is as true of elderly adults as it is of younger adults (*see* Personality Stages; Stress and Coping with Stress).

Widowhood and Widowerhood

Widowhood and widowerhood refer to the state of a woman or man, respectively, who has not remarried after the death of a spouse. Widowerhood has been found to be much more depressing for older men than widowhood is for older women. Older women appear to adapt to loss of a spouse more readily than do older men. Canadian researchers examined the relationship between psychological well-being and religiosity and spirituality of spouses (aged sixty-five to eighty-seven) who had been widowed or widowered from six months to two years. Widows were found to have better well-being than widowers. Religious and spiritual beliefs had a greater positive effect on the well-being of widows than on the well-being of widowers.

Researchers in Hong Kong found that the frequency of communication with and contact with family members and friends was positively related to the degree of life satisfaction (*see* Life Satisfaction) for widows. However, for widowers the degree of life satisfaction was unrelated to the frequency of interactions with other people. Apparently, maintaining a high level of interpersonal relationships is a more important goal for widows than it is for widowers.

There are more widows than widowers in the United States, partly because longevity is greater for women and partly because men aged sixty-five and older are less likely than a woman of the same age range to survive long after the death of a spouse (*see also* Survival after Death of a Spouse or Significant Other). Another contributing factor is the greater probability of remarriage by widowers (often with younger women) than by widows. Widows who either remarry or consider remarrying tend to be younger than those who do not. Few widowers remarry soon after their wives' deaths, but many of them do eventually remarry. Widowers are more likely to leave the home shared with their late spouses than are widows. Widowers are also nearly three times as likely as widows to relocate in another state entirely.

The first stage of widowhood or widowerhood is usually that of grief. Evidence indicates that grief persists for at least thirty months (and often longer) after the death of a spouse for most widows and many widowers. However, elderly men are more likely than elderly women to repress their emotional distress after the death of a spouse. Such distress may contribute to the earlier death after widowerhood for men than after widowhood for women. Researchers at the University of Southern California found that men who survive the initial eighteen months of widowerhood are likely to live the same life span they would have without the death of their spouse.

The resolution of grief or bereavement is generally viewed as depending on the coping strengths of the individual experiencing the bereavement as well as the nature of the social network available to that individual. Experts recommend accepting the reality of death, accepting the pain it yields, and beginning to adjust to life without the deceased. For more information about living with grief, contact Web sites http://www.aarp.org/griefandloss or http://www.compassionatefriends.org.

Gerontologists continue to debate whether grief is experienced more intensely by widows or by widowers. After six or so months, grief, and the loneliness that accompanies it, is typically followed by a reorganization of the widow's or widower's life. The reorganization requires a role transition from being a member of a husband-wife team to being on one's own. Most of the research by gerontologists has focused on the social networks of the widow or widower that may either aid or hinder the role transition. This research has revealed that a network of friends is of greater aid than is a network of family members. Research at Portland State University has provided information as to why this difference probably exists. Widows and widowers perceive friends to be more flexible in their relations with them than are family members. Family members are perceived as frequently placing unwanted commitments on the widow or widower (for example, frequent babysitting of grandchildren).

In general, elderly widows and widowers express lower life satisfaction than do elderly nonwidows and nonwidowers of the same age. Interestingly, however, widows and widowers tend to possess greater self-efficacy (*see* Self-Efficacy) than nonwidows and nonwidowers. Perhaps managing on one's own enhances their knowledge of their own capabilities, and it increases their self-confidence.

Bereaved widows and widowers are also likely to view their late spouses more positively and their marriage as having been more satisfactory than do nonbereaved elderly married people. The results of a survey of bereaved and nonbereaved older people in California indicated further that the more positive widows and widowers view their marriage in retrospective, the more likely they were to feel depressed. By contrast, the opposite was true for elderly people who were still married. That is, they were more likely to feel depressed when they viewed their ongoing marriage as being less satisfactory.

Widows who have remarried tend to express fewer concerns about financial matters, home maintenance, and so on than either widows who did not remarry or widows who considered remarriage but did not do so. Moreover, widows who remarry tend to report fewer concerns about these matters than they can recall having during the period after their first husband's death. By contrast, widows who consider remarriage (but do not remarry) tend to report, on average, more concerns than they had after their husband's death.

Of further interest is the possible difference between the bereavement experienced by elderly widows and widowers whose spouses died suddenly and unexpectedly and the bereavement experienced by elderly widows and widowers whose spouses died from natural causes and whose death was therefore largely expected. Surveys have indicated that the survivors of suicide and other sudden, unexpected deaths (for example, from an automobile accident) differed from survivors of natural deaths in the greater intensity of emotional distress. Widows and widowers of spouses who suffered from a lingering terminal illness tend to experience anticipatory grieving that accompanies the illness. Such anticipation of grief seems to ease their emotional strain after the spouse's death. Anticipatory grieving probably accounts for the fact that the depression and anxiety experienced six or so months after a spouse's death is less for elderly survivors than it is for young survivors.

Widowhood and widowerhood are commonly associated with declining health because they occur most often in late adulthood when health problems are often present. However, a decline in health after a spouse's death need not be inevitable. The deceased husband or wife may have been the one who encouraged his or her spouse to engage in health-promoting behaviors (for example, regular exercising). Some surviving spouses may have other sources of encouragement that prod health behaviors and help compensate for the loss of the spouse. Close relatives and friends need to encourage healthy behaviors in recently widowed or widowered relatives— and to encourage them to avoid health-risky behaviors. *See also* Divorce; Nutrition and Diet.

Winter Storms

Winter storms may place adults of all ages in a dangerous position. The potential hazard is likely to be especially great for older adults. There are a number of precautions they should take to avoid hypothermia (*see* Temperature Sensitivity) or a serious fall. If at all possible, they should stay indoors during the storm. If they do have to go out outdoors, they should wear several layers of lightweight clothing rather than a single heavy coat, and they should wear gloves or mittens, ear muffs, and a hat. They should cover their mouths to protect their lungs. They should walk very slowly on snowy or icy sidewalks. After the storm, if they must shovel snow, they should be very careful and take frequent breaks to avoid overexertion.

Wisdom

The definition of *wisdom* in a dictionary is likely to read something like "the ability to judge soundly and deal well with facts, especially as they relate to life and conduct." Wisdom does seem to be related to intelligence, especially to that form of intelligence known as crystallized intelligence (*see* Intelligence) in which life's experiences add to our accumulated knowledge. However, intelligence is usually used in reference to knowledge of words (vocabulary), knowledge about famous people ("Who wrote *Hamlet?*"), knowledge about famous events ("When did the Civil War begin?"), knowledge about geography ("What's the largest city in Ethiopia?"), and so on—the kind of knowledge we find being tested daily on such television shows as *Jeopardy*.

Wisdom means a different kind of knowledge but one, nevertheless, likely to accumulate with years of living. Researchers at the Max Planck Institute in Berlin have been vigorously conducting research on wisdom. As they define it, wisdom consists of an expert knowledge system dealing with the pragmatics of life, such as life planning and life management. They believe that not all elderly people excel in wisdom, relative to younger people, but they also believe that the percentage of older people who excel in wisdom is significantly greater than the percentage of younger people who excel.

Their research studies lend considerable support to their belief. Participants of various ages are given problems that deal with such topics as life planning and asked how the problem might be resolved. For example, in one of the problems the dilemma facing a sixty-year-old widow is described. She had recently received a business degree and had opened her own business, an activity very important to her. However, she heard that her son had been left with two small children in his care. What should she do—close her business and move in with her son to care for the children, or arrange for financial aid for her son to cover the cost of child care?

The quality of the solutions proposed has been found to be higher for older adults than for younger adults. Researchers in Australia discovered that the elderly women in their study who were superior at resolving such problems had an internal locus of control (*see* Control over Life's Events), relative to those elderly women who were less proficient in finding effective solutions. The researchers at the Max Planck Institute did find that the quality of solutions was slightly higher for young adults when the problem was one facing a young adult. Wisdom does seem to be a mental ability that increases with age, rather than declines (as is also true for the kinds of knowledge considered to be part of crystallized intelligence).

Wisdom seems to have three basic components or dimensions. The first is a cognitive dimension demanding understanding of the significance of an event and the deeper meaning of an event ("I always try to get to the heart of the matter"). The second is a reflective dimension enabling the wise person to look at events from many different perspectives ("I try to imagine how I would feel if I were in her place"). The third is an affective dimension calling for sympathy and compassion ("I feel protective of someone who is the underdog").

Women's Health Initiative

The Women's Health Initiative was a fifteen-year research study that began in 1991 to investigate the most common causes of death, disability, and poor quality of life in postmenopausal women, specifically cardiovascular disease, cancer, and osteoporosis. The study involved 161,808 generally healthy women who were past menopause. They ranged in age from fifty to seventy-nine at the time of their enrollment, with an average age of sixty-three years. The percentage of minority women was 17.5. A major part of the study was to evaluate the effects of estrogen-replacement therapy (hormone-replacement therapy) on heart disease, osteoporosis and fractures, and breast and colon cancers (*see* Breast Cancer; Colon Cancer; Estrogen Replacement Therapy [Hormone Replacement Therapy]; Fractures [Hip]; Osteoporosis). Another part of the study evaluated the purported benefits of a low-fat diet on women's health (*see* Nutrition and Diet).

Word Associations

For each of the following words, give the first word that comes to mind: *table, king, bread*. A fairly safe prediction is that the words you gave were *chair, queen,* and *butter*. These are examples of word associations. When *table, king,* and *bread* are given to a group of people, most of the members of the group will respond with *chair, queen,* and *butter*. The most popular, that is, the most frequently given, association to a given word is called the *primary associate*. *Table, king,* and *bread* are examples of words that have strong (highly probable) primary associates.

This is true regardless of the adult age level of the group members giving the associates. It is also true that most word associates are of a particular form known as a *paradigmatic associate*. This is again true for both younger and normally aging older adults. A paradigmatic associate is one that is of the same grammatical group or form as the word to which it is given (for example, both nouns, as in the case of *queen* to *king*). Paradigmatic associates may also usually replace each other in a sentence without a major change in the meaning of that sentence. For example, "The _____ sat on the throne"—either *king* or *queen* may fill the blank meaningfully. Not all words have strong primary associates. Consider the word *deep*. Associates are likely to include *shallow, dark,* and *water. Shallow* is the primary associate, but it is given by fewer than 20 percent of a group of adults, again regardless of the members' age level.

Incidentally, *water* as an associate is an example of what is called a *syntagmatic associate*. A syntagmatic associate is of a different grammatical class than the word to which it is associated (for instance, noun and adjective for *water* and *deep*), and they do not replace each other in a sentence. Both normally aging older adults and younger adults give relatively few syntagmatic associates. By contrast, children and patients with Alzheimer's disease give frequent syntagmatic associates.

The pronounced similarity of word associations among adults of different ages suggests that there is little change in the organization or structure of our mental dictionaries or lexicons with normal aging (*see* Lexicon). Another type of word association adds to our conviction that normal aging has little, if any, effect on the structure of the lexicon. Here, participants are given taxonomic categories, such as "a metal" and "a four-footed animal," and they are asked to name several instances or exemplars of each category. Categorical names are an important part of the organization of related words in our lexicons. Most people will respond with *iron, copper,* and *gold* when asked to name metals and *dog, cat,* and *horse* when asked to name four-footed animals. This is as true for normally aging elderly adults as it is for younger adults.

Work

Work consists of gainful employment in the workforce. It is to be distinguished from other productive but nonpaid work or activity such as volunteer work or family caregiver (*see* Activity [Productive]; Participation in Voluntary Organizations and Volunteer Work).

According to the U.S. Department of Labor, the percentage of men older than the age of sixty-five who participated in the labor force decreased from nearly 50 percent in 1950 to about 17 percent in 1991. On the other hand, from 1995 to 1997 workers in their fifties increased by 12 percent compared to an increase of 3.8 percent for workers of all ages combined. In fact, the percentage of workers who are age fifty-five and older is expected to increase to 36.8 percent in the year 2006 compared to 31.3 percent in the year 1998. The decline in the number of workers over age sixty-five is especially pronounced for blue-collar workers. Various surveys have indicated that they retire at a younger age than do white-collar workers, with the average for service workers falling between the two.

Although the decline has been less pronounced for women, a similar trend of decreasing work involvement with age is apparent. This means that the ratio of retired elderly people to employed younger people has been steadily increasing. The net effect has been to increase the tax burden on those in the labor force to finance programs directly relevant to elderly people (for example, Social Security and Medicare). Baby boomers are expected to be encouraged to work after age sixty-five, and 80 percent of those surveyed said they want to work after retirement.

According to the 2000 U.S. Census, 14 percent of people age sixty-five and older were in the civilian workforce. Among those working, women were less likely than men to work in executive, administrative, and managerial occupations (12 percent versus 19 percent), but more likely than men to work in administrative-support jobs (28 percent versus 6 percent).

In one large survey of men aged sixty-nine to eighty-four, about one in five had worked some time during the past year. The reasons given for working were good health and a strong dislike for retirement. Of those surveyed who were not working, very few indicated a desire to be working. The probability of employment was found to be related positively to educational level (the higher the level, the greater the likelihood of employment), negatively related to amount of income (the higher the income, the lower the likelihood of employment), and negatively related to age (the higher the age, the lower the likelihood of employment)

In a survey of people born between 1931 and 1941, researchers at Indiana University found that, regardless of race or sex, persons with a disability are less likely to work than persons without a disability, and when employed, disabled individuals worked for lower pay than the nondisabled. These conditions were especially acute for older minority men and women, and particularly for older disabled Hispanic women.

The trend toward fewer working older people has taken place even though the legal minimum mandatory retirement age increased from sixty-five to seventy in 1978 and has since been eliminated altogether for many workers. Why, then, are so many older people withdrawing from the labor force? One of the more frequent reasons people give for withdrawal is their health status. Men who report their health to be poor do retire an average of more than a year earlier than men who report their health to be at least good. However, it seems unlikely that poor health is the major reason for the decline of older people in the labor force. In general, the health status of older people has been increasing, not decreasing, over the past forty years. Many older people may cite declining health as the reason for their retirement because they believe it to be a more socially acceptable reason than the real reason (for example, wanting more leisure time).

A more important reason for retiring at age sixty-five (and often earlier) is the financial benefit often received for so doing. About 90 percent of retired people have at least some of their retirement income from Social Security. People who retire beyond age sixty-five are penalized in terms of their Social Security benefits relative to what they would receive if they had retired at age sixty-five or younger. The same is true for people receiving private pensions on retirement (about 35 percent of retirees do). That is, it is financially to their benefit to retire earlier than later.

Evidence regarding the relationship between age and job satisfaction is conflicting. In general, the evidence indicates either no relationship or a moderate increase in job satisfaction with age. Older workers do tend to perceive their jobs as having characteristics that more closely match their own needs than do younger workers. This is a likely reason that absenteeism from the job, both voluntary and involuntary, has been found to be related inversely to age. That is, older workers are absent less frequently than are younger workers. This seems to be true at least until workers approach some fixed retirement age. A study by researchers at the University of

Kansas Medical Center revealed that the closer male workers came to that age, the more burdensome those jobs became in terms of tension and fatigue experienced at work.

Interestingly, researchers at the National Institute of Mental Health discovered that the intellectual complexity of work over the years affects intellectual functioning. Over a twenty-year period they found that workers engaged in work that requires thought, independent judgment, and decision making tend to raise their level of mental functioning. This was found to be especially true for workers who were older at the start of the twenty-year period.

The Age Discrimination in Employment Act has existed since the late 1960s. However, it may be difficult to prove age discrimination (*see* Age Discrimination at Work). It is also difficult to avoid ageism (*see* Ageism) by employers in evaluating older employees. Some older employees may have job-related skills that show moderate declines with normal aging. However, increasing experience on the job may often lead to the acquisition of compensatory skills (*see* Expertise) that are overlooked by employers. Employers need to have a better understanding of normal aging and the fact that age changes do not necessarily result in major negative behavioral consequences. Future generations of older employees may have little difficulty with age discrimination given the likelihood that they are aging more successfully than earlier generations. That is, they may be avoiding many negative effects of aging by having lived a healthier lifestyle. Of course, members of future generations may be retiring at a much younger age than those of the present generation.

If you need help on a work issue you believe involves age discrimination, call the Equal Employment Opportunity Commission in Washington, D.C. (800-669-4000), to connect with one of its fifty field offices. An alternative is to contact AARP Foundation Litigation Unit, Building A-4, 601 E Street Northwest, Washington, DC 20049 (Web site is http://www.aarp.org). *See also* entries on Retirement.

Working Memory

Memory researchers believe that a very important part of the human memory system is a component they call *working memory.* Working memory functions like a "mental box" that is divided into two parts. The first part is a store for holding prior information briefly (*see* Short-Term Memory); the second part is a place for performing various mental operations. Consider what you are doing when you add the numbers nine, five, and seven. The first two numbers are summed to give fourteen. This information is held in the store component of working memory while you identify the next number and add it to give twenty-one (this is accomplished with the operations component). The operations component is especially important for long-term memory. It is here that new information is encoded and placed in the long-term store, and it is also here where a memory search is conducted to recall or recognize information previously placed in the long-term store.

Working memory is believed to have a limited capacity for the storage of prior information and for conducting such mental operations as encoding new information for memorization. Most researchers of memory aging believe that the capacity of working memory diminishes during the course of the adult life span, becoming moderately less in late adulthood than in early adulthood. Whether capacity diminishes with aging only for storage or only for conducting mental operations, or for both, is not fully understood. However, the evidence to date suggests that on average storage capacity decreases only slightly, and the operations capacity decreases somewhat more.

Working memory's overall capacity is usually determined by measuring a participant's reading span. The participant is first given a sentence that must be answered true or false, while at the same time remembering the last word in the sentence. For example, consider "Beaches are often found by an ocean" as the sentence. "True" is the correct answer, and *ocean* is the word to be remembered. If the last word is remembered correctly, the participant is then given two consecutive sentences, each to be answered true or false, and each to have its last word remembered. For example, the participants may read the sentences "Cats are members of the canine family" and "A rose is a flower found in many gardens." The sentences are answered "false" and "true" respectively, and *family* and *gardens* are the words to be remembered. If both last words are remembered correctly, then the participant receives three consecutive sentences, with three last words to be remembered.

This procedure continues until the number of sentences in the series is too large to permit memory of all of the last words. The largest number of sentences that can be spanned without a memory error defines the participant's reading span. The reading span of elderly participants has been found to average about one sentence less than that of young adult participants, presumably reflecting the decrease in working memory's capacity with aging.

Individual differences among elderly participants in their reading spans have been found to be related to their scores on various memory tasks, such as the recall of a story's content. Older participants with greater span scores (and presumably greater working-memory capacities) are more proficient memorizers than elderly participants with smaller span scores (and presumably smaller working-memory capacities).

A decline in working memory's capacity is not necessarily an inevitable consequence of normal aging. There is evidence to indicate that working memory is one of the abilities that is positively affected by long-term regular physical exercise (*see* Exercise [Relationship to Physical/Mental Performances]). Elderly people who have been regular exercisers for years tend to have larger reading span scores than elderly people who have had less active physical lives. The extent to which highly active mental lives may slow any age-related declines in working memory's capacity is unknown, but is probably equally substantial.

Worries

A survey of adults age sixty-five and older revealed that the most frequently expressed worry (reported by 56 percent of those surveyed) is over our country's social problems. Worries about their own aches and pains were expressed by nearly half of those surveyed (43 percent).

Worst Things about Getting Old

What is the worst thing about getting to be old? This question was asked of people age sixty-five and older in a study called *Images of Aging in America.* The most frequent response (given by 32 percent of those surveyed) was health problems. Others responded with such concerns as being close to death (12 percent) and dependency on others (5 percent).

What are the main concerns younger Americans have about growing old? A survey by *Parade* magazine and ResearchAmerica of a cross section of one thousand young adult Americans provides an answer to this question. The main concern about growing old (expressed by 37 percent) was declining health. The second greatest concern (expressed by 29 percent) was financial problems. More than 60 percent expressed some fear of losing their mental ability as compared to only 29 percent who feared their physical ability would diminish. More than 83 percent stated that they are doing activities to help them stay healthy as they age.

Index of Entries and Cross-References

AAMI. *See* Age-associated memory impairment

AARP, 1. *See also* Accidents (automobile); Alcoholism (incidence and causes); Computers; Drivers (improving their skills); Elderhostel; Magazine reading; Participation in voluntary organizations and volunteer work

Abdominal aortic aneurysm. *See* Cardiovascular diseases

Abilities (Physical and Mental) and Activity, 1-3. *See also* Activity (mental) and mental performance; Exercise (relationship to physical/mental performances); Expertise; Motor skill learning; Reading and Reading skills; Verbal ability; Wechsler Intelligence Tests

Abnormal Aging, 3. *See also* Senile dementia

Absenteeism. *See* Work

Absent mindedness. *See* Prospective memory

Abuse. *See* Elder abuse

Accidents (airplane). *See* Accidents (automobile); Functional age

Accidents (at Home), 3

Accidents (at Work), 3

Accidents (Automobile), 4-7. *See also* Alzheimer's disease; Drivers (improving their skills); Handedness

ACE inhibitors. *See* Blood pressure (high and low)

Acetaminophen. *See* Arthritis; Pain medications (analgesics)

Acetylcholine. *See* Alzheimer's disease; Brain and aging; Senile dementia

Acid reflux. *See* Aspirin; Esophageal cancer

Action Memory, 7-9

Activities of Daily Living, 9-11. *See also* Alzheimer's disease; Centenarians; Diabetes; Disability (assistance with activities of daily living); Disability (incidence and assistance); Fractures (hip); Locomotion; Mini-Mental State Exam; Participant selection for research studies; Well-being (psychological)

Activity Diversity (Cognitive Benefits), 11

Activity (Mental) and Mental Performance, 11-13. *See also* Disuse principle; Plasticity theory

Activity (Physical), 13. *See also* Slowing-down principle

Activity (Productive), 13-14

Activity Theory, 14-15

Actonel. *See* Osteoporosis

Acupuncture, 15. *See also* Sleep therapy

Acute respiratory syndrome. *See* Chronic respiratory diseases

Adapting a Home for Elderly Residents, 16. *See also* Computerized homes; Falls

Adapting to Fading Eyesight, 16. *See also* Visual disorders (coping with macular degeneration)

Adrenalin. *See* Arousal

Adult Day Care Centers, 16-17. *See also* Respite care

Advance Directives, 17-18. *See also* Euthanasia

Advance organizers. *See* Reading and reading skills

Advertising. *See* Consumers of merchandise in stores

Advice. *See* Unsolicited support and advice

Aftereffects (Visual), 18-19. *See also*

Stimulus persistence
Age-Associated Memory Impairment, 19–20
Age Change versus Age Difference, 20–21. *See also* Cross-sectional method; Longitudinal method; Sequential method
Age (different definitions). *See* Biological age; Functional age; Old (defining late adulthood); Subjective age
Age Discrimination at Work, 22. *See also* Work
Age Discrimination in Employment Act. *See* Age discrimination at work; Old (defining late adulthood); Work
Ageism, 22–24. *See also* Ageism exists in some words; Myths about aging
Ageism Exists in Some Words, 24
Age Simulation, 24–25
Age spots in the skin. *See* Body build and body characteristics
Agitative Behaviors by Nursing Home Residents, 25. *See also* Alzheimer's disease
Agnosia. *See* Multi-infarct dementia
AIDS (Acquired Immunodeficiency Syndrome), 26
Alcoholics Anonymous. *See* Alcoholism (treatment)
Alcoholism (Incidence and Causes), 26–27. *See also* Stress and coping with stress
Alcoholism (Treatment), 27. *See also* Psychotherapy
Alcohol (Physical and Mental Effects), 27–29
Alendronate. *See* Osteoporosis
Alexander technique. *See* Posture
Allergies, 29
Alpha-beta blockers. *See* Blood pressure (high and low)
Alpha blockers. *See* Blood pressure (high and low)
Alternative Medical Treatments, 29. *See also* Acupuncture
Alternatives to living with an adult child or in a nursing home. *See* Assisted living facilities; Home care
Altruism (Adult Age Differences) 29–30. *See* also Altruism (health benefits for seniors)
Altruism (Health Benefits for Seniors), 29–30. *See also* Altruism (Adult Age Differences)
Aluminum. *See* Alzheimer's disease
Alzheimer's Association, 31
Alzheimer's Disease, 31–37. *See also* Abnormal aging; Age associated memory impairment; Alcohol (physical and mental effects); Bathing; Brain and aging; Caregiving (type of mentally impaired patient); Depression (incidence, symptoms, causes); Falls; False memory; Lexicon; Motion perception; Senile dementia; Sleep disorders; Smoking; Socially inappropriate behavior; Urinary incontinence; Wandering; Word associations
Amantadine. *See* Influenza
Ambien. *See* Sleep disorders
Amnesia. *See* Alcohol (physical and mental effects); Forgetting
Amyloid beta-protein. *See* Alzheimer's disease
Anagram Solving, 37
Analgesics. *See* Pain medications (analgesics)
Androgyny, 37–38. *See also* Gender and sex differences in aging
Anemia, 38–39. *See also* Angiodysplasia; Stomach cancer; Syncope
Aneurysm. *See* Cardiovascular diseases
Angina. *See* Cardiovascular diseases
Angiodysplasia, 39. *See also* Anemia
Angiogenesis inhibitors. *See* Cervical cancer
Angioplasty. *See* Cardiovascular diseases; Peripheral arterial disease and claudication
Anorexia nervosa. *See* Neurosis
Antiaging Products—Do They Really Work? 39. *See also* Antioxidants; Growth hormone (physical effects)
Antibodies. *See* Why aging? (biological theories of aging)
Antidiuretic hormone. *See* Urination
Anti-inflammatory drugs. *See* Alzheimer's disease; Arthritis; Cardiovascular diseases
Antioxidants, 39–40. *See also* Chocolate; Prostate cancer; Why aging? (biological theories of aging)
Anus. *See* Bowels
Anxiety, 40–41. *See also* Alzheimer's

disease; Neurosis; Posttraumatic stress disorder
APDE-4. *See* Alzheimer's disease
Aphasia, 41. *See also* Stroke
Apnea. *See* Sleep disorders
Apraxia. *See* Stroke
Aprotinin. *See* Cardiovascular diseases
Arcus senilis. *See* Visual disorders
ARDS. *See* Chronic respiratory diseases
Area Agencies on Aging. *See* Food and meal services
Arimidex. *See* Breast cancer
Arithmetic Ability, 41–42
Arixtra. *See* Cardiovascular diseases
Army Alpha and Army Beta Intelligence Tests, 42–43
Aromasin. *See* Breast cancer
Arousal, 43–44
Arteriosclerosis. *See* Cardiovascular diseases.
Arthritis, 44–47. *See also* Activities of daily living; Acupuncture; Alzheimer's disease; Leisure activities
Aspirin, 47. *See also* Arthritis; Cardiovascular diseases; Hearing; Pain medications (analgesics); Stroke
Assertiveness. *See* Personality traits
Asset Health Dynamics among the Oldest Old (AHEAD), 47–48
Assisted Living Facilities, 48. *See also* Home care; Nursing home admissions
Assistive Devices, 49. *See also* Canes and crutches; Wheelchairs
Asthma, 49–50
Atherosclerosis. *See* Cardiovascular diseases
Athlete's foot. *See* Foot problems
Atrial fibrillation. *See* Stroke
Attention and Stroke Recovery, 50
Attention (Overview), 50–51. *See also* Attention and stroke recovery; Divided attention; Selective attention; Vigilance
Attitudes (Political and Social), 51–52. *See also* Cohort (generational) effect; Humor; Rigidity
Attribution, 52–53. *See also* Work
Autobiographical Memory, 53–54
Automaticity of memory. *See* Episodic memory
Automatic Teller Machines (ATMs), 54. *See also* Scams

Automobile driving. *See* Accidents (automobile); Dark adaptation; Drivers (having passengers); Drivers (improving their skills); Driving (activity after cessation or reduction; Driving (identifying cognitively unqualified drivers); Driving (why many seniors limit or quit driving)
Aversion therapy. *See* Psychotherapy
Avian flu. *See* Influenza

Baby Talk (Elderspeak), 55. *See also* Speech perception
Back Pain, 55. *See also* Activities of daily living
Bacterial pneumonia. *See* Pneumonia
Balance. *See* Dizziness; Falls; Locomotion
Balanced Budget Act of 1997. *See* Medicare
Balance Impairment and Cognitive Demand, 55–56. *See also* Falls, Locomotion
Baldness. *See* Facial appearance
Baltimore Longitudinal Study. *See* Cornell Medical Index; National Institute on Aging
Barium enema X-ray examination. *See* Colon cancer
Barriers to Health in Older Men, 56. *See also* Longevity
Basal cell cancer. *See* Skin cancer
Basal ganglia. *See* Brain and aging
Basal metabolic rate. *See* Body build and body characteristics
Bathing, 56–57. *See also* Bruises
Bean sprouts. *See* Alzheimer's disease
Beck Depression Inventory. *See* Depression (diagnostic tests)
Bed Rest, 57
Bed Sores, 57–58
Beer. *See* Alcohol (physical and mental effects)
Behavior modification. *See* Classical conditioning; Operant conditioning; Psychotherapy; Psychotherapy with nursing home residents; Sleep therapy; Smoking
Beliefs about Aging Affect Physical Health, 58
Benign paroxysmal vertigo. *See* Dizziness
Benign prostate hyperplasia. *See* Prostate gland

Benign senescent forgetfulness. *See* Age associated memory impairment

Benzodiazepine. *See* Sleep disorders

Bereavement. *See* Widowhood and widowerhood

Beta amyloid. *See* Alzheimer's disease

Beta blockers. *See* Cardiovascular diseases

Beta-carotene. *See* Antioxidants; Visual disorder

Bifocals, 58

Biliary dyskinesis. *See* Gall bladder diseases

Bingo, 59

Biofeedback. *See* Pain management; Psychotherapy; Urinary incontinence

Biological Age, 59

Biological clock. *See* Why aging? (Biological theories of aging)

Biology of aging. *See* Brain and aging; Old (defining late adulthood); Physiological functions; Why aging? (Biological theories of aging)

Biopsy. *See* Skin cancer

Bipolar psychosis. *See* Psychosis

Bird flu. *See* Influenza

Bisphosphonates. *See* Paget's disease

Bladder Cancer, 59–60

Bladder control and urination. *See* Physiological functions; Urinary incontinence; Urination

Bladder (Overactive), 60

Blessed Mental Status Test, 60

Blister. *See* Foot problems

Blood Pressure (High and Low), 60–61. *See also* Cardiovascular disease and mental performance; Cardiovascular diseases; Hypertension; Loneliness; Postural change and orthostasis; Sleep disorders; Stroke

Body Build and Body Characteristics, 61–63

Body Mass Index, 63

Body Odor, 63

Bone loss. *See* Osteoporosis; Paget's disease

Boredom, 63–64

Bowel incontinence. *See* Bowels

Bowels, 64–65

Brain and Aging, 65–69. *See also* Alzheimer's disease; Plasticity theory

Brain aneurysm. *See* Cardiovascular diseases

BRCAT. *See* Breast cancer

Breast Cancer, 69–71. *See also* Cancer (general information); Estrogen-replacement therapy (Hormone replacement therapy); Nutrition and diet; Osteoporosis

Breasts. *See* Body build and body characteristics; Breast cancer

Breathing capacity. *See* Old (defining late adulthood); Physiological functions

Bridge. *See* Activity (mental) and mental performance; Expertise

Brimonidine Tartrate. *See* Visual disorders

Broca's area of the brain. *See* Aphasia

Bronchial pneumonia. *See* Pneumonia

Bruises, 72

Bunions. *See* Foot problems

Bypass surgery. *See* Cardiovascular diseases

Cabbage. *See* Breast cancer

Calcium channel blockers. *See* Blood pressure (high and low)

Calcium citrate. *See* Osteoporosis

Calcium oxalate. *See* Physiological functions

Canada Fitness Study. *See* Strength and stamina

Cancer (General Information), 73–74. *See also* Alcohol (physical and mental effects); Health risk behaviors; Why aging? (biological theories of aging)

Canes and Crutches, 74. *See also* Assistive devices

Canine Ambassador Program. *See* Pet therapy

Cantaloupe. *See* Osteoporosis

Carbon Monoxide Poisoning, 74

Carboplatin. *See* Testicular cancer

Cardiac arrest. *See* Cardiovascular diseases

Cardiac cath. *See* Cardiovascular diseases

Cardiopulmonary resuscitation (CPR). *See* Cardiovascular diseases

Cardiovascular Disease and Mental Performance, 74–75

Cardiovascular Diseases, 75–81. *See also* Blood pressure (high and low); Cardiovascular diseases (psychological interventions); Cholesterol; Defibrillators; Growth hormone (physical effects); Hostility; Longitudinal studies of aging's effects on health and cognition; Stroke; Syncope; Teeth, gums, and mouth

Cardiovascular Diseases (Psychological Interventions), 81

Cardura. *See* Prostate gland

Caregivers (Early Adulthood), 81

Caregivers (Elderly Parents), 81–82

Caregivers (Family and Friends), 82–85. *See also* Caregivers (hassles in administering medications); Caregivers (how African American and white caregivers differ); Participation in voluntary organization and volunteer work; Racial and ethnic differences in aging; Respite care; Sleep complaints; Stress and coping with stress

Caregivers (Hassles in Administering Medications), 86

Caregivers (How African American and White Caregivers Differ), 86

Caregivers (Long Distance), 86

Caregivers (Negative Reactions of Recipients of Care), 86–87

Caregivers (Paid Workers), 87

Caregivers (Positive Effects of Caregiving), 87–88

Caregivers (Secondary), 88

Caregiving (Type of Mentally Impaired Patient), 88

Carotid artery. *See* Stroke

Carrots, 88

Cataracts. *See* Accidents (automobile); Visual disorders

Catechins. *See* Chocolate

Categorical instances. *See* Word associations

CAT scans. *See* Alzheimer's disease; Brain and aging

Causes of Death, 89

Cautiousness, 89. *See also* Recognition memory versus recall memory; Verbal learning

Cellular aging. *See* Why aging? (biological theories of aging)

Centenarians, 90. *See also* Longevity (what determines a long life?); Surgery survival

Center for Epidemiological Studies Depression Scale. *See* Depression (Diagnostic tests)

Centers for Disease Control and Prevention. *See* Arthritis

Cerebellum. *See* Brain and aging; Classical conditioning

Cerebral anemia. *See* Syncope

Cerebral arteriosclerosis. *See* Multi-infarct dementia

Cerebral cortex. *See* Alzheimer's disease; Brain and aging

Cerebral hemispheres. *See* Brain and aging; Divided attention

Cervical Cancer, 90–91

Chess. *See* Expertise

Chicken Pox. *See* Shingles

Children View Aging Negatively, 91–92

Chocolate, 92

Cholesterol, 92–93. *See also* Cardiovascular diseases; Nutrition and diet

Chronic bronchitis. *See* Chronic respiratory diseases

Chronic fatigue syndrome. *See* Fatigue (clinical syndrome)

Chronic pain. *See* Pain (chronic); Pain management

Chronic obstructive pulmonary disease, See Chronic respiratory diseases

Chronic Respiratory Diseases, 93–94

Chunking in memory. *See* Expertise; Short-term memory

Cisplatin. *See* Hearing

Classical Conditioning, 94–96. *See also* Psychotherapy

Claudication. *See* Peripheral arterial disease and claudication

Clergy (What Do They Know about Aging), 96

Clinical Dementia Rating Scale, 97

Clinical Psychology, 97

Clinical trials. *See* Drug tests (clinical trials)

Clock Drawing Test, 97–98

Coalition of Advocates for the Rights of the Infirm (CARIE). *See* Elder abuse

Codeine. *See* Pain medications (analgesics)

Coffee, 98

Cognitive Impairment (Incidence), 98

Cognitive (Mental) Stages of Development, 98–99

Cognitive therapy. *See* Psychotherapy: Sleep therapy

Cohort (Generational) Effect, 99–100. *See also* Attitudes (political and social);

Cross-sectional method; Longitudinal method; Personality traits

Collagen. *See* Body build and body characteristics; Facial appearance

College Investments, 100–101

Colon Cancer, 101–2

Colonoscopy. *See* Colon cancer

Color Perception, 102–3

Common Cold, 103

Compensatory model. *See* Stress and coping with stress

Complaints about memory. *See* Memory Complaints

Complex vigilance. *See* Vigilance

Compliance with medications. *See* Medication compliance and comprehension

Computed Axial Tomography (CAT) scans. *See* Alzheimer's disease; Brain and aging

Computerized Homes, 103

Computer programming. *See* Motor skill learning

Computers, 104. *See also* Internet, Internet (differences between users and nonusers), Motor skill learning

Concept Learning, 104–5

Conformity, 105–6

Congestive heart failure. *See* Cardiovascular diseases

Conservatism. *See* Attitudes (political and social); Cohort (generational) effects; Family values and traditionalism; Humor

Constancies of Perception, 106–7

Constipation. *See* Bowels; Physiological functions

Constrain-induced movement. *See* Stroke

Consumer Directive Care for Disabled Elders, 107–8

Consumer Fraud, 108. *See also* Scams

Consumers of Merchandise in Stores, 108

Contextualism. *See* Why aging? (Psychological theories of aging)

Continuity versus Discontinuity in Adult Development, 109

Control over Life's Events, 110–11. *See also* Retirement (adjustment to); Wisdom

Convergent versus divergent thinking. *See* Originality

Conversation Memory, 111–12

Coping behavior. *See* Stress and coping with stress

Coping with Frailty, 112

Copper. *See* Visual disorders

Cornell Medical Index, 112–13

Corns and calluses. *See* Foot problems

Cough. *See* Common cold

Coumadin. *See* Stroke

Countercontrol method. *See* Sleep therapy

COX-2 inhibitors. *See* Arthritis; Pain medications (analgesics)

Cranberries. *See* Urination

Creativity, 113–15. *See also* Originality

Cremation, 115

Crestor. *See* Cholesterol

Creutzfeldt-Jakob disease. *See* Senile dementia

Crime Prevention, 115–16

Crimes (Victim of and Fear of), 116

Crossover effect in mortality. *See* Racial and ethnic differences in aging

Cross-sectional Method, 116–18

Crystallized intelligence. *See* Intelligence; Wechsler Intelligence Tests

Cultural Differences in Memory, 118–19

Curiosity, 119

Daily Help, 120

Dancing, 120

Dark Adaptation, 120–21

Daydreaming, 121–22. *See also* Boredom

DBS (deep brain stimulation). *See* Parkinson's disease

Death and Dying, 122–24. *See also* Personality and mortality; Stress and coping with stress; Widowhood and widowerhood

Decision-making, 124. *See also* Accidents (automobile); Advance directives; Cancer (general information); Cautiousness; Expertise; Managerial ability; Stress and coping with stress; Work

Deep sleep. *See* Sleep

Defibrillators, 124

Deja vu. *See* Implicit memory

Delayed Rewards, 124–25

Delirium, 125

Delta waves. *See* Sleep

Dementia. *See* Alzheimer's disease; Multi-infarct dementia; Parkinson's disease;

Senile dementia

Demerol. *See* Pain medications (analgesics)

Demography of Aging, 125–27

Dentures. *See* Teeth, gums, and mouth

Depression (Diagnostic Tests), 127–28

Depression (Incidence, Symptoms, Causes), 128–30. *See also* Alzheimer's disease; Caregivers (family and friends); Death and dying; Learned helplessness; Pessimism about your physical health and depression; Religion in later life; Retirement (adjustment to); Sibling relationships; Widowhood and widowerhood

Depression (nonclinical). *See* Depression (performances with)

Depression (Performances with), 130. *See also* Activity (productive); Memory training

Depression (Prognosis), 130

Depression (Treatment), 131–32. *See also* Psychotherapy; Reminiscence

Depth Perception, 132–33

Deteriorating Neighborhoods, 133

Detrol. *See* Bladder (overactive)

Diabetes, 133–34. *See also* Alzheimer's disease; Health status and mental performance; Stroke; Teeth, gums, and mouth; Visual disorders

Diabetic retinopathy. *See* Visual disorders

Dialecticism. *See* Why aging? (Psychological theories of aging)

Dialysis. *See* End state renal disease

Diary Keeping, 134

Diary Studies of Memory Failures, 134–35. *See also* Everyday memory

Diastolic blood pressure. *See* Blood pressure (high and low)

Dichotic listening. *See* Divided attention

Digitalis. *See* Cardiovascular diseases

Digestion. *See* Physiological functions

Digital tonometer. *See* Visual disorders

Digit span. *See* Memory span

Digoxin. *See* Cardiovascular diseases

Dipyridamole. *See* Medications

Disability (Adaptation), 135

Disability (Assistance with Activities of Daily Living), 135–36

Disability (Educational Level), 136

Disability (Effect of Social Support), 136. *See also* Obesity (effects on longevity and disability)

Disability (Incidence and Assistance), 136–37. *See also* Accidents (at home); Religion in later life; Walkers; Wheel chairs

Disability (Psychological and Social Consequences), 137–38. *See also* Activities of daily living; Depression (incidence, symptoms, causes); Religion in later life; Retirement communities; Work

Discourse Memory, 138–39. *See also* Continuity versus discontinuity in adult development

Diseases (Acute and Chronic), 139–40

Disengagement Theory, 140. *See also* Activity theory

Distance perception. *See* Depth perception

Disuse Principle, 141–42. *See also* Activity (mental) and mental performance

Diuresis. *See* Nocturia

Diuretics. *See* Blood pressure (high and low); Cardiovascular diseases; Hearing; Heat stroke; Postural change and orthostasis

Diverticulitis, 142. *See also* Physiological functions

Divided Attention, 142–43. *See also* Attention and stroke recovery; Attention (overview); Bingo

Divorce, 144–45. *See also* Longevity; Marriage and marital satisfaction; Norms; Parenthood in later Life; Stress and coping with stress

Dizziness, 145–46. *See also* Falls; Postural change and orthostasis; Syncope

DNA. *See* Why aging? (biological theories of aging)

Domestic violence. *See* Elder abuse

Dopamine. *See* Brain and aging; Parkinson's disease

Double jeopardy hypothesis. *See* Racial and ethnic differences in aging

Dreaming. *See* Nightmares; Sleep

Drinking problems. *See* Alcoholism; Alcohol (physical and mental effects)

Drivers (Having Passengers), 146

Drivers (Improving Their Skills), 146. *See also* Accidents (automobile)

Driver's License Renewal, 146–47

Driving. *See* Accidents (automobile); Dark

adaptation; Drivers (having passengers); Drivers (improving their skills); Driving (activity after cessation or reduction); Driving (identifying cognitively unqualified drivers); Driving (why seniors limit or quit driving)

Driving (Activity after Cessation or Reduction), 147

Driving (Identifying Cognitively Unqualified Drivers), 148

Driving (Why Many Seniors Limit or Quit Driving), 148–49

Drug Abuse, 149

Drug Tests (Clinical Trials), 149–50

Dry mouth. See Teeth, gums, and mouth

Durable power of attorney. See Advance directives

Dynamic acuity. See Vision

Dysarthria. See Voice

Dyspareunia. See Menopause and ovulation

Dysphagia. See Swallowing

Dyspnea. See Physiological functions

Dysrhythmia. See Cardiovascular diseases

Echocardiography. See Stroke

Echoic memory. See Sensory memory

Ecological Validity, 151. See also Everyday memory; Reasoning

Educational Level, 151–53. See also Alzheimer's disease; Sexual behavior (heterosexual); Wechsler Intelligence Tests

EKG. See Cardiovascular disease

Elder Abuse, 153–55

Elderhostel, 155–56

Elderspeak. See Baby talk (elderspeak)

Electroconvulsive therapy (ECT). See Depression (treatment)

Embolus. See Cardiovascular diseases

Emotional intelligence. See Emotions

Emotion-focused coping. See Stress and coping with stress

Emotions, 156–58. See also Caregivers (positive effects of caregiving); Depression (incidence, symptoms, causes); Divorce; Emotions and memory, Friendships; Well-being (psychological)

Emotions and Memory, 158

Emphysema. See Chronic respiratory diseases

Empty nest. See Parenthood in later life

Enbrel. See Arthritis

Endentulous. See Teeth, gums, and mouth

Endometrial hyperplasia. See Uterine cancer

Endovascular repair therapy. See Cardiovascular diseases

End-State Renal Disease, 158–59

Enlighten model. See Stress and coping with stress

Entitlements, 159–60. See also Medicare

Environmental Press, 160. See also Residence

Epinephrine. See Arousal

Episodic Memory, 161–63

Equity theory. See Friendships

Esophageal Cancer, 163

Essential hypertension. See Hypertension

Estate Taxes, 163

Estrogen. See Estrogen replacement therapy (Hormone replacement therapy)

Estrogen Replacement Therapy (Hormone Replacement Therapy), 164. See also Alzheimer's disease; Breast cancer; Cardiovascular diseases; Cholesterol; Colon cancer; Gallbladder diseases; Osteoporosis; Stroke; Uterine cancer

Euthanasia, 164–65

Event based prospective memory. See Prospective memory

Everyday Memory, 165–66. See also Diary studies of memory failures

Evista. See Breast cancer; Osteoporosis

Excessive heat or cold. See Temperature sensitivity

Exelon. See Depression (Treatment)

Exercise and depression. See Depression (treatment)

Exercise and nursing home residents. See Exercise (relationship to physical/mental performances)

Exercise (Relationship to Physical/Mental Performances), 167–69. See also Abilities (physical and mental) and activity; Activity (physical); Bingo; Brain and aging; Depression (performances with); Diabetes; Falls; Health risk behaviors; Self-efficacy; Walking; Working memory

Exercise Capacity, 166–67

Exercise Types, 169–70. *See also* Walking
Expertise, 171–72
Explicit memory. *See* Implicit memory
Extended family. *See* Parenthood in later life
Extroversion. *See* Personality traits
Eyewitness Testimony, 173

Face Memory, 174. *See also* Eyewitness testimony
Facial Appearance, 174–75. *See also* Hiding your age
Facts of Aging Quiz, 175–76
Fad diets. *See* Nutrition and diet
Fainting. *See* Postural change and orthostasis; Syncope
Falls, 176–79. *See also* Dizziness; Foot problems; Fractures (hip); Locomotion
False Memory, 179–80. *See also* Recognition memory versus recall memory; Selective control of memory
Family therapy. *See* Psychotherapy
Family values and Traditionalism, 180
Famvir. *See* Shingles
Fatigue and Mental Performance, 180
Fatigue (Clinical Syndrome), 180
Fatigue (Physical), 181. *See also* Computers
Fear of dying. *See* Death and dying
Fear of falls. *See* Falls
Femara. *See* Breast cancer
Fibrillation. *See* Cardiovascular diseases
Fibroids. *See* Uterine cancer
Fibromyalgia. *See* Arthritis
Field dependence—field independence. *See* Personality style
Field of vision. *See* Accidents (automobile); Vision
Finger Movements and Exercise, 181
Finger pinch. *See* Finger movements and exercise
Fire, 181
Five-fluorouracil. *See* Colon cancer
Flashbulb memories. *See* Source memory
Flavanols. *See* Chocolate
Flaxseed, 182
Flexible sigmoidoscopy. *See* Colon cancer
Floaters in the eye. *See* Visual disorders
Flomax. *See* Prostate gland
Fluid Intake, 182. *See also* Bladder cancer; Fluid intake (cold weather); Fluid intake (differences between younger and older adults)
Fluid Intake (Cold Weather), 183
Fluid Intake (Differences between Younger and Older Adults), 183
Fluid intelligence. *See* Intelligence; Primary Mental Abilities (PMA) Test; Wechsler Intelligence Tests
Food and Meal Services, 183–84
Food identifications. *See* Taste
Food stamps. *See* Food and meal services
Foot problems, 184–85. *See also* Accidents (automobile)
Forgetting, 185–87
Form Perception, 187–88
Fosamax. *See* Paget's disease
Foster Grandparent Program, 189
Fovea. *See* Visual disorders
Fox, Michael J. *See* Parkinson's disease
Fractures (Hip), 189–90. *See also* Falls; Osteoporosis
Frailty as a Clinical Syndrome, 190. *See also* Falls; Frailty (identifying degrees); Frailty incidence and causes); Nutrition and diet; Slowing-down principle
Frailty (Identifying Degrees), 190–91
Frailty (Incidence and Causes), 191
Framingham Study of Heart Disease. *See* Longitudinal studies of aging's effects on health and cognition
Free radicals. *See* Why aging? (biological theories of aging)
French paradox. *See* Antioxidants; Portion size and heart health
Frequency-of-Occurrence Memory, 191–92. *See also* Episodic memory
Friendships, 192–93. *See also* Loneliness; Successful aging
Frontal lobe deficit. *See* Brain and aging; Frontal lobe functioning (improving it in dementia), Source memory
Frontal Lobe Functioning (Improving It in Dementia), 193
Frontal lobes. *See* Brain and aging
Functional Age, 193–94
Functional reasoning. *See* Reasoning
Functional status. *See* Self-rated functioning
Funerals, 195

Gait. *See* Falls; Locomotion

Gallbladder Diseases, 196
Gallstones. *See* Gallbladder diseases
Gamblers (Differences between Younger and Older Gamblers), 196–97
Gamma-aminobutyric acid. *See* Brain and aging
Gamma secretase. *See* Alzheimer's disease
Gardasil. *See* Cervical cancer
Gardening. *See* Leisure activities; Osteoporosis
Garlic, 197
Gender and Sex Differences in Aging, 197–98. *See also* Accidents (automobile); Activities of daily living; Activity (productive); Alcoholism (incidence and causes); Alzheimer's disease; Androgyny; Barriers to health in older men; Bladder cancer; Bladder (Overactive); Caregivers (family and friends); Control over life's events; Crime prevention; Crimes (victim of and fear of); Disability (incidence and assistance); Disability (psychological and social consequences); Divorce; Elder abuse; Emotions; Facial appearance; Falls; Food and meal services; Friendships; Generativity; Grandparenting; Hearing; Health promotion programs; Health status and mental performance; Hiding your age; Homeless older people; Humor; Life Expectancy; Longevity; Longitudinal studies of aging's effects on health and cognition; Magazine reading; Marriage and marital satisfaction; Motion perception; Multi-infarct dementia; Nutrition and diet; Osteoporosis; Participation in voluntary organizations and volunteer work; Religion in later life; Self-esteem; Senior centers; Sex differences and scientific ability; Sexual behavior (heterosexual); Sleep complaints; Sleep disorders; Smell; Stomach cancer; Strength and stamina; Stroke; Survival after death of a spouse or significant other; Temperature sensitivity; Tuberculosis; Urinary incontinence; Visual disorders; Well-being (psychological); Widowhood and widowerhood
General Well-Being Schedule. *See* Well-being (psychological)
Generativity, 199. *See also* Personality stages
Geriatric Depression Scale, 199. *See also* Depression (diagnostic tests)
Geriatrics, 199
Gerontological psychology. *See* Gerontology
Gerontology, 200
Ginkgo, 200. *See also* Alzheimer's disease
Glare. *See* Accidents (automobile); Vision; Visual disorders
Glaucoma. *See* Visual disorders
Glucosamine chondroitin. *See* Arthritis
Goals, 200–201. *See also* Marriage and marital satisfaction
Goldmann tonometer. *See* Visual disorders
Gout. *See* Arthritis
Grandparenting, 201–3. *See also* Consumers of merchandise in stores
Grandparents Raising Their Own Grandchildren, 203–4
Grapefruit. *See* Cholesterol
Grape Juice, 204. *See also* Cardiovascular diseases
Graying hair. *See* Facial appearance
Grief. *See* Widowhood and widowerhood
Group therapy. *See* Psychotherapy
Growth Hormone (Physical Effects), 204–5
Guardianship and Conservatorship, 205
Gyri. *See* Brain and aging

Hair. *See* Facial appearance
Hamilton Rating Scale for Depression. *See* Depression (diagnostic tests)
Hammertoe. *See* Foot problems
Handedness, 206
Hands, 206–7
Handwriting, 207. *See also* Speed of behavior
Hay fever. *See* Diseases (acute and chronic)
Health Literacy, 207
Health Maintenance Organizations (HMOs), 207–8. *See also* Medicare
Health Promotion Programs, 208
Health Risk Behaviors, 208–9. *See also* Influenza
Health (self-ratings). *See* Health status and mental performance

Health span. *See* Life span

Health Status and Mental Performance, 209–10. *See also* Cardiovascular disease and mental performance

Healthy People 2010, 346. *See* Racial and ethnic differences in aging

Hearing, 210–12. *See also* Activities of daily living; Gender and sex differences in aging; Tinnitus; Untreated hearing impairment (effects on spouses)

Heart beat. *See* Heart rate

Heart disease and heart attacks. *See* Cardiovascular diseases

Heart Rate, 213

Heart transplant. *See* Cardiovascular diseases

Heart valves. *See* Cardiovascular diseases

Heat exhaustion. *See* Heat stroke

Heat Stroke, 213

Heel spurs. *See* Foot problems

Height and weight. *See* Body build and body characteristics

Hemoglobin. *See* Anemia

Hemorrhagic stroke. *See* Stroke

Herbal medicines. *See* Alternative medical treatments

Herceptin. *See* Breast cancer

Heredity versus Environment as Determiners of Functional Health. 214.

Heterocyclic antidepressants. *See* Depression (treatment)

Hiding your age, 214. *See also* Facial appearance

High blood pressure. *See* Blood pressure (high and low)

Hip fractures. *See* Falls; Fractures (hip); Osteoporosis

Hippocampus. *See* Alzheimer's disease; Brain and aging

Hip Replacement, 214–15

Historical time effect. *See* Longitudinal method

Hold and don't hold intelligence tests. *See* Wechsler Intelligence Tests

Holiday Greeting Cards, 215

Home Care, 215. *See also* Assisted living facilities

Homeless Older People (Reasons for Their Homelessness), 215–16

Homeless Older People (Who Are they?), 216

Home Maintenance, 216

Home Medical Devices, 216–17

Home Ownership, 217

Homosexuality, 217–18

Hormone replacement therapy. *See* Estrogen replacement therapy (hormone replacement therapy)

Hospice Care, 219

Hospital Infections, 219

Hostility, 219

Household Expenditures, 219–20

How Much Longer Do Seniors Want To Live? 220. *See also* Centenarians

Human Growth Hormone (Antiaging Effects), 220. *See also* Growth hormone (physical effects)

Human papillomavirus. *See* Cervical cancer

Humor, 220–21

Huntington's disease. *See* Senile dementia

Huperzine A. *See* Alzheimer's disease

Hypertension, 221–22. *See also* Blood pressure (high and low); Cardiovascular disease and mental performance; Cardiovascular diseases; Hypertension and mental functioning; Psychotherapy

Hypertension and Mental Functioning, 222

Hypochondria. *See* Neurosis

Hypotension. *See* Blood pressure (high and low)

Hypothermia. *See* Temperature sensitivity; Winter storms

Hypovolemia. *See* Blood pressure (high and low)

Hypoxemia. *See* Sleep disorders

Ibuprofen. *See* Arthritis; Pain medications (analgesics); Spinal stenosis

Iconic memory. *See* Sensory memory; Span of apprehension

Identity crisis. *See* Personality stages

Illiteracy. *See* Health literacy

Illusions, 223–24. *See also* Age simulation

Imagery, 224–25. *See also* Episodic memory; Verbal learning

Images of Aging in America. *See* Worst things about getting old

Immune Responses and Stress, 225

Immune system. *See* Arthritis; Immune responses and stress; Pneumonia; Why aging? (biological theories of aging)

Immunological theory of aging. *See* Why
aging (biological theories of aging)

Immunotherapy. *See* Skin cancer

Implicit Memory, 225–27

Impotence. *See* Sexual behavior (heterosexual)

Inactivity. *See* Activity (physical); Inactivity
of middle-aged and older women

Inactivity of Middle-Aged and Older
Women, 227

Incidental Memory, 228. *See also* Action
memory; Conversation memory

Income of Elderly People, 228. *See also*
Entitlements

Incontinence. *See* Urinary incontinence

Inderal. *See* Tremor (essential)

Indiplon. *See* Sleep disorders

Indomethacin. *See* Arthritis

Inferential reasoning. *See* Reasoning

Inflammatory breast cancer. *See* Breast
cancer

Influenza, 229–30. *See also* Influenza vaccines

Influenza Vaccines, 230

Ingrown toenails. *See* Foot problems

Inhibitory processes. *See* Selective attention; Socially inappropriate behavior

Insect Bites and Stings, 230–31

Insomnia. *See* Sleep disorders

Institutionalization (effects of). *See* Pet
therapy

Instrumental activities of daily living. *See*
Activities of daily living

Insulin. *See* Alzheimer's disease; Diabetes

Integrity versus despair. *See* Personality
stages

Intelligence, 231–33. *See also* Army Alpha
and Army Beta Intelligence Tests;
Cardiovascular disease and mental
performance; Longitudinal studies of
aging's effects on health and cognition; Practical intelligence; Twins;
Wechsler Intelligence Tests

Intentional Forgetting, 233

Intentional memory versus incidental
memory. *See* Action memory;
Conversation memory; Discourse
memory; Episodic memory;
Frequency-of-occurrence memory;
Memory for television programs;
Source memory; Spatial memory;

Temporal memory

Internet, 233. *See also* Computers;
Internet (differences between users
and nonusers); Web sites (useful for
medical information)

Internet (Differences between Users and
Nonusers), 233

Interpersonal Tensions, 234. *See also*
Stress and coping with stress

Interventions (for improving lives of
older adults). *See* Abilities (physical
and mental) and activity; Agitative
behaviors by nursing home residents;
Alzheimer's disease; Bathing;
Cardiovascular diseases (psychological
interventions); Caregivers (family and
friends); Classical conditioning;
Dancing; Depression (treatment);
Dysarthria; Falls; Foot problems;
Hospice care; Memory training;
Operant conditioning; Pet Therapy;
Plasticity theory; Postural change and
orthostasis; Psychotherapy;
Psychotherapy with nursing home residents; Reminiscence; Respite care;
Sexual behavior (heterosexual); Sleep
disorders; Sleep therapy; Smoking;
Stress and coping with stress; Stroke;
Temperature sensitivity; Transfer of
learning/training; Urinary inconti-
nence; Visual disorders; Weather (tor-
nado); Winter storms

Intrinsic factor. *See* Anemia

Introversion. *See* Personality traits

IRA, *see* College investments; Retirement
(planning)

Iron deficiency anemia. *See* Anemia

Irregular heart beat. *See* Cardiovascular
diseases

Irritable bowel syndrome. *See* Bowels

Ischemic Heart disease, 234. *See also*
Cardiovascular diseases

Job Loss, 235

Job Training,235

Jurors, 235–36

Keyword method. *See* Memory training

Kidney Cancer, 237

Kidneys. *See* End-state renal disease;
Physiological functions

Kidney stones. *See* Physiological functions

Knee Replacement, 237

Knowledge about your own memory. *See* Metamemory

Knowledge (general) about the world. *See* Longitudinal studies of aging's effects on health and cognition; Semantic memory; Wechsler Intelligence Tests

Korsakoff's disease. *See* Alcohol (physical and mental effects); Implicit memory

Kurzweil National Federation of the Blind Reader. *See* Visual disorders

Labyrinthitis. *See* Dizziness

Lacrimal glands. *See* Tear secretion

Laser surgery. *See* Visual disorders

Late-onset schizophrenia. *See* Psychosis

Laughter (Is It the Best Medicine for Seniors?), 238

Learned Helplessness, 239

Learning (Overview), 239–40. *See also* Classical conditioning; Concept learning; Maze learning; Motor skill learning; Operant conditioning; Spatial learning; Verbal learning

Learning-how-to-learn. *See* Transfer of learning/training

Lecithin. *See* Alzheimer's disease

Legal Advice, 240

Leg cramps. *See* Peripheral arterial disease and claudication

Leisure Activities, 241–42. *See also* Leisure activities (why some decline in late adulthood)

Leisure Activities (Why Some Decline in Late Adulthood), 242

Leukemia, 242

Levodopa. *See* Parkinson's disease

Lexicon, 242–44. *See also* Semantic memory; Spelling; Word associations

Licorice, 244

Life Expectancy, 244–45

Life Insurance, 245

Life Satisfaction, 245–47. *See also* Activity theory; Disability (psychological and social consequences); Frailty; Generativity; Goals; Mental health and mental health services; Neuroticism; Participation in voluntary organizations and volunteer work; Racial and ethnic differences in aging: Religion in later life; Retirement (adjustment to); Retirement communities; Retirement (theories of life satisfaction); Senior centers; Subjective age; Urinary incontinence; Well-being (psychological); Widowhood and Widowerhood

Life Span, 247–48

Lifting Heavy Objects, 248

Lighthouse Research Institute. *See* Visual disorders

Lipitor. *See* Cholesterol

Lipofuscin. *See* Brain and aging; Why aging? (biological theories of aging)

Liver Cancer, 248

Living wills. *See* Advance directives

Lobar pneumonia. *See* Pneumonia

Locomotion, 249. *See also* Accidents (automobile); Falls

Loneliness, 249–50

Longevity, 250–52. *See also* Educational level; Longevity (what determines a long life?); Sleep

Longevity (What Determines a Long Life?), 252. *See also* Longevity; Obesity (effects on longevity and disability); Sleep

Longitudinal Method, 252–54

Longitudinal Studies of Aging's Effects on Health and Cognition, 254–56

Long-term Care, 256

Long-term memory. *See* Episodic memory

Loyola Generativity Scale. *See* Generativity

Lucentis. *See* Visual disorders

Lumpectomy. *See* Breast cancer

Lung Cancer, 256–57. *See also* Smoking

Lupus. *See* Arthritis

Lycopene. *See* Nutrition and diet; Prostate cancer; Tomatoes

MacArthur Foundation Study of Successful Aging. *See* Successful Aging

Macular degeneration. *See* Visual disorders; Visual disorders (coping with macular degeneration)

Magazine Reading, 258

Magnetic Resonance Imaging. *See* Brain and aging

Male pattern baldness. *See* Facial appearance

Mammaglobin. *See* Breast cancer

Mammography (digital). *See* Breast cancer

Mammography (film). *See* Breast cancer

Managerial Ability, 258

Marriage and Marital Satisfaction, 259–60. *See also* Caregivers (positive effects of caregiving); Divorce; Well-being (psychological); Widowhood and widowerhood

Mastectomy. *See* Breast cancer

Mattis Dementia Rating Scale, 260

Maturity (Psychological), 260

Mayer-Salovey-Caruso Emotional Intelligence Test. *See* Emotions

Maze Learning, 260–61. *See also* Spatial learning

Meals on Wheels. *See* Food and meal services

Meat (well-done). *See* Breast cancer

Medicaid, 261. *See also* Adult day care centers

Medical model. *See* Stress and coping with stress

Medical Records, 261–62

Medicare, 262–63. *See also* Entitlements; Health Maintenance Organizations (HMOs); Medicaid; Medicare fraud; Medicare hospital patients

Medicare Fraud, 263–64

Medicare Hospital Patients, 264

Medicare Prescription Drug Benefit Program. *See* Medicare

Medication Compliance and Comprehension, 264–66. *See also* Overmedication

Medications, 266–67

Medication Sharing, 267

Medulla. *See* Brain and aging

Melancholia. *See* Depression (incidence, symptoms, causes)

Melanoma. *See* Skin cancer

Melatonin. *See* Sleep disorders

Memory Complaints, 267–68. *See also* Depression (performances with); Diary studies of memory failures; Memory training

Memory for Newsworthy Events, 268–69

Memory for stories and articles. *See* Continuity versus discontinuity in adult development; Discourse memory

Memory for Television Programs, 269

Memory (Overview), 269–72. *See also* Action memory; Autobiographical memory; Conversation memory; Diary studies of memory failures; Discourse memory; Emotions and memory; Episodic memory; Everyday memory; Face memory; False memory; Frequency-of-occurrence memory; Gender and sex differences in aging; Implicit memory; Memory for newsworthy events; Memory for television programs; Memory span; Memory training; Metamemory; Picture memory; Prospective memory; Recognition memory versus recall memory; Selective control of memory; Semantic memory; Smell; Source memory; Spatial memory; Temporal memory; Time of day and memory performance; Very long-term memory; Working memory

Memory Span, 272–73. *See also* Arousal

Memory Strategies. *See* Metamemory

Memory Training, 273–75. *See also* Metamemory

Ménière's Disease. *See* Dizziness

Menopause and Ovulation, 275–76

Mental activity. *See* Activity (mental) and mental performance

Mental dictionary. *See* Lexicon

Mental Health and Mental Health Services, 276–77

Mental rotation. *See* Imagery

Mental Status Questionnaire, 277

Metabolism. *See* Body build and body characteristics; Nutrition and diet; Old (defining late adulthood); Physiological functions

Metamemory, 277–79. *See also* Diary studies of memory failures; Everyday memory; Metamemory in Adulthood (MIA) Questionnaire and Metamemory Functioning Questionnaire (MFQ)

Metamemory in Adulthood Questionnaire (MIA) and Metamemory Functioning Questionnaire, 279

Metaphors, 279–80

Methadone. *See* Pain medications (analgesics)

Method of loci. *See* Memory training

Middle-age spread. *See* Body build and body characteristics; Nutrition and diet

Midlife Crisis, 280

Migration (Moving), 280–81

Mild cognitive dementia (MCD). *See* Age-associated memory impairment; Senile dementia

Mindwandering. *See* Daydreaming

Mini-Mental State Exam, 181. *See also* Activities of daily living; Participant selection for research studies; Senile dementia

Minocycycline. *See* Arthritis

Mirapex. *See* Arthritis; Parkinson's disease; Sleep disorders

Mixed connective tissue disease. *See* Arthritis

Mnemonics. *See* Action memory; Memory training; Verbal learning

Mobility. *See* Locomotion

Modifying Negative Health Behaviors, 281–82

Mood induction. *See* Emotions

Moral model. *See* Stress and coping with stress

Morphine. *See* Pain medications (analgesics)

Motion Perception, 282

Motor Behavior, 282

Motor Skill Learning, 283–85. *See also* Abilities (physical and mental) and activity

MRI. *See* Brain and Aging

Multifactorial Memory Questionnaire (MMQ), 285

Multi-Infarct Dementia, 285–86. *See also* Caregiving (type of mentally impaired patient); Stroke

Muscles. *See* Strength and stamina

Mycoplasma. *See* Pneumonia

Myocardial infarction. *See* Cardiovascular disease

Myths about Aging, 286. *See also* Consumers of merchandise in stores; Curiosity; Daydreaming; Death and dying; Diseases (acute and chronic); Emotions; Exercise types; Homosexuality; Neurosis

Nails, 287

Narcolepsy. *See* Sleep disorders

Nardil. *See* Depression (treatment)

National Heart, Lung, and Blood Institute, 287

National Institute on Aging, 287–88

Natural Disasters (Distress Experiences), 288–89

Negative attitudes toward elderly people. *See* Ageism

Negative life events. *See* Stress and coping with stress

Negative Stereotype and Memory, 289

NEO Inventory. *See* Personality traits

Nerve blocks. *See* Pain management

Nerve growth factor. *See* Alzheimer's disease; Brain and aging

Nerve signal transmission. *See* Physiological functions

Nerve wind up theory. *See* Pain medications (analgesics)

Neurofibrillary tangles. *See* Alzheimer's disease; Brain and aging

Neuropsychology. *See* Age-associated memory impairment

Neurosis, 289. *See also* Neuroticism; Self-rated health

Neuroticism, 290. *See also* Cornell Medical Index; Personality traits

Neurotransmitters. *See* Alzheimer's disease; Brain and aging

Nightmares, 290

Nitroglycerin. *See* Cardiovascular diseases

Nocturia, 290. *See also* Prostate gland

Nolvadex. *See* Breast cancer

Nonprescription drugs. *See* Medications

Nonspecific transfer. *See* Transfer of learning/training

Norepinephrine. *See* Brain and aging

Normative Aging Study. *See* Cornell Medical Index; Longitudinal studies of aging's effects on health and cognition

Norms, 291–92. *See also* Wechsler Intelligence Tests

Norpramin. *See* Depression (treatment)

NSAIDS. *See* Arthritis; Cardiovascular diseases; Pain medications (analgesics)

Nuclear stress test. *See* Cardiovascular diseases

Nucleus basalis of Meynert. *See* Alzheimer's disease; Brain and aging

Nun Study, 292–93. *See also* Alzheimer's disease; Self-rated functioning

Nurses Health Study. *See* Longitudinal studies of aging's effects on health and cognition

Nursing Home Administrators. *See* Searching for a quality nursing home

Nursing Home Admissions, 293

Nursing Home Deficiencies, 293–94
Nursing Home Discharge Outcomes, 294
Nursing Home Infections, 294
Nursing Home Residents (Contacts with Family and Friends), 294–95
Nursing Home Residents (Number), 295
Nursing Home Residents (Their Rights), 295
Nursing Homes Staff (Resident Dependency), 296
Nutrition and Diet, 296–98. See also Antioxidants; Bladder cancer; Breast cancer; Cholesterol; Fractures (hip); Prostate cancer; Stroke

OARS. See Older Americans Research and Services Questionnaire
Obesity, 299. See also Nutrition and diet; Obesity (childhood obesity predicts adult obesity); Obesity (effects on longevity and disability); Sleep disorders
Obesity (Childhood Obesity Predicts Adult Obesity), 299
Obesity (Effects on Longevity and Disability), 299–300
Obstacle avoidance. See Falls
Occult blood test. See Colon cancer
Occupational therapists. See Leisure activities
Odor identification. See Smell
Old (Defining Late Adulthood), 300–301
Older Americans Act. See Senior centers
Older Americans Research and Services Questionnaire (OARS), 301
Omega-3 fatty acids. See Cholesterol
Openness. See Personality traits
Operant Conditioning, 302. See also Pain management; Psychotherapy; Psychotherapy with nursing home residents; Smoking
Opiate analgesics. See Pain medications (analgesics)
Optimism versus pessimism. See Personality style; Pessimism about your physical health and depression
Oral cancer. See Teeth, gums, and mouth
Orgasms. See Sexual behavior (heterosexual)
Originality, 302–3. See also Creativity
Orthostasis. See Postural change and orthostasis

Osteoarthritis. See Arthritis
Osteoarthritis Severity Scale Items. See Arthritis
Osteopenia, 303
Osteoporosis, 303–4. See also Estrogen-replacement therapy (hormone replacement therapy); Fractures (hip); Menopause and ovulation; Osteopenia
Ototoxic drugs. See Hearing
Ovarian Cancer, 304–5
Overmedication, 305
Oxaliplatin. See Colon cancer
OxyContin. See Pain medications (analgesics)

Pacemaker. See Cardiovascular diseases
Paget's Disease, 306
Pain, 306–7
Pain (Chronic), 307
Painless heart attack. See Cardiovascular diseases
Pain Management, 307–8
Pain Medications (Analgesics), 308–9
Paired-associate learning. See Verbal learning
Palliative treatment. See Pancreatic cancer
Pancreas. See Diabetes
Pancreatic Cancer, 309
Pap smear test. See Cervical cancer
Paradoxical sleep. See Sleep
Paranoia. See Alzheimer's disease; Psychosis
Parent-Child Conflicts, 309–10
Parenthood in Later Life, 310–11
Parkinson's Disease, 311–12. See also Brain and aging; Depression (treatment)
Paroxysmal positional vertigo. See Dizziness
Participant Selection for Research Studies, 312
Participation in Research, 312–13
Participation in Voluntary Organizations and Volunteer Work, 313–14
Partners in Caregiving: The Dementia Services Program, 314
Patient controlled analgesics. See Pain management
Patient Self-determination Act. See Advance directives
Patronizing Communication, 314
Pattern recognition. See Form perception

Pavlovian conditioning. *See* Classical conditioning

Peer Review Organization (PRO). *See* Medicare hospital patients

Pegword method. *See* Memory training

Pentoxil. *See* Peripheral arterial disease and claudication

Perception. *See* Color perception; Constancies of perception; Dark adaptation; Depth perception; Form perception; Illusions; Motion perception; Speech perception

Performance intelligence. *See* Wechsler Intelligence Tests

Periodontal disease. *See* Teeth, gums and mouth

Periostal. *See* Teeth, gums, and mouth

Peripheral Arterial Disease and Claudication, 314–15

Permastore. *See* Very long-term memory

Pernicious anemia. *See* Anemia

Personality and Mortality, 315

Personality (Overview), 316–17. *See also* Control over life's events; Personality and mortality; Personality stages; Personality style; Personality traits; Twins

Personality Stages, 316–17

Personality Style, 317–18

Personality Traits, 318–20. *See also* Caregivers (family and friends); Centenarians; Control over life's events; Curiosity

Perspiration. *See* Heat stroke

Pessimism about Your Physical Health and Depression, 320

Pets (at home). *See* Pet therapy

Pet Therapy, 320–21

Philadelphia Geriatric Center Affect Rating Scale. *See* Emotions

Phlebitis. *See* Cardiovascular diseases

Phobia. *See* Classical conditioning; Psychotherapy

Phonemic regression. *See* Speech perception

Physical activities of daily living. *See* Activities of daily living

Physical activity. *See* Activities of daily living; Activity (physical)

Physical Attractiveness, 321

Physicians (Communication with), 321–22. *See also* Barriers to health in older men

Physiological Functions, 322–23. *See also* Old (defining late adulthood)

Pick's disease. *See* Senile dementia

Picture Memory, 323–24

Picture superiority effect. *See* Picture memory

Piles. *See* Body build and body characteristics

Pineal gland. *See* Sleep disorders

Plasticity Theory, 324. *See also* Abilities (physical and mental) and activity; Brain and aging; Reasoning; Stroke; Why aging? (psychological theories of aging)

PMA Test. *See* Primary Mental Abilities (PMA) Test

Pneumococcus Pneumonia. *See* Pneumonia

Pneumonia, 324–25. *See also* Influenza

Polymalgia rheumatica. *See* Arthritis

Polyunsaturated fat. *See* Cholesterol

Pomegranate juice. *See* Nutrition and diet

Pons. *See* Brain and aging

Portion Size and Heart Health, 326

Positive growth in late adulthood. *See* Why aging? (psychological theories of aging)

Positron Emission Tomography (PET) scans. *See* Alzheimer's disease; Brain and aging

Posttraumatic Stress Disorder, 326–27

Postural Change and Orthostasis, 327–28

Posture, 328–29. *See also* Falls

Potassium. *See* Nutrition and diet

Potassium bicarbonate supplements. *See* Osteoporosis

Poverty income level. *See* Entitlements; Income of elderly people

Practical intelligence, 329. *See also* Intelligence; Problem solving; Racial and ethnic differences in aging

Practice effects on mental performances. *See* Disuse principle; Transfer of learning/training

Prayer. *See* Religion in later life

Prednisone. *See* Shingles

Prefrontal lobes. *See* Brain and aging

Presbycusis. *See* Hearing

Presbyopia. *See* Vision

Presenile dementia. *See* Alzheimer's disease

Primary memory. *See* Short-term memory

Primary Mental Abilities (PMA) Test, 329–30. *See also* Longitudinal studies of aging's effects on health and cognition, 329–30

Prisoners (Elderly), 330

Proactive interference. *See* Forgetting

Problem-focused coping. *See* Stress and coping with stress

Problem Solving, 330–31. *See also* Daydreaming; Originality; Practical intelligence

Problems Perceived by Elderly People, 331

Problems Physicians Have with Older Patients, 332

Progeria, 332

Progesterone. *See* Menopause and ovulation

Propoxyphene. *See* Medications

Propranolol. *See* Posttraumatic stress disorder

Proscar. *See* Prostate gland

Prospective Memory, 332–34

Prostate Cancer, 335–36. *See also* Nutrition and diet; Prostate gland

Prostate Gland, 336–37. *See also* Prostate cancer; Sexual behavior (heterosexual)

Prostate-specific antigen (PSA). *See* Prostate cancer

Proverbs (Interpretation), 337

Prozac. *See* Depression (treatment)

Psychoanalytic therapy. *See* Psychotherapy

Psychosis, 338–39

Psychotherapy, 339–42. *See also* Depression (treatment); Humor; Psychotherapy with nursing home residents; Reminiscence; Sleep therapy; Smoking; Urinary incontinence

Psychotherapy with Nursing Home Residents, 342–43

PTSD. *See* Posttraumatic stress disorder

Public Assistance, 343

Public School Support, 343

Pulmonary embolism. *See* Cardiovascular diseases

Quackery, 344

Quantitative changes versus qualitative changes in development. *See* Continuity versus discontinuity in adult development

Racial and Ethnic Differences in Aging, 345–48. *See also* Activity (productive); Adult day care centers; Caregivers (family and friends); Educational level; Food and meal services; Grandparenting; *Healthy People 2010;* Homeless older people; Life expectancy; Life satisfaction; Locomotion; Marriage and marital satisfaction; Mini-Mental State Exam; Nursing home admissions; Osteoporosis; Participation in voluntary organizations and volunteer work; Prostate cancer; Racial differences in functional decline; Religion in later life; Retirement (racial inequity); Senior centers; Sleep complaints; Smoking; Stomach cancer; Stroke; Suicide; Testicular cancer; Tuberculosis; Visual disorders; Well-being (psychological); Work

Racial Differences in Functional Decline, 348–49

Radiation therapy. *See* Breast cancer

Radical prostatectomy. *See* Prostate cancer

Raloxifene. *See* Breast cancer; Osteoporosis

Reaction Time, 349–50. *See also* Accidents (automobile); Age change versus age difference

Reading and Reading Skills, 350. *See also* Abilities (physical and mental) and activity; Lexicon; Magazine reading

Reading span. *See* Working memory

Reality orientation. *See* Psychotherapy with nursing home residents

Reasoning, 350–51. *See also* Proverbs (interpretation)

Recognition Memory Versus Recall Memory, 351–53. *See also* Action memory; Episodic memory; False memory

Relationship with Physician (Duration), 353

Relenza. *See* Influenza

Reliability. *See* Variability of behavior

Religion and Meaning in Life, 353–54

Religion in later life, 354–56. *See also* Death and dying; Grandparenting; Religion and meaning in Life; Smoking; Widowhood and widowerhood

Reminiscence, 356–57. *See also*

Autobiographical memory;
Daydreaming; Psychotherapy
Remote memory. *See* Very long-term
memory
Remotivation therapy. *See* Psychotherapy
with nursing home residents
REM sleep. *See* Sleep
Renova. *See* Facial appearance
Reorientation therapy. *See* Psychotherapy
with nursing home residents
Requip. *See* Parkinson's disease; Sleep dis-
orders
Residence, 357. *See also* Environmental
press
Resignation. *See* Stress and coping with
stress
Respect for Elderly People, 357–58
Respiration. *See* Physiological functions
Respite Care, 358
Restless leg syndrome. *See* Sleep disorders
Retirees and Re-entry into the Workforce,
358
Retirement (Adjustment to), 359
Retirement Communities, 359–60
Retirement (Contacts with Adult
Children), 360–61
Retirement (Involuntary), 361
Retirement (Life after), 361–62 *See also*
Goals; Marriage and marital satisfac-
tion; Work
Retirement (Locations), 363
Retirement (Planning), 364–65
Retirement (Racial Inequity), 365
Retirement (sex differences). *See*
Retirement (theories of life satisfac-
tion)
Retirement (Theories of Life
Satisfaction), 365
Retirement (Timing), 366. *See also* Work
Retirement (Uncertainty), 366
Retroactive interference. *See* Forgetting
Retrospective memory. *See* Episodic mem-
ory; Prospective memory
Rheumatoid arthritis. *See* Arthritis
rhuMAb-E25. *See* Asthma
Right ear advantage. *See* Divided atten-
tion
Rights of residents of long-term care facil-
ities. *See* Nursing home residents
(their rights)
Rigidity, 367. *See also* Attitudes (political
and social)

RNA. *See* Why aging? (biological theories
of aging)
Rod and Frame Test. *See* Personality style
Roles Seniors Play, 367–69
Rollators. *See* Walkers
Ropinirole. *See* Parkinson's disease
Roth (IRA). *See* Retirement (planning)
Rural Older People and (Characteristics
and Problems They Face), 368–69

Saccadic eye movements. *See* Vision
Safe Return Program. *See* Wandering
Salagen. *See* Teeth, gums, and mouth
Salt Intake, 370. *See also* Stroke
SAMe. *See* Depression (treatment)
Sarcopenia, 370
Saturated fat. *See* Cholesterol
Scams, 370–71. *See also* Consumer fraud
Schizophrenia. *See* Psychosis
Sciatica. *See* Spinal stenosis
Sclerotherapy. *See* Body build and body
characteristics
SDAT. *See* Alzheimer's disease
Searching For a Quality Nursing Home,
371–72
Seattle Longitudinal Study. *See*
Longitudinal studies of aging's effects
on health and cognition
Secondary hypertension. *See*
Hypertension
Secondary memory. *See* Episodic memory
Sedentary Lifestyle of Many Older
Women, 372
Seizures, 373
Selective Attention, 373–75. *See also*
Accidents (automobile); Attention
(overview); Personality style
Selective Control of Memory, 375
Self-care (health). *See* Self-rated function-
ing
Self-Concept, 376
Self-Efficacy, 376. *See also* Activities of
daily living; Control over life's events;
Falls; Widowhood and widowerhood
Self-Esteem, 379. *See also* Baby talk (elder-
speak); Disability (psychological and
social consequences); Religion in later
life; Reminiscence; Retirement
(adjustment to)
Self-Evaluations and Adjustment to
Stressful Transitions, 377–78
Self-Rated Functioning, 378

Self-rated health. *See* Health status and mental performance

Selegiline transdermal patch. *See* Depression (treatment)

Semantic Memory, 378–79. *See also* Lexicon

Seminom cancer. *See* Testicular cancer

Senile Dementia, 379–80. *See also* Accidents (automobile); Alzheimer's disease; Multi-infarct dementia; Parkinson's disease

Senile dementia of the Alzheimer's type. *See* Alzheimer's disease

Senile plaques. *See* Alzheimer's disease; Brain and aging

Senior Centers, 380–81. *See also* Services (formal)

Senior Olympics, 381

Seniors in the Community: Risk Evaluation for Eating and Nutrition Questionnaire, 381–82

Senses. *See* Hearing; Smell; Taste; Temperature sensitivity; Touch; Vision

Sensory Functioning and Mental Functioning (Relationship), 382

Sensory Memory, 382–83

Sensory training. *See* Psychotherapy with nursing home residents

September 11, 2001. *See* Natural disasters

Sequential Method, 383

Serial learning. *See* Verbal learning

Serial position effects. *See* Verbal learning

Serotonin. *See* Brain and aging

Services (Formal), 384

Serzone. *See* Depression (treatment)

Sex Differences and Scientific Ability, 384

Sexual Behavior (Heterosexual), 384–87. *See also* Homosexuality

Sexual dysfunctioning. *See* Sexual behavior (heterosexual)

Shape constancy. *See* Constancies of perception

Shingles, 387–88

Shortness of breath. *See* Physiological functions

Short-term Memory, 388–90. *See also* Memory span; Working memory

Short Test of Functional Health Literacy. *See* Health Literacy

Sibling Relationships, 390–91

Sigmoidoscopy. *See* Colon cancer

Signs and Forms, 391

Simple vigilance. *See* Vigilance

Sinemet. *See* Parkinson's disease

Sinusitis. *See* Diseases (acute and chronic)

Size constancy. *See* Constancies of perception

Sjogren's Syndrome. *See* Teeth, gums, and mouth

Skin. *See* Bathing; Body build and body characteristics; Bruises; Skin cancer

Skin Cancer, 391–92

Skipping Meals, 392

Sleep, 392–94. *See also* Sleep complaints; Sleep disorders; Sleep (inefficient);Sleep therapy

Sleep Complaints, 394

Sleep Disorders, 394–97. *See also* Sleep (inefficient); Visual disorders (sleep problems)

Sleep (Inefficient), 397

Sleep-maintenance insomnia. *See* Sleep disorders

Sleep-onset insomnia. *See* Sleep disorders

Sleep Therapy, 398. *See also* Acupuncture

Slowing-Down Principle, 398–99. *See also* Longevity; Reaction time; Short-term memory; Speed of behavior; Verbal fluency

Smallpox, 399–400

Smell, 400–401

Smoking, 401–2. *See also* Chronic respiratory diseases; Lung cancer; Visual disorders

Snoring. *See* Sleep disorders

Social activity and longevity. *See* Activity theory; Longevity

Social gerontology. *See* Gerontology

Social interactions. *See* Friendships; Social networks

Socially Inappropriate Behavior, 402–3

Social Networks, 403. *See also* Friendships

Social Security benefits. *See* Entitlements

Somatotropin. *See* Growth hormone (physical effects)

Sominex. *See* Sleep disorders

Sonogram. *See* Prostate cancer

Source Memory, 403–4. *See also* Episodic memory

Span of Apprehension, 404–5

Spatial Ability, 405–6. *See also* Abilities (physical and mental) and activity; Gender and sex differences in aging; Sex differences and scientific ability;

Spatial learning; Spatial memory

Spatial Learning, 406–7

Spatial Memory, 407–8. *See also* Episodic memory

Specific transfer. *See* Transfer of learning/training

Speech impairments. *See* Voice

Speech Perception, 408–10. *See also* Hearing

Speed of Behavior, 410. *See also* Slowing–down principle

Spelling, 410–11

Sphincter muscle. *See* Bowels

Spider veins. *See* Body build and body characteristics

Spinal Stenosis, 411

Spreading activation. *See* Lexicon

Squamous cell cancer. *See* Skin cancer

Stages of mental development. *See* Cognitive (mental) stages of development

Standard deviation. *See* Variability of Behavior

Static acuity. *See* Vision

Steroids. *See* Asthma

Stimulus control method. *See* Sleep therapy

Stimulus Persistence, 411. *See also* Aftereffects (visual)

Stomach Cancer, 411–12

Strength and Stamina, 412–13. *See also* Abilities (physical and mental) and activity

Streptomycin. *See* Hearing

Stress and Coping with Stress, 413–14. *See also* Alcoholism (incidence and causes); Alcohol (Physical and mental effects); Caregivers (elderly parents); Caregivers (family and friends); Continuity versus discontinuity in adult development; Divorce; Drug abuse; Humor; Learned helplessness; Mental health and mental health services; Posttraumatic stress disorder; Religion in later life; Reminiscence; Self-evaluations and adjustment to stressful transitions; Visual disorders (coping with macular degeneration)

Stress incontinence. *See* Urinary incontinence

Stress test. *See* Cardiovascular diseases

Stroke, 416–19. *See also* Blood pressure (high and low); Cardiovascular diseases; Cholesterol; Multi-infarct dementia

Stroop effect. *See* Lexicon

Subjective Age, 420,

Successful Aging, 420. *See also* Reminiscence; Successful aging: an alternative perspective

Successful Aging: An Alternative Perspective, 420. *See also* Successful aging

Suicide, 421–22

Sulci. *See* Brain and aging

Sundown syndrome. *See* Sleep disorders

Support groups. *See* Caregivers (family and friends)

Surgery Survival, 422

Survival after Death of a Spouse or Significant Other, 422. *See also* Widowhood and widowerhood

Swallowing, 422–23

Sweepstakes scam. *See* Scams

Switching Tasks, 423. *See also* Hypertension and mental functioning

Syllogisms. *See* Reasoning

Symptoms (physical and psychological). *See* Cornell Medical Index

Syncope, 423

Syntagmatic associations. *See* Word associations

Syntax, 424

Systematic desensitization therapy. *See* Psychotherapy

Tacit knowledge. *See* Practical intelligence

Tacrine. *See* Alzheimer's disease

Talkativeness. *See* Verbosity

Tamiflu. *See* Influenza

Tamoxifen. *See* Breast cancer

Targis microwave therapy. *See* Prostate gland

Taste, 425–27

Tea, 427

Tear Secretion, 427–28

Teeth, Gums, and Mouth, 428–29

Telemarketing scams. *See* Scams

Telephone, 429

Television Viewing, 429–30

Telomere. *See* Why aging? (Biological theories of aging)

Temperature Sensitivity, 430–31

Temporal discounting. *See* Delayed rewards

Temporal Memory, 431–32. *See also* Action memory; Episodic memory; Verbal learning

Tequin. *See* Pneumonia

Terminal Drop Phenomenon, 432

Terminal Illness, 432–33

Testicular Cancer, 433

Testosterone. *See* Alzheimer's disease; Antiaging products—do they really work? Facial appearance; Menopause and ovulation; Sexual behavior (heterosexual)

Tetanus, 433

Text memory. *See* Discourse memory

Thalamus. *See* Brain and aging

Theories of aging. *See* Why aging? (biological theories of aging); Why aging? (psychological theories of aging)

ThinPrep Pap smear test. *See* Cervical cancer

Thrombolytic stroke. *See* Stroke

Time-based prospective memory. *See* Prospective memory

Time Estimation, 433–34

Time-Lag Comparison, 434

Time of Day and Memory Performance, 435

Tinnitus, 435–36. *See also* Hearing

Tip-of the-tongue state. *See* Verbal ability

Tissue plasminogen activator. *See* Stroke

TNF inhibitors. *See* Arthritis

Toilet Seats, 436

Tomatoes, 436

Total hip orthoplasty. *See* Hip replacement

Touch , 436

TPA (tissue plasminogen activator). *See* Stroke

Trail Making Test, 437. *See also* Depression (performances with); Hypertension and mental functioning; Switching tasks

Transfer of Learning/Training, 437–38. *See also* Forgetting

Trans fats. *See* Cholesterol; Nutrition and diet

Transient ischemic attacks. *See* Stroke

Transrectal ultrasound endoscope. *See* Prostate cancer

Transurethral resection. *See* Prostate cancer

Traveling, 439. *See also* Crime prevention; Elderhostel; Vaccinations and shots for traveling

Trekking poles. *See* Walking

Tremor (Essential), 439–40

Tremors. *See* Brain and aging; Parkinson's disease; Tremor (essential)

Triad. *See* Crime prevention

Triglycerides. *See* Cardiovascular diseases

Tuberculosis, 440

Twins, 440–41

Tylenol: Extra strength. *See* Pain medications (analgesics)

Tylenol PM. *See* Pain medications (analgesics); Sleep disorders

Type A versus type B behavior. *See* Retirement (Involuntary)

Typing. *See* Expertise

Underdiagnosis of Illnesses, 442

Unsolicited Support and Advice, 442

Untreated Hearing Impairment (Effects on Spouses), 442–43

Unusual Uses Test. *See* Originality

Urge incontinence. *See* Urinary incontinence

Urinary Incontinence, 443–45

Urination, 445. *See also* Physiological functions; Prostate gland; Urinary incontinence

Urodynamics. *See* Urinary incontinence

Uterine Cancer, 445–46

Vaccination for cervical cancer. *See* Cervical cancer

Vaccinations and Shots for Traveling, 447. *See also* Influenza vaccines; Pneumonia; Tetanus

Vaccine for pneumonia. *See* Pneumonia

Valuation of life concept. *See* How much longer do seniors want to live?

Variability of Behavior, 447–48

Varicella-zoster. *See* Shingles

Varicose veins. *See* Body build and body characteristics

Vasodilators. *See* Blood pressure (high and low)

Ventricular resynchronizer. *See* Cardiovascular diseases

Verbal Ability, 448–49. *See also* Gender and sex differences in aging; Syntax; Verbosity

Verbal Fluency, 450

Verbal Learning, 450–52

Verbosity, 452

Vertigo. *See* Dizziness

Very Long-Term Memory, 453

Vestibular system. *See* Dizziness

Veterans Health Study. *See* Longitudinal studies of aging's effects on health and cognition

Viagra. *See* Sexual behavior (heterosexual)

Victoria Longitudinal Study. *See* Longitudinal studies of aging's effects on health and cognition

Vigilance, 454–55. *See also* Attention (overview)

Vioxx. *See* Pain medications (analgesics)

Vision, 455–56. *See also* Accidents (automobile); Activities of daily living; Bifocals; Color perception; Constancies of perception; Dark adaptation; Depth perception; Falls; Form perception; Illusions; Visual disorders

Visual Disorders, 456–59. *See also* Diabetes, Visual disorders (coping with macular degeneration);

Visual Disorders (Coping with Macular Degeneration), 459

Visual Disorders (Sleep Problems), 459–60

Visudyne. *See* Visual disorders

Vitamin B12 deficiency anemia. *See* Anemia

Vitamin D Supplements, 460. *See also* Osteoporosis

Vitamins. *See* Anemia, Antioxidants; Breast cancer; Cardiovascular diseases; Cholesterol; Fractures (hip); Nutrition and diet; Osteoporosis; Prostate gland; Visual disorders; Vitamin D supplements

Vocabulary. *See* Abilities (physical and mental) and activity; Intelligence; Verbal ability; Wechsler Intelligence Tests

Vocal polyps. *See* Voice

Voice, 460

Volunteer organizations and work. *See* Participation in voluntary organizations and volunteer work

Voters, 461

Wales study of physical activity. *See* Activity (physical)

Walkers, 462

Walking, 462–63

Walking equipment. *See* Foot problems

Wandering, 463. *See also* Alzheimer's disease

Warner syndrome. *See* Progeria

Warnings, 463–64

Water intake. *See* Fluid intake

Wear and tear principle of biological aging. *See* Why aging? (biological theories of aging)

Weather (Tornado), 464

Web Sites (Use for Medical Information), 464

Wechsler Intelligence Test, 465–66. *See also* Educational level

Wechsler Memory Scale, 467

Well-Being (Psychological), 467–68. *See also* Life satisfaction; Neuroticism; Religion in later life

Werner syndrome. *See* Progeria

Wernicke's area of the brain. *See* Aphasia

Wheelchairs, 469

White House Conferences on Aging, 469–70

Why Aging (Biological Theories of Aging), 470–71

Why Aging? (Psychological Theories of Aging), 472. *See also* Personality stages

Widowhood and Widowerhood, 473–75. *See also* Divorce; Life satisfaction; Nutrition and diet; Touch

Winter Storms, 475

Wisdom, 475–76. *See also* Abilities (physical and mental) and activity; Life satisfaction; Practical intelligence; Problem solving

Women's Health Initiative, 476–77. *See also* Fractures (hip); Nutrition and diet; Osteoporosis; Stroke

Word Associations, 477–78

Work, 478–80. *See also* Accidents (at work); Activity (productive); Age discrimination at work; Articles on Retirement; Participation in voluntary organizations and volunteer work

Working Memory, 480–82. *See also* Episodic memory; Posture; Short-term memory

Worries, 482

Worst Things about Getting Old, 482

Wrinkles. *See* Body build and body charac-
    teristics

Xalatan. *See* Visual disorders
Xerostoma. *See* Teeth, gums, and mouth

YAVIS syndrome. *See* Ageism

Yellowing of the lens. *See* Age simulation;
    Color perception; Illusions
Yogurt. *See* Pneumonia

Zinc. *See* Visual disorders
Zung Self-Rating Scale. *See* Depression
    (diagnostic tests)

Index of Entries by Broad Topics

Abnormal Aging and Impairments with Aging

Abnormal aging, 3
Activities of daily living, 9–11
Adapting a home for elderly residents, 16
Adapting to fading eyesight, 16
Adult day care centers, 16–17
Age-associated memory impairment, 19–20
Agitative behaviors by nursing home residents, 25
Alzheimer's Association, 31
Alzheimer's disease, 31–37
Aphasia, 41
Bed sores, 57–58
Beliefs about aging affect physical health, 58
Bifocals, 58
Blessed Mental Status Test, 60
Caregivers (hassles in administering medications), 86
Clinical Dementia Rating Scale. 97
Computerized homes, 105
Coping with frailty,112
Creutzfeldt-Jakob disease. *See* Senile dementia
Delirium, 125
Depression (diagnostic tests), 127–28
Depression (incidence and causes), 128–30
Depression (performances with), 130
Depression (prognosis), 130
Depression (treatment), 131–32
Deteriorating neighborhood, 133
Disability (adaptation), 135
Disability (incidence and assistance), 136–37
Diseases (acute and chronic), 139–40
Drug abuse, 149
Drug tests (clinical trials), 149–50
Elder abuse, 153–55
Falls, 176–79
Frailty as a clinical syndrome, 190
Frailty (identifying degrees), 190–91
Frailty (incidence and causes), 191
Grandparents raising their own grandchildren, 203–4
Huntington's disease. *See* Senile dementia
Immune responses and stress, 225
Interpersonal tensions, 234
Korsakoff's disease. *See* Alcohol (physical and mental effects)
Mattis Dementia Rating Scale, 260
Mild cognitive dementia. *See* Senile dementia
Multi-infarct dementia, 285–86
Natural disasters (distress experiences), 288–89
Neurosis, 289
Neuroticism, 290
Nursing home residents (their rights), 295
Parkinson's disease, 311–12
Pick's disease. *See* Senile dementia
Progeria, 332
Psychosis, 338–39
Retirement (uncertainty), 366
Senile dementia, 379–80
Sleep disorders, 394–97
Visual disorders, 456–59
Visual disorders (coping with macular degeneration), 459–60
Visual disorders (sleep problems), 459–60
Wandering, 463
Warnings, 463–64
Weather (tornado),464
Werner syndrome. *See* Progeria

Adjustment to Aging, Stress and Coping with Stress

Assisted living facilities, 48
Death and dying, 122–24
Divorce, 144–45
Environmental press, 160
Euthanasia, 164–65
Funerals, 195
Generativity, 199
Home care, 215
Hospice care, 219
Learned helplessness, 239
Marriage and marital satisfaction, 259–60
Parent-child conflicts, 309–10
Parenthood in later life, 310–11
Posttraumatic stress disorder, 326–27
Retirees (and re-entry into the workforce), 358
Retirement (adjustment to), 359
Retirement (involuntary), 361
Retirement (theories of life satisfaction), 365
Stress and coping with stress, 413–14
Why aging? (psychological theories of aging), 472
Widowhood and widowerhood, 473–75

Behavior (Physical, Mental, and Social)

Activities of daily living, 9–11
Activity (mental) and mental performance, 11–13
Activity (physical), 13
Activity (productive), 13–14
Activity theory, 14–15
Altruism (adult age differences), 29–30
Altruism (health benefits for elders), 29–30
Androgyny, 37–38
Attitudes (political and social), 51–51
Attribution, 52–53
Automatic teller machines (ATMs), 54
Baby talk (elderspeak), 55
Bathing, 56–57
Bingo, 59
Boredom, 63–64
Computers, 104
Conformity, 105–6
Consumers of merchandise in stores, 108
Control over life's events, 110–11
Crime prevention, 115–16
Crimes (victim of and fear of), 116
Curiosity, 119

Daydreaming, 121–22
Decision-making, 124
Delayed rewards, 124–25
Disability (psychological and social consequences), 137–38
Disengagement theory, 140
Drivers (improving their skills), 146
Driver's license renewal, 146–47
Driving (activity after cessation), 147
Drug abuse, 149
Elderhostel, 155–56
Exercise capacity, 166–67
Exercise (relationship to physical/mental performances), 167–69
Exercise types, 169–70
Falls, 176–79
Family values and traditionalism, 180
Fatigue (clinical syndrome), 180
Finger movements and exercise, 181
Foster Grandparent Program, 189
Friendships, 192–93
Goals, 200–201
Grandparenting, 201–3
Handwriting, 207
Health risk behaviors, 208–9
Hiding your age, 214
Home maintenance, 216
Homosexuality, 217–18
Hostility, 219
Humor, 220–21
Inactivity of middle-aged and older women, 227
Internet, 233
Internet (differences between users and nonusers), 233
Learned helplessness, 239
Leisure activities, 241
Leisure activities (why some decline in late adulthood), 242
Lifting heavy objects, 248
Locomotion, 249
Magazine reading, 258
Managerial ability, 258
Migration (moving), 280–81
Motor behavior, 282
Nightmares, 290
Parenthood in later life, 310–11
Participation in research, 312–13
Participation in voluntary organizations and volunteer work, 313–14
Patronizing communication, 314
Religion and meaning in life, 353–54

Religion in later life, 354–56
Reminiscence, 356–57
Respect for elderly people, 357–58
Retirement (contacts with adult children), 360–61
Retirement (life after), 361–62
Retirement planning, 364–65
Retirement (timing),
Rigidity, 366
Roles seniors play, 367–69
Scams, 370–71
Sedentary lifestyles of many older women, 372
Self-efficacy, 376
Sexual behavior (heterosexual), 384–87
Sibling relationships, 390–91
Sleep, 392–94
Sleep complaints, 394
Smoking, 401–2
Socially inappropriate behavior, 402–3
Social networks, 403
Suicide, 421–22
Television viewing, 429–30
Traveling, 439
Unsolicited support and advice, 442
Voters, 461
Walking, 462–63
Work, 475–80

Biology of Aging and Physical Changes with Aging

Alzheimer's disease, 31–37
Back pain, 55
Balance impairment and cognitive demands, 55–56
Bifocals, 58
Biological age, 59
Body build and body characteristics, 61–62
Body mass index, 63
Body odor, 63
Brain and aging, 65–69
Diseases (acute and chronic), 139–40
Drug tests (clinical trials), 149–50
Exercise (relationship to physical/mental performance), 167–69
Exercise types, 169–70
Facial appearance, 174–75
Fatigue and mental performance, 180
Fatigue (physical), 181
Fluid intake, 182
Fluid intake (cold weather), 183

Fluid intake (differences between young and older adults), 183
Foot problems, 184–85
Frontal lobe dysfunctioning (improving it in dementia), 193
Growth hormone (physical effects), 204–5
Handedness, 206
Hands, 206–7
Hiding your age, 214
Human growth hormone (antiaging effects), 220
Locomotion, 249
Menopause and ovulation, 275–76
Nails, 287
Physical attractiveness, 321
Physiological functions, 322–23
Postural change and orthostasis, 327–28
Posture, 328–29
Prostate gland, 336–37
Sarcopenia, 370
Sexual behavior (heterosexual), 384–87
Strength and stamina, 412–13
Swallowing, 422–23
Tear secretion, 427–28
Teeth, gums, and mouth, 428–29
Urination, 445
Voice, 460
Why aging? (biological theories of aging), 470–71

Emotion, Mood States, and Personality

Anxiety, 40–41
Arousal, 43–44
Control over life's events, 110–11
Crime (victim of and fear of), 116
Depression (diagnostic tests), 127–28
Depression (performances with), 130
Depression (prognosis), 130
Depression (treatment), 131–32
Emotion and memory, 158
Emotions, 156–58
Falls, 176–79
Geriatric Depression Scale, 199
Hostility, 219
Learned helplessness, 239
Loneliness, 249–50
Neuroticism, 290
Pain, 306–7
Personality and mortality, 315
Personality (overview), 316–17
Personality stages, 316–17

Personality style, 317–18
Personality traits, 318–20
Pessimism about physical health and depression, 320
Self-esteem, 379
Well-being (psychological), 467–68
Widowhood and widowerhood, 473–75
Worries, 482

General Information about Aging
Activity theory, 14–15
Advance directives, 17–18
Age change versus age difference, 20–21
Ageism, 22–24
Ageism exists in some words, 24
Age simulation, 24–25
Bathing, 56–57
Biological age, 59
Centenarians, 90
Children view aging negatively, 91–92
Clergy (what they know about aging), 96
Cohort (generational) effect, 99–100
College, investments, 100–101
Continuity versus discontinuity in adult development, 109
Cremation,115
Demography of aging, 125–27
Diary keeping, 134
Disengagement theory, 140
Ecological validity, 151
Educational level, 151–53
Entitlements, 159–60
Estate taxes, 161
Euthanasia, 164–65
Facts of Aging Quiz, 175–76
Fire, 181
Food and meal services, 183–84
Functional age, 193–94
Gender and sex differences in aging, 197–98
Guardianship and conservatorship, 205
Holiday greeting cards, 215
Homeless older people (reasons for their homelessness), 215–16
Home ownership, 217
How much longer do seniors want to live? 220
Income of elderly people, 228
Jurors, 235–36
Life expectancy, 244–45
Life insurance, 245
Life span, 247–48

Longevity, 250–52
Long-term care, 256
Myths about aging, 286
Norms, 291–92
Nursing home administrators. *See* Searching for a quality nursing home
Nursing home admissions, 293
Nursing home deficiencies, 293–94
Nursing home infection, 294
Nursing home residents (contacts with family and friends), 294–95
Nursing home residents (number), 295
Nursing home residents (their rights), 295
Nursing homes staff (resident dependency), 296
Old (defining late adulthood), 300–301
Plasticity theory, 324
Prisoners (elderly), 330
Public assistance, 342
Public school support, 343
Racial and ethnic differences in aging, 345–48
Residence, 357
Retirees and re-entry into the workforce, 358
Retirement communities, 359–60
Retirement (involuntary), 361
Retirement (life after), 361–62
Retirement locations, 363
Retirement (racial inequity), 365
Retirement (theories of life satisfaction), 365
Retirement (timing), 366
Senior Olympics, 381
Services (formal), 384
Subjective age, 420
Successful aging, 420
Successful aging: an alternative perspective, 420
Toilet seats, 436
Twins, 440–41
Why aging? (biological theories of aging), 470–71
Why aging? (psychological theories of aging), 472

Mental Capabilities and Functions
Abilities (physical and mental) and activity, 1–3
Activity (mental) and mental performance, 11–13

Activity theory, 14–15
Alcohol (physical and mental effects),
     27–29
Anagram solving, 37
Arithmetic ability, 41–42
Attention (overview), 50–51
Cardiovascular disease and mental per-
     formance, 74–75
Cognitive impairment (incidence), 98
Cognitive (mental) stages of develop-
     ment, 98–99
Creativity, 113–15
Disability (educational level), 136
Divided attention, 142–43
Driving (identifying cognitively unquali-
     fied drivers), 148
Driving (why many seniors limit or quit
     driving), 148–49
Educational level, 151–53
Exercise (relationship to physical/mental
     performances, 167–69
Expertise, 171–72
Fatigue and mental performance, 180
Gender and sex differences in aging,
     197–98
Health status and mental performance,
     209–10
Imagery, 224–25
Intelligence, 221–23
Learning
     Classical conditioning, 94–96
     Concept learning, 104–5
     Learning (overview), 239–40
     Maze learning, 260–61
     Motor skill learning, 283–85
     Operant conditioning, 302
     Spatial learning, 406–7
     Transfer of learning/training, 437–38
     Verbal learning, 450–52
Memory
     Action memory, 7–9
     Age-associated memory impairment,
          19–20
     Autobiographical memory, 53–54
     Conversation memory, 111–12
     Cultural differences in memory,
          118–19
     Diary studies of memory failures,
          134–135
     Discourse memory, 138–39
     Disuse principle, 141–42
     Emotion and memory, 158

Episodic memory, 161–63
Everyday Memory, 165–66
Eyewitness testimony, 173
Face memory, 174
False memory, 179–80
Forgetting, 185–87
Frequency-of-occurrence memory,
     191–92
Implicit memory, 225–27
Incidental memory, 228
Intentional forgetting, 233
Lexicon, 242–44
Memory complaints, 267–68
Memory for newsworthy events,
     268–69
Memory for television programs, 269
Memory (overview), 269–72
Memory span, 272–73
Memory training, 273–75
Metamemory, 277–79
Negative stereotype and memory, 289
Picture memory, 323–24
Prospective memory, 332–34
Recognition memory versus recall
     memory, 351–53
Selective control of memory, 375
Semantic memory, 378–79
Sensory memory, 382–83
Short-term memory, 388–90
Source memory, 403–4
Spatial memory, 407–8
Temporal memory, 431–32
Very long-term memory, 453
Working memory, 480–82
Metaphors, 279–80
Originality, 302–3
Perception
     Aftereffects (visual), 18–19
     Constancies of perception, 106–7
     Dark adaptation, 120–21
     Depth perception, 132–33
     Form perception, 187–88
     Illusions, 223–24
     Motion perception, 282
     Speech perception, 408–10
     Stimulus persistence, 411
     Practical intelligence, 329
Problem solving, 330–31
Proverbs (interpretation), 337
Reaction time, 349–50
Reading and reading skills, 350
Reasoning, 350–51

Selective attention, 373–75
Self-concept, 376
Self-efficacy, 376
Senses
    Hearing, 210–12
    Pain, 306–7
    Smell, 400–401
    Taste, 425–27
    Temperature sensitivity, 430–31
    Touch, 436
    Untreated hearing impairment
        (effects on spouses), 442–43
    Vision, 455–56
    Visual disorders, 456–59
Sensory functioning and mental function-
    ing (relationship), 382
Signs and Forms, 391
Slowing-down principle, 398–99
Span of apprehension, 404–5
Spatial ability, 405–6
Speed of behavior, 410
Spelling, 410–11
Switching tasks,423
Syntax, 424
Telephone, 429
Time estimation, 433–34
Verbal ability, 448–49
Verbal fluency, 450
Verbosity, 452
Vigilance,
Wisdom, 475–76
Word associations, 477–78

Mental and Diagnostic Tests
Army Alpha and Army Beta intelligence
    tests, 42–43
Blessed Mental Status Test, 60
Clinical Dementia Rating Scale, 97
Clock Drawing Test, 97–98
Cornell Medical Index, 112–13
Depression (diagnostic tests), 127–28
Drug tests (clinical trials), 149–50
Geriatric Depression Scale, 199
Longitudinal studies of aging's effects on
    health and cognition, 254–56
Mattis Dementia Rating Scale, 260
Mental Status Questionnaire, 277
Metamemory in Adulthood (MIA)
    Questionnaire and Metamemory
    Functioning Questionnaire (MFQ),
    279
Mini-Mental State Exam, 181

Multifactorial Memory Questionnaire
    (MMQ), 285
Norms, 291–92
Older Americans Research and Services
    Questionnaire (OARS), 301
Primary Mental Abilities (PMA) Test,
    329–30
Seniors in the Community: Risk
    Evaluation for Eating and Nutrition
    Questionnaire, 381–82
Trail Making Test, 437
Wechsler Intelligence Tests, 465–66
Wechsler Memory Scale, 467

**Nature of Aging Research and Major
Research Studies**
Baltimore Longitudinal Study. See
    National Institute on Aging
Cohort (generational) effect, 99–100
Cross-sectional method, 116–18
Ecological validity, 151
Framingham Study of Heart Disease. See
    Longitudinal studies of aging's effects
    on health and cognition
Longitudinal method, 352–54
MacArthur Foundation Study of
    Successful Aging. See Successful aging
Normative Aging Study. See Longitudinal
    studies of aging's effects on health and
    cognition
Nurses Health Study, See Longitudinal
    studies of aging's effects on health and
    cognition
Nun study, 292–93
Participant selection for research studies,
    312
Participation in research, 312–13
Seattle Longitudinal Study, See
    Longitudinal studies of aging's effects
    on health and cognition
Sequential method, 383
Time-lag comparisons, 434
Veterans Health Study. See Longitudinal
    studies of aging's effects on health and
    cognition
Victoria Longitudinal Study. See
    Longitudinal studies of aging's effects
    on health and cognition
Women's Health Initiative, 476–77

Negative Life Events
Accidents (at home), 3

Accidents (at work), 3
Accidents (automobile), 4–7
Age-associated memory impairment, 19–20
Arthritis, 44–47
Bed sores, 57–58
Cancer (general information), 73–74
Carbon monoxide poisoning, 74
Cardiovascular diseases, 75–81
Diseases (acute and chronic), 139–40
Divorce, 144–45
Domestic violence. *See* Elder abuse
Elder abuse, 153–55
Falls, 176–79
Fracture (hip), 189–90
Gamblers (differences between younger and older gamblers), 196–97
Homeless older people (who are they?), 216
Job loss, 235
Midlife crisis, 280
Parent-child conflicts, 309–10
Problems perceived by elderly people, 331
Rural older people (characteristics and problems they face), 368–69
Skipping meals, 392
Sleep complaints, 394
Sleep disorders, 394–97
Sleep (inefficient), 397
Surgery survival, 422
Survival after death of spouse or significant other, 422
Urinary incontinence, 443–45
Widowhood and widowerhood, 473–75
Worries, 482
Worst things about getting old, 482

Organizations, Programs, and Services
AARP, 1
Adult day care centers, 16–17
Alzheimer's Association, 31
Asset Health Dynamic among the Oldest Old (AHEAD), 47–48
Crime prevention, 115–16
Elderhostel, 155–56
Entitlements, 159–60
Food and meal services, 183–84
Foster Grandparent Program, 189
Geriatrics, 199
Gerontology, 200
Health Maintenance Organizations (HMOs), 207–8
Health promotion programs, 208
Hospice care, 210–11
Legal advice, 240
Mental health and mental health services, 276–77
National Institute on Aging, 287–88
Participation in voluntary organizations and volunteer work, 313–14
Partners in Caregiving: The Dementia Services Program, 314
Retirement communities, 359–60
Senior centers, 380–81
Services (formal), 384
Veterans Administration. *See* Longitudinal studies of aging's effects on health and cognition
White House Conferences on Aging, 469–70

Physical and Mental Health
Advance directives, 17–18
AIDS (Acquired immune deficiency syndrome), 26
Alcoholism (incidence and causes), 26–27
Alcohol (physical and mental effects), 27–29
Allergies, 29
Anemia, 38–39
Antioxidants, 39–40
Arthritis, 44–47
Aspirin, 47
Asthma, 49–50
Balance impairment and cognitive demand, 55–56
Barriers to health in older men, 56
Bladder cancer, 59–60
Bladder (overactive), 60
Blood pressure (high and low), 60–61
Bowels, 64–65
Bruises, 72
Cancer (general information), 73–74
Carbon monoxide poisoning, 74
Cardiovascular disease and mental performance, 74–75
Cardiovascular diseases, 75–81
Causes of death, 80
Cervical cancer, 90–91
Chocolate, 92
Cholesterol, 92–93
Chronic respiratory diseases, 93–94

Claudication. *See* Peripheral arterial disease and claudication

Coffee, 98

Colon cancer, 101–2

Common cold, 103

Cornell Medical Index, 112–13

Death and dying, 122–24

Defibrillators, 124

Delirium, 125

Diabetes, 133–34

Diseases (acute and chronic), 139–40

Diverticulitis, 142

Dizziness, 145–46

Drug abuse, 149

Drug tests (clinical trials), 149–50

End-state renal disease, 158–59

Esophageal cancer, 163

Estrogen replacement therapy (hormone replacement therapy), 164

Exercise (relationship to physical/mental health performances) 167–69

Fluid intake, 182

Foot problems, 184–85

Fractures (hip), 189–90

Frailty as a clinical syndrome, 190

Gall bladder diseases, 196

Garlic, 197

Ginkgo, 200

Grape juice, 204

Health literacy, 207

Health promotion programs, 208,

Health risk behaviors, 208–9

Health status and mental performance, 209–10

Heart rate, 213

Heat stroke, 213

Heredity versus environment as determiners of functional health, 214

Hip replacement, 214–15

Home medical devices, 216–17

Hospice care, 219

Hospital infections,,219

Hypertension, 221–22

Hypertension and mental functioning, 222

Immune responses and stress, 225

Influenza, 229–30

Influenza vaccines, 230

Insect bites and stings, 230–31

Ischemic heart disease, 234

Kidney cancer, 237

Knee replacement, 237

Laughter (is it the best medicine for seniors?), 238

Leukemia, 242

Licorice, 244

Life satisfaction, 245–47

Liver cancer, 248

Longevity (what determines a long life?), 252

Lung cancer, 256–57

Maturity (psychological), 260

Medicaid, 261

Medical records, 261–62

Medicare, 262–63

Medicare fraud, 263–64

Medicare hospital patients, 264

Medication compliance and comprehension, 264–66

Medications, 266–67

Medication sharing, 267

Menopause and ovulation, 275–76

Mental health and mental heath services, 276–77

Modifying negative health behaviors, 281–82

Neurosis, 289

Nocturia, 290

Nursing home deficiencies, 293–94

Nursing home discharge outcomes, 294

Nursing home infections, 294

Nutrition and diet, 296–98

Obesity, 299

Obesity (childhood obesity predicts adult obesity), 299

Obesity (effects on longevity and depression), 299–300

Osteopenia, 303

Osteoporosis, 303–4

Ovarian cancer, 304–5

Overmedication, 305

Paget's disease, 306

Pain, 306–97

Pain (chronic), 307

Pain management, 307–8

Pain medications (analgesics), 308–9

Peripheral arterial disease and claudication, 314–15

Physicians (communication with), 321–22

Physiological functions, 322–23

Pneumonia, 324–25

Portion size and heart health, 326

Posttraumatic stress disorder, 326–27

Postural changes and orthostasis, 327–28

Problems physicians have with older patients, 332
Progeria, 332
Prostate cancer, 335–36
Prostate gland, 336–37
Psychosis, 338–39
Quackery, 344
Racial differences in functional declines, 348–49
Relationship with physician (duration of), 353
Religion in later life, 354–56
Respite care, 358
Salt intake, 370
Sarcopenia, 370
Seizures, 373
Self-concept, 376
Self-esteem, 379
Sexual behavior (heterosexual), 384-87
Shingles, 387-88
Skin cancer, 391-92
Sleep disorders, 394=397
Smallpox, 399-400
Spinal stenosis, 411
Stomach cancer, 411-12
Stroke, 416-19
Suicide, 421-33
Surgery survival, 422
Syncope, 423
Tea, 427
Teeth, gums, and mouth, 428-29
Terminal drop phenomenon, 432
Terminal illness, 432-33
Testicular cancer, 433
Tetanus, 433
Tinnitus, 435-36
Tomatoes, 436
Tremor (essential), 439-40
Tuberculosis, 440
Underdiagnosis of illness, 442
Untreated hearing impairment (effect on spouses), 442-43
Urinary incontinence, 443-45
Uterine cancer, 445-46
Vaccinations and shots for traveling, 447
Visual disorders, 456-59
Vitamin D supplements, 460
Web sites (use for medical information), 464
Well-being (psychological), 467–68
Werner syndrome. See Progeria

Professions Relevant to Aging
Biological gerontology. See Gerontology
Clinical psychology, 97
Geriatrics, 199
Neuropsychology. See Age Associated Memory Impairment
Psychological gerontology. See gerontology
Social gerontology. See Gerontology

Therapy, Treatment, and Interventions
Activity diversity (cognitive benefits), 11
Acupuncture, 15
Adult day care centers, 16–17
Alcoholism (treatment), 27
Alternative medical treatments, 29
Antiaging products—do they really work? 39
Antioxidants, 39–40
Assistive devices, 49
Asthma, 49–50
Attention and stroke recovery, 50
Bed rest, 57
Beliefs about aging affect physical health, 58
Canes and crutches, 74
Caregivers (early adulthood), 81
Caregivers (elderly parents), 81–82
Caregivers (family and friends), 82–85
Caregivers (how African American caregivers and white caregivers differ), 86
Caregivers (long distance), 86
Caregivers (negative reactions of recipients of care), 86–87
Caregivers (paid workers), 87
Caregivers (positive effects of caregiving), 87–88
Caregivers (secondary), 88
Caregiving (type of mentally impaired patient), 88
Classical conditioning, 94–96
Consumer directive care for disabled elders, 107–8
Daily help, 120
Dancing, 120
Disability (assistance with activities of daily living), 135–36
Disability (effect of social support), 136
Disability (incidence and assistance), 136–37
Disability (psychological and social consequences), 137–38

Disuse principle, 141–42
Drivers (improving their skill), 146
Estrogen replacement therapy (hormone replacement therapy), 164
Falls, 176–79
Flaxseed, 182
Frontal lobe dysfunctioning (improving it in dementia), 193
Garlic, 197
Grape juice, 204
Home medical devices, 216–17
Influenza vaccines, 235–230
Job training, 235
Memory training, 273–75
Mnemonics. *See* Memory training
Modifying negative health behaviors, 281–82
Nursing home staff (resident dependency), 296

Operant conditioning, 302
Pain management, 307–8
Pet therapy, 320–21
Psychotherapy, 339–42
Psychotherapy with nursing home residents, 342–43
Reminiscence, 356–57
Respite care, 358
Self-care (health). *See* self-rated functioning
Sexual behavior (heterosexual), 384–87
Sleep therapy, 398
Smoking, 401–2
Toilet seats, 436
Transfer of learning/training, 437–38
Urinary incontinence, 443–45
Vaccinations and shots for traveling, 447
Walkers, 462
Wheelchairs, 469

About the Authors

Donald H. Kausler, Curators' Professor Emeritus of Psychology at the University of Missouri–Columbia, is the author of several books, including *Learning and Memory in Normal Aging.* His son Barry C. Kausler is a media producer and writer based in Columbia. His daughter Jill A. Krupsaw is a registered nurse in Little Rock, Arkansas.